# The Natural Pregnancy Book

# The Natural Pregnancy Book

## Herbs, Nutrition, and Other Holistic Choices

### · Aviva Jill Romm ·

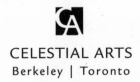

CELESTIAL ARTS
Berkeley | Toronto

Celestial Arts
an imprint of Ten Speed Press
P.O. Box 7123
Berkeley, California 94707
www.tenspeed.com

Distributed in Australia by Simon and Schuster Australia, in Canada by Ten Speed Press Canada, in New Zealand by Southern Publishers Group, in South Africa by Real Books, and in the United Kingdom and Europe by Publishers Group UK.

Library of Congress Cataloging-in-Publication Data
Romm, Aviva Jill.
The natural pregnancy book : herbs, nutrition, and other holistic choices / Aviva Jill Romm.
    p. ; cm.
Includes bibliographical references and index.
ISBN-13: 978-1-58761-178-0 (pbk.) / ISBN-10: 1-58761-178-3 (pbk.)
1. Pregnancy—Popular works. 2. Holistic medicine—Popular works. 3. Alternative medicine—Popular works.
    [DNLM: 1. Pregnancy—physiology—Popular Works. 2. Pregnancy—psychology—Popular Works. 3. Holistic Health—Popular Works. 4. Natural Childbirth—Popular Works. 5. Phytotherapy—methods—Popular Works. WQ 150 R766n 2003] I. Title.
RG525.R675   2003
618.2'4—dc21                                                      2003003779

Cover design by Leslie Waltzer, Crowfoot Design
Text design by Toni Tajima

First printing, 2003
Printed in Canada

5  6  7  8  9  10  —  11  10  09  08  07

This book is dedicated to all of the women who have,
over the centuries, kept women's wisdom alive—it is because of their courage
that I am here today; to my husband, Tracy Romm, and to our children,
Iyah, Yemima, Forest, and Naomi; to my sister-in-law, Felicity Romm,
and her children, Serenity, Caleb, and Keziah Romm, for their incredible strength;
and finally, to the spirit of my brother-in-law, Chip Romm.

# Contents ❧

# Acknowledgments

THIS BOOK COULD NOT HAVE BEEN WRITTEN without the unfailing support of my mate, Tracy Romm. Tracy is truly a midwife's advocate, a man who understands what it means for me to leave home in the middle of the night to wipe a woman's brow, say a few encouraging words, and be honored to greet a new member of our human family—while he scrambles to juggle his own work schedule to accommodate my work. He also knows what it takes to "midwife" a book—and he has been my unfailing assistant in the process. He has joyfully played with, fed, read to, and nurtured our four children during the numerous hours it took to write this book—and in the intervening years since the first edition was published. And he has encouraged me to keep writing because he cares so much about those who might benefit—the next generations, as well as our own.

I am overjoyed by and thankful for the presence of my four children—my son, Iyah Khalil, my stalwart supporter and ardent encourager; and my three daughters, Yemima Shanti, who at six said, "Mom, you're an awesome woman!" and at fourteen says "Mom, you get more beautiful every day," and my Forest Grace and Naomi Shoshannah, who played the most magical games by my side as I typed away on these keys when they were babies, and who now during these revisions have grown into strong and competent young people. These four people have shared me generously with the world, and I am honored to be their mom.

I would like to thank all of the midwives, herbalists, and healers who have been my teachers, friends, and inspiration—too numerous to mention, but you know who you are! A special place in my heart is reserved for Sarahn Henderson, my soul sister, midwife, and teacher; Lizzie McDaniels-Feigenbaum, for beginning this journey with me and still being here; Lisa Olko, for being there after my own babies were born, and for letting me be there for her; and Kim Land, my confidante and friend extraordaire. I also want to offer a special word of honor to Ina May Gaskin for being my original inspiration—it was her book *Spiritual Midwifery,* which found its way to me when I was fifteen, that really opened my eyes to being a midwife— and to Jeannine Parvati Baker for welcoming me into the herbal and midwifery sisterhood. Also, thanks to Michael Tierra for incredible amounts of encouragement and support in the herbal community over the years, as well as to Rosemary Gladstar and Susun Weed for support for my books since the beginning.

Thanks to Elaine Gill and the staff at The Crossing Press for originally recognizing that this book needed to be published and for having full faith in me, and to the folks at Celestial Arts for making my dreams come true by bringing this book into the fold. Also, thanks go to Dr. Richard Clofine for careful review of the manuscript.

Finally, I am eternally grateful to the families that have welcomed me into the sacred space of their pregnancies, and who have called me, with joy, their midwife.

# Foreword *by Ina May Gaskin* ♥

WHEN I WAS PREGNANT FOR THE FIRST TIME BACK IN 1965, I naively supposed there must be a book that would answer the questions that continuously bubbled up in my mind. How was I to stay within the twelve- to fifteen-pound weight gain allowed by my obstetrician and not be constantly hungry? Why was this weight limit necessary? What should I expect when I went into labor? How was I to learn how to take care of a baby? How did maternal instincts develop? (I thought I was sadly lacking in this department because I hadn't played with baby dolls as a child.) I searched both the university and public libraries in my town for the book I wanted but came up with nothing.

My obstetrician was of little or no help in answering my questions because he always seemed to be in a hurry—even though I never saw anyone else in his waiting room. In fact, for all I knew, I was the only pregnant woman in that small midwestern town where I was attending graduate school. Not once during this pregnancy did I talk to anyone (besides my obstetrician) who was either pregnant or claimed to know anything about pregnancy. Obtaining a midwife was totally out of the question—in fact, doing that never once occurred to me, because I was unaware there was any such being in all of the United States.

It was at my last prenatal visit before going into labor that my obstetrician informed me that since this was my first baby, I would be having a forceps delivery.

When I protested, he interrupted to tell me that a natural birth of a first-time mother was likely to result in a brain-damaged baby. Unconvinced, I decided the best strategy for avoiding a forceps delivery—I knew from reading historical novels that forceps could cause brain damage—was to be the quietest woman ever to have a baby in that hospital.

It didn't work. My baby was pulled out by forceps, despite how silently I labored. She wasn't brain damaged, but she and I were both negatively affected for many years by the psychological separation that stemmed from our physical separation for nearly twenty-four hours after her birth, and I felt that her birth had been something that had happened to me instead of something that I had done.

Young mothers these days do not have to worry about unnecessary forceps deliveries because this fashion in obstetrics, once so widely and uncritically accepted in our country, is now as extinct as the pterodactyl. There are now far more books available on pregnancy and childbirth than most women have time to read or money to buy, and childbirth classes are available to probably the majority of women in the United States. Husbands, partners, family members, and even friends are allowed in the labor and delivery rooms of most hospitals, and it is a common, if mistaken, perception that childbirth is now handled in the best way possible.

The reality is far less reassuring. For one thing, not all of the books are that helpful. Many contain misleading information or even misinformation. As for interventions in the process of pregnancy, labor, and birth, it is now possible—even likely—for American women to have unnecessary ultrasonography during pregnancy, unnecessary inductions, unnecessary intravenous feedings, unnecessary electronic fetal monitoring, and unnecessary anesthesia during labor. Needless cesarean sections reached epidemic proportions in the United States during the 1970s and have remained at historically high levels ever since, despite the strenuous efforts of consumer organizations such as the International Cesarean Awareness Network (ICAN) to lower them and despite the repeated recommendations by the obstetricians' own professional organization, the American College of Obstetricians and Gynecologists (ACOG).

Because, after forty years of concerted efforts to revive the profession of midwifery in the United States, there are still only a few thousand midwives available to attend the four million births that happen annually, not every woman is going to be able to find a midwife to provide her prenatal care and to attend her birth.

Regardless of whether you have a midwife, or if you are one of the women who cannot obtain midwifery care, Aviva's book is going to be a comfort to you. She understands as a mother and as a midwife what you are going through; and she has an uncommon gift of writing down her knowledge in a way that is accessible and graceful. Read it and be nurtured.

# Preface

THIS BOOK WAS CONCEIVED NEARLY TWENTY YEARS AGO in the kitchen of a dear friend's home. At that time she and I, both midwives and each the mother of a young child, were beginning a lifetime journey of uncovering and rediscovering a great wealth of information about childbearing and child raising. We were gleaning information from a variety of sources: anthropological research, medical and lay texts, our work as mothers and midwives, the experiences of other midwives and mothers, and most significantly what we were learning from our intuition, from each other as women friends, from our partnerships with our mates, and from our babies. We had seen that pregnancy did not have to be ten (lunar) months of drudgery, discomfort, and exhaustion. We were finding that pregnancy and motherhood could be highly creative times, filled with confidence, perceptiveness, awe, and appreciation for the beauty of our changing physical shape, and the extension of this in the form of our growing children.

Standing in the doorway of that kitchen on an early spring day, a moment ripe for beginnings, I found an inspiration and made the commitment to carry this inspiration inside me, to gestate and nurture my discoveries until, like a baby after a full-term pregnancy, a book would be ready to emerge, to be born—a book to share the joy and strength I was gaining from my experiences. That so many women see pregnancy as a burden to be endured, a time fraught with insecurity and doubt, seemed a great loss. Aware of the transformative potential of the written word, I became determined to contribute a positive, supportive narrative about pregnancy by a woman and mother, for women.

I now have four children. I've had healthy pregnancies, strong labors, and beautiful births. I've nursed and deeply enjoyed each of our children. Each pregnancy has reaffirmed my conviction that natural health care is the bedrock of my continuing wellness and that of our children. In addition to my own pregnancies, I have had the honor to know and assist many women and families on the mostly joyous, sometimes tumultuous, and occasionally painful path of pregnancy. I have watched with joy in the past five or so years since this book was first published, as women have become increasingly aware of the options of natural birth and home birth, and of the potential value of natural therapies as safe alternatives to some of the conventional medical treatments of common pregnancy complaints. It is a pleasure to update this book to include what now is not only the art of natural healing but the emerging science as well.

## Part I

# Your Pregnancy

## Chapter 1

# The Basics

*The Natural Pregnancy Book* is written for all women, regardless of how extensively they want to use natural remedies. Women who simply wish to have a relaxed and healthy pregnancy and to be knowledgeable about this process can gain a great deal from the sections on nutrition, movement, and relaxation. Women with jobs outside the home can learn how to stay healthy and well nourished. Women who choose to forgo careers in order to be with their children full-time will find support and validation for that choice. Women who are not yet pregnant but would like to be can use this book as part of their preparation for entering pregnancy in optimal health.

Grandmothers, aunts, sisters, friends, and partners of pregnant women can read this book to re-create the support systems that women have relied upon for generations, both during pregnancy and after the baby is born. This book will enable these women to be a positive and nourishing influence for the pregnant woman.

Women who are interested in what is known in our country as "alternative healing," "holistic medicine," "complementary medicine," or "natural health" will find this book one they turn to again and again for practical methods of relieving common pregnancy discomforts and promoting optimal health in pregnancy.

Most of this book is addressed to women, because pregnancy, although it offers a transformational experience for their male partners, is a woman's experience, one that a woman can, and I believe should, claim as her own. With this ownership of pregnancy, hopefully will come a sense of pride and self-respect that will give women the confidence to make choices and be the creative agents of their prenatal care. It is my profound hope that our culture will evolve to respect the rich potential for growth also available to men through their participation in pregnancy, and that men will respectfully avail themselves of this possibility. Ideally, men will become cooperative partners with a healthy respect for the primacy of the needs of the pregnant women and their babies. Optimally a partnership emerges in which both partners are finely attuned to each other's needs, with everyone benefiting, including the child. Pregnancy is an opportunity for both partners to join together on the joyous path of building a lasting family.

*"The open heart, freed from fear, experiences the world in all its mystery and brilliance. All of us need to practice awe-robics, like Lily Tomlin's character, Trudy."*

*—Diane Mariechild*

Pregnancy is a time rich in possibility for relationship building between the parents and baby, even while the baby is still gestating. Hopefully, involved partners will read much of this book. Chapter 13 is written specifically for fathers. I also mean it to include partners in nontraditional relationships. Due to my lack of experience with lesbian couples, I cannot speak directly to their needs. To these women, I apologize and hope that this book is still valuable to them.

## A Brief History of Birthing Practices

Approximately four million women in the United States give birth every year. Of these women, the majority (96 percent or about 3,840,000 women) choose physicians to attend them. (Not accounted for in this figure of four million are those women who miscarry or choose an abortion. They too overwhelmingly choose physicians for their care.) Only 4 percent (about 160,000 women) receive care from midwives and only 1 percent of those (1,600) women choose home births.

Prior to the twentieth century, in the United States home birth and natural childbirth were the norm. After that time, the midwife's role was usurped by medical doctors with final control assumed by obstetricians. The idea was conveyed that doctors and hospitals were safer and more desirable than midwives and home births. However, the fact is that in those days there was greater danger of women dying in childbirth in hospitals due to puerperal fever, primarily because physicians failed to wash their hands between patients.

With this shift toward hospitals and obstetricians, women became more passive and less active in giving birth to their babies. Technology encouraged such passivity, for instance, with the standard obstetric tables with the stirrups high in the air, wrist straps to hold the woman immobile, twilight sleep to keep them unconscious, and excessive use of forcep deliveries and cesarean sections.

In the late 1960s, prompted in part by the civil rights and women's rights movements, women began to demand equality. At the same time, various methods (Leboyer, Dick Read, and Lamaze) were promulgated, emphasizing a more natural approach to birth. Women began to ask their partners to participate in their pregnancies and births, and it became commonplace for men to do so. Nevertheless, with all these advances, women were still cast in stereotypical roles, compliant as before.

In the 1970s and 1980s, technology was emphasized more in obstetrical care. Due to legal and financial considerations on the part of many doctors, hospitals, medical supply houses, and insurance companies, prenatal and intrapartum testing became requisite for all pregnant women, rather than optional for those at higher risk. Women as a whole did not question this growing number of interventions or their consequences.

Well into the 1980s, most women were still not informed about pregnancy and birth, and obstetrics all but absolved them of their responsibility. They were still patronized, frequently drugged, strapped down for birth, and subject to isolating and inconsiderate treatment. Babies, directly after birth, were still held upside down and slapped, and whisked away from their mothers. Few women breastfed their babies.

Despite some gains in equal rights in the workplace and home, women were still not decision makers in their pregnancies and birthing experiences. Women lost the political control over childbearing that existed when it was a private, women's experience, and instead let the medical establishment become the authority.

Never before have pregnant women been expected to subject themselves to the level of prenatal testing, screening, and diagnosis as now. Because of our tendency to believe unquestioningly in medical experts, we allow ourselves and our babies to undergo practices that we are told are safe, but medical literature often cites as harmful. This book offers suggestions for a different model of care, but also documents medical techniques that women might choose or need. This book is a compilation of the best that the tradition of midwifery has to offer in noninvasive methods for promoting and maintaining pregnancy wellness. It is a woman-to-woman guide to pregnancy care.

I believe that pregnancy is a natural process of which our bodies are perfectly capable, and that pregnancy is a process of initiation and growth into a value system that respects and honors women's creative power.

This book is woman centered and feminist for two reasons. First, I firmly believe that women are the only true authorities about the female reproductive cycle. It is through the voices and experiences of women, the true authorities, that we gain the most valuable knowledge about pregnancy, birth, and mothering. I aim to bring attention to these women's voices and experiences. Second, as feminists we are puzzled as to how we can keep women's rights in childbearing without tying women to a false view of reproduction as a biological imperative. Devaluing childbearing in the effort to prove women's equality to men is harmful for all women. This may seem irrelevant to many women who do not consider themselves feminists, but such values have deeply affected all women to the point where many shun the idea that pregnancy, birth, and mothering are valuable experiences.

It is essential to acknowledge the importance of the pregnancy experience for the growth not only of the baby but for the woman as well. This book invites women to claim our bodies' processes as a part of our strength, not of our weakness, and to work together for the empowerment of women. I believe that reclaiming pregnancy should be part of our collective effort for broad-reaching social changes in all aspects of women's health care.

While this book offers many alternatives to conventional medical care, it is not antimedical, antihospital, or antiobstetrician. As a midwife I have seen truly necessary medical interventions and have been thankful for their skillful employment, have met dedicated and caring physicians, nurses, and nurse-midwives, and have seen great improvements in hospitals. What I take issue with is the inappropriate use of technology and the attitude that pregnancy is an illness.

I wish to create a new view of pregnancy. Pregnant women are viewed, culturally, as weak (they are discouraged from physical work), girlish (evidenced by childish-looking maternity clothes and the patronizing attitudes of some doctors), and irrational (demonstrated by strange food cravings and heightened emotional sensitivity). This book strives to help women reframe their thinking in order to regain their natural authority. Through the development of our own voice and story, trust in our ability to understand common medical rationale and practices, and confidence in our capability for competent decision making, we can feel more fully empowered to transform the cultural stereotypes that undermine the potential for positive growth and transformation inherent in the pregnancy experience.

*The Natural Pregnancy Book* is devoted not only to helping women gain trust and respect for their birthing abilities, but also to planting the idea that babies are sensitive and aware in the womb. The physical nourishment and emotional caring that babies receive in the womb lays the foundation for their physical as well as their emotional and social health. Children who feel cared for and wanted have a greater likelihood of developing into confident and caring adults. If babies can hear and respond to music while in the womb (this has been scientifically documented), then certainly they can sense love or rejection. So it is that from early in gestation, we can begin to teach our children to trust and respect their bodies by setting the example of doing so for ourselves.

It is my sincerest hope that those who read this book will be inspired to listen to and respect their bodies and, in doing so, find a sense of well-being and confidence that will assist them throughout their lives. May this be a gift that we pass on to our daughters and sons, that they too may respect themselves, and each other.

## What I Mean by Natural

With the popularization of "natural childbirth" through such childbirth education methods as the Lamaze method, it has become common to consider any birth that occurs vaginally (as opposed to a cesarean section) as a natural birth, regardless of whether there have been interventions or the use of medications. While it is a disservice to a woman to feel guilty if she ultimately decides to have an epidural, to call such a birth "natural" trivializes the common use of drugs and interventions during both pregnancy and birth, and dilutes the likelihood of women recognizing that it is possible and empowering to experience a pregnancy and birth free of unnecessary intrusions or interventions. When I use the word *natural,* I am referring to untampered-with and unhindered biological processes, techniques that support such healthy biological functioning, and substances that are primarily derived from unrefined sources.

A natural approach to pregnancy necessitates that you respect the forces of your body—those that cause conception to occur and that also cause your baby to grow in your womb—and that you try to work in harmony with those forces by bringing elements from the natural world (for example, foods in their natural state and herbs) into your pregnancy experience.

# Alternative Childbirth and the Resurgence of Midwifery

In the mid-1970s, a small but determined number of women began to question the type of treatment they were receiving from the medical profession in their pregnancy and birth experiences. Coincident with the rise of the women's self-help movement and the so-called back-to-the-land movement, women began to turn to a more traditional and natural approach to pregnancy and birth, relying more on trust in natural cycles for reassurance of their wellness than on medical advice and testing. A resurgence in midwifery care, home birth, and the use of practical self-care began. Some of the earliest pioneers of this movement include Ina May Gaskin, Sheila Kitzinger, Jeannine Parvati Baker, Elizabeth Davis, Raven Lang, Nan Koehler, Suzanne Arms, and Rahima Baldwin, as well as the midwives who founded the Childbirth Providers of African Descent—Shafia Monroe, Sondra Abdullah Zaimah, Ayanna Ade, and Rashida Mujtabah—and countless other women whose persistent and courageous efforts have kept natural birth options open for all of us.

With the growth of this alternative childbirth movement, midwives and mothers had available to them both the best natural traditions and the best advanced obstetrical knowledge on which to draw. In fact, many midwives were women who wanted to provide other women with the type of care that they wished they had received during pregnancy. Women began to teach childbirth education classes, and some of them, such as sociologist and anthropologist Sheila Kitzinger and midwife and educator Rahima Baldwin, founded international organizations to inform and empower pregnant women. A handful of supportive physicians also provided assistance for those desiring a more natural approach to pregnancy and birth.

By the 1980s, the alternative childbearing movement had gained momentum, and though less than 1 percent of all women chose home births, midwifery was no longer a thing of the past. With the resurgence of midwifery came a resurgence of the prejudice against women healers and the attendant persecution of midwives. In many areas of the United States, traditional midwives have been arrested, harassed, and faced with restraint-of-trade charges, and have endured emotional and economic hardships as a result of court cases and legal fees. Of course, the families of these practitioners have suffered greatly as well. Even certified nurse-midwives, fully trained and sanctioned by the medical establishment, are forced to practice strictly under the auspices of an obstetrician. It is determined by individual obstetricians, as well as the regulating organization of nurse-midwives, just how much autonomy a nurse-midwife is allowed.

In an effort to consolidate knowledge and create internal midwifery standards, as well as to provide a consistent forum for education, in 1982 midwives across the United States formed the Midwives Alliance of North America, an organization that now has an international membership and is working to foster public acceptance and recognition of independent midwifery not only as a respected profession, but also as an option available to a greater spectrum of women. This is in keeping with the belief that midwifery is political and social work that extends beyond small circles of "back-to-nature" women who choose to have babies at home. Midwives are committed to the care of pregnant women and are working to create a political environment in which all women have the option of receiving the kind of care and support midwives offer—professional care that is nurturing and designed to meet the needs of individual women.

The alternative childbirth movement has had a significant impact on women's experiences of childbirth, even for those choosing to give birth conventionally and in the hospital. Practices such as rooming-in, the presence of fathers, friends, and children at births, and the development of birthing suites and birthing centers are all testimony to the efforts of the alternative childbirth movement. The growing popularity of organic foods during pregnancy, exercise and yoga for prenatal relaxation and toning, and attention to holistic and spiritual health, including the use of herbs, massage, and meditation, also reflect the influence of the alternative birth movement on mainstream pregnancy and birthing practices.

> *Midwives are committed to the care of pregnant women and are working to create a political environment in which all women have the option of receiving the kind of care and support midwives offer—professional care that is nurturing, designed to meet the needs of individual women.*
>
> *—A. J. R.*

## Looking to the Future

Even though changes can be seen in how our country views pregnancy, most women still hand over that responsibility to the medical profession, awaiting validation at regular intervals that their bodies are—or are not—working. We wait for confirmation of pregnancy from a doctor or a home pregnancy test because we have lost trust in the sensations and messages that arise from within us. We think we need someone to tell us that we're pregnant, that our babies are growing, that our pelvis is big enough, and so on. Despite the enormous contribution and progress of the women's self-help movement, most women have no idea what their cervix looks or feels like, what nutrients they need for a healthy pregnancy, or what their uterus does to help the baby get born. We have so thoroughly externalized information about our bodies, and have become so doubtful of our bodies' abilities, that we see pregnancy and birth as fully medical events—almost as if it is the ultrasounds, alpha-fetoprotein tests, and chorionic villi samples that make the baby healthy. Yet ultrasounds have not been proven safe for babies, alpha-fetoprotein tests have an exceptionally high false positive margin, and chorionic villi sampling has resulted in babies with missing limbs.

I am not suggesting that we abandon all prenatal testing. I do question the routine use of invasive testing and the way such testing affects the ability of a woman to form a strong, intuitive connection with her baby. I also wonder how a woman can give birth naturally or trust herself to be a mother if she can't trust her body to grow a healthy baby. At a time when a woman should be developing into a confident parent, the medical profession in general deals a severe blow to that developing confidence by making her dependent upon its experts for guidance.

Further, women who choose to forgo such invasive prenatal testing are frequently subjected to guilt, especially if a problem does arise. All women should be encouraged to trust their bodies' ability to nurture a child and should be free to request or forgo medical interventions during pregnancy without emotional coercion. True freedom means being able to say no, as well as being able to say yes.

I propose that women consider what it would be like to regain confidence in ourselves, beginning with the experiences that our bodies present to us through our reproductive cycles, if not before. Regaining confidence in our bodies, it seems to me, is the most challenging aspect in overcoming what we have lost in our complex history of childbearing.

It is within our grasp as women and mothers to determine what pregnancy and prenatal care will be in the twenty-first century. Will we become convinced that technological intervention is wiser than our bodies' natural processes? Or will we welcome these processes and come to view our bodies—indeed, ourselves—with respect for our strengths, power, and beauty?

## Chapter 2

# Becoming Body-Centered

*O*n TV and in other media, our culture can be seen as body-image centered, not body-centered. Most of us therefore relate to our bodies not by what we feel but by how we think we look to others. We base our feelings about our bodies on our appearance. This often leads to dangerous patterns. Dieting, for example, has become a major focus for many women. Studies report that in the 1980s and 1990s there was an explosion of eating disorders, particularly in teenage girls. An estimated eight million American women are reported as anorexic, bulimic, or compulsive dieters.

Commercials and advertisements offer an array of products that will make our bodies cleaner, more convenient, and more pleasant smelling. What are the effects on our psyches of such an implied contempt for the female body and the view of its functions as fundamentally dirty? It is only when we decide not to sanitize our bodies in order to make them conform to external standards that we become capable of understanding the language of our bodies.

In *Women's Bodies, Women's Wisdom,* Dr. Christiane Northrup, an obstetrician and gynecologist and a specialist in holistic health for women, writes, "The state of a woman's health is indeed completely tied up with the culture in which she lives and her position in it, as well as in the way she lives her life as an individual. We cannot hope to reclaim our bodily wisdom and inherent ability to create health without first understanding the influence of our society on how we think and care for our bodies." How we think about and care for our bodies is the basis for how we feel during pregnancy. Therefore, it is important to look at some of the underlying beliefs and attitudes that women in our culture are exposed to and too often internalize. By understanding and redefining your relationship with your body, you will be improving the likelihood that you experience pregnancy as a positive and magical process.

Not only does popular media cause us to distrust our bodies' natural processes, but the medical profession, into whose hands most of us were literally born, has conditioned us to rely on its experts for answers to our questions about our bodies. Conventional medicine subordinates our subjective knowing, emphasizing that our ability to heal is not an innate human capacity but a result of medical training and techniques. We are taught that normal processes such as birth, menopause, and death are processes that require medical supervision and intervention. It is not encouraged, or even acknowledged, that we have the ability to be healthy without constant medical assistance. We learn that fatigue, hunger, sadness, stress, headaches, menstrual cramps, the sensations of childbirth, and most other physical feelings that are uncomfortable or unpleasant can be suppressed. We are not taught that these feelings are the language of our bodies, and that our bodies speak to us more and more strongly until we are finally forced to sit up and listen. This happens usually when we ignore little messages until they turn into discomforts, then symptoms, then outright diseases. But we can change this conditioning by listening to our bodies.

## Learning to Listen to Your Body

Each of us receives messages daily from our body, informing us when, what, and how much to eat, when to sleep, when to exercise our muscles, when to have a bowel movement, and so on. Your body is quick to detect, through cellular responses of assimilation and rejection, when you are nourishing yourself and when you are harming yourself. This is true of not only foods and substances that you ingest, but also situations in which you find yourself, and thoughts and feelings you have. You can feel these responses, if you pay attention, in your nerves and muscles. For example, you may find that areas of your body tense up in a stressful situation, or that you sneeze in a room where a cat has recently been if you are allergic to cats.

The concept of being body-centered is not meant to imply separation of the body, mind, and emotions. In fact, all of these faculties are inextricably connected and interwoven in the organism we call a *human*. On a literal and biological level, one cannot say that the mind begins here and ends there, as if the mind were only the brain, and the body everything below the brain. Actually, nerve pathways, hormones, and genetic messages course throughout the body, connecting the messages of the brain, and vice versa, from the entire body to the brain—the brain is part of the whole body. Feelings occur when internal, physiological processes trigger various emotional responses, as well as when external situations trigger biological and emotional reactions.

Becoming body-centered is in no way meant to imply that you shouldn't exercise your intellect—quite the contrary. However, it is possible for your thoughts to subvert your emotions and physical sensations in a culture where we are taught to do so. Being body-centered means unlearning the process of subverting your body, while still using your intelligence. You can learn to override and transform the culturally imposed and inauthentic voices that tell you how you should think and how you should be so that you know and accept who and how you truly are.

All women would benefit by listening to their bodies, and ideally women will learn this skill prior to pregnancy. However, if you are new to this idea, pregnancy is a particularly ripe time for learning to do so because it is a time when your body manifests many new and noticeable messages.

Learning to listen to your body, like learning any language, takes time, commitment, and practice. People who are fluent in numerous languages often comment that the best way to learn a new language is to be totally immersed in hearing it, such as by spending time in a foreign country or at least by surrounding oneself with native speakers of that language. Pregnancy, though not separate from the continuity of a woman's life, is a unique experience permitting a time of total immersion in the language of the body with many heightened physical sensations. Women are also apt to speak more freely with one another about their bodies when they are pregnant than they are at any other time, providing you with an opportunity to be around other women who are also trying to understand the language of their own bodies. Women who have already had children, "native speakers" if you will, are often eager to share their experiences. Spending time with women who have had natural and healthy experiences may help you gain comfort and confidence in listening to the unique language of your own body.

Pregnant women not only experience dramatic physical transformations, but also emotional and social transformations as our perceptions of ourselves as mothers grow, and as our social roles and responsibilities change. However, unless we reflect about our attitudes toward our bodies and make a commitment to loving and trusting our bodies, we run the risk of carrying harmful patterns into our pregnancies. For example, a woman with an eating disorder may not allow herself and her baby to gain enough weight to nurture herself and her baby for a healthy pregnancy, birth, and postpartum. A woman who feels she is fat or not beautiful may become very depressed when her body seems to be getting bigger as pregnancy progresses. This depression, unpleasant in itself, can also lead to physical problems such as poor dietary habits, bad posture, and further problems such as constipation or lower backache. This is just a simple example of how poor self-image, based on comparing oneself to a cultural ideal, may be harmful during pregnancy.

Perhaps the most practical way to begin listening to your body is to pay attention to the most common messages you receive daily: hunger, thirst, fatigue, and elimination. Try to notice when you begin to feel the sensations that alert you to eat, drink, rest, or go to the bathroom. What are these sensations? When do you notice them? And most important, how do you respond to them?

- Do you eat when you're hungry, or do you think about whether you should eat and then skip a meal, afraid that if you eat too much you might get fat?

- Do you urinate when you feel the urge to, or like so many women, do you wait until a more convenient time or until you just can't wait any longer? Many women do the latter, not realizing that this can cause urinary tract infections, to which women are especially susceptible during pregnancy.

- Do you allow yourself to rest or sleep when you feel fatigued, or do you keep pushing yourself to do more until you collapse at the end of the day? Or do you push your body further with the help of coffee, chocolate, or sugar? Do you get down on yourself for being tired, thinking that you should be getting more done?

- Do you recognize that you may be feeling weepy, irritable, nauseated, faint, cold, and clammy, or that you have a headache because your blood sugar is too low and you need to eat a solid meal?

- Did you know that particular food cravings are your body's way of calling out for specific nutrients? For example, you may be craving sweets because you need more energy, but your body really needs more protein, which will provide you with more lasting energy.

Like many women, you may realize that you are not listening to your body. Just by deciding to be more alert to your own needs, you'll find yourself recognizing and responding to your body's signals more readily, and you will feel better for doing so. Keeping a journal can be a useful method for charting specific urges or sensations, as well as your responses and reactions. Remember that it takes time and patience to learn any language, but that you and your baby both deserve optimal care and loving attention.

## Feelings and Fears about Your Body

Another aspect of being body-centered is to admit to yourself how you truly feel about your body. If you stand before a mirror unclothed, do you find yourself criticizing parts of your body? Do you criticize your nose, breasts, thighs, or buttocks? Try to understand where those critical messages came from—were you criticized as a child or as a teenager by other kids, or do you compare yourself to the images on magazine covers? Try to replace those old, critical voices with positive messages called "affirmations"—for example, "I love my body for growing my baby so well" or "I love these breasts, which will provide my baby with warm and nourishing milk." You not only can create a greater appreciation of your body by doing this, but also can actually improve your health by giving yourself positive affirmations about your inherently miraculous, beautiful, and unique self.

It is also helpful to acknowledge fears that you have about your body—for example, if you carry an undercurrent of fear that you won't be able to breastfeed, or are afraid that your cervix won't dilate adequately in labor. All of us have heard stories of such problems, and sometimes we internalize other people's experiences. Being in a constant state of low-level fear can directly affect wellness and increase the likelihood of that problem occurring. If you harbor fears, or suspect you might, talk to your body in a loving way, saying something positive instead. Give yourself permission to accept and love your body just as it is, and trust that your body is perfectly designed for health. For example, if you fear that your cervix won't dilate adequately in labor, one of the things you can do is tell yourself daily, "My cervix will soften and open to birth my beautiful baby." You can visualize your cervix as a flower bud, gently and steadily opening, and you can put visual reminders of your opening cervix around your home: photographs of fully opened blossoms, or of the planet Saturn with its wide rings encircling the round planet much the way your cervix will eventually open around your baby's head.

The basic idea is that if you have a negative body image you can work actively to transform yourself into someone who feels genuinely good about herself and her abilities. You can use a journal for writing loving affirmations to your body. Expressive artwork, such as drawing, is also a way to create positive images for yourself.

The most useful skill any of us have for responding to the messages that arise is feeling. From our earliest experiences, we are taught to squelch our emotions ("it's not nice to be angry," "don't cry"—sometimes followed by "or I'll give you something to cry about" or "you're a scaredy-cat") and to follow our intellect. We have also been taught that unpleasant physical sensations are a nuisance, and have been encouraged to suppress such sensations with medication or by putting on a happy face. We were not taught that emotions are a signal of our comfort or discomfort in a given situation or environment, and that our physical sensations let us know what is going on in our bodies. We were also never taught that our physical sensations can reflect our emotions. The best way to regain this knowledge is simply to stop and feel. If you have a headache coming on, you don't have to reach for the aspirin, or even herbs, nor do you have to analyze why you have a headache. By becoming very still and relaxed, and paying attention to your body from this still place, you will find that you can gain an awareness of exactly what you need to do for yourself— perhaps eat, drink water, rest, or remove yourself from a stressful situation. Perhaps an herbal remedy will help, or speaking with a friend or health-care provider. However, first you need to get in touch with that part of you that is your best authority. Try paying attention to how you feel emotionally about the sensations or discomforts you are having, and see what information you get from allowing yourself to feel your feelings. No one knows you better than you!

## Moving Your Body Joyously

Becoming body-centered requires us to be oriented to our physical needs, and this includes spending time enjoying and nurturing our bodies. Bodies need to be moved, sometimes slowly and gracefully, sometimes quickly and with some force. Activities such as yoga, dance, swimming, walking briskly, volleyball, tennis, cross-country skiing, horseback riding, tai chi, you name it (as long as it is safe if you are already pregnant) are all ways to move your body joyously and exuberantly. They fill your body with vitality, stimulate your circulation (which improves cardiovascular functioning), oxygenate the body, enliven your mind, and lift and prevent depression. You not only improve your health and prepare your body for the very physical work of birth, but you also enrich your body awareness and self-esteem.

Regular massage is also a way to get in touch with and enjoy your body as you let tension melt away. In addition, massage is a form of passive exercise for the recipient, with many of the benefits of physical exercise, such as improved circulation and removal of waste products from the muscles. Scheduling problems and the high cost for professional massage need not prohibit you from exploring this possibility for nurturing your body. Your mate or a friend can give you a massage. Even as little as twenty minutes of massage on an occasional basis will be beneficial. See chapter 7 for further discussions and explanations of both movement and massage techniques for pregnancy.

As you learn to release tension from your body and develop appreciation and respect for your body, you will gradually find yourself better able to respond to and nourish yourself. And you will discover that as you take better care of yourself, you will feel happier and healthier, and that your self-esteem and positive body image will come from within. You will like yourself just for being who you are.

## Reclaiming Women's Wisdom

Women's wisdom is a term used to encompass the practices and beliefs that women have developed over centuries and that still benefit women today. Among these are midwifery, nourishing and therapeutic methods of food preparation, herbalism, healing touch, and many other kinds of healing that can enrich our lives. Women have often been the primary physicians for their families, tribes, and villages. These are the main healing modalities that I draw upon in this book.

Women's wisdom is also based on the stories that women tell about their lives and what we can learn from these stories. Women's wisdom allows us to bring our whole selves into the treatment rather than fragmenting parts of ourselves. Likewise, in women's ways of healing, there is the awareness that healing must occur in the person's life, not just in her body, and that physical healing alone cannot occur until the underlying factors of illness and discomfort are addressed. These factors may be as simple as finding more time in your own life, say thirty minutes twice a week, to nurture yourself in whatever way suits you.

Women's wisdom also embraces our subjective knowledge based on feelings and personal experience. This intuition may include dreaming about your baby before conception and sensing who the child will be, and transpersonal knowing, such as having abdominal cramps only to discover that your best friend or sister is in early labor. These are all without logical explanation; they are sympathetic experiences that allow us to realize the psychic aspects of our connection to our bodies and to each other.

These experiences remind us that there is more to life than meets the eye, and that there really is no separation between the mind, body, and spirit.

Women have always been considered more psychic, more closely related to the mysterious aspects of life due to menstruation, pregnancy, and ability to birth our young. Our culture has discredited this multisensory awareness, considering it unreliable, even nonexistent. Women's wisdom, like much of the work that women do, is based on the human aspects of life and valuing emotional and sensory experiences. Women have long recognized the deep psychic connections between a mother and child, knowing, for example, even from thousands of miles away, when a child is well or in danger. Breastfeeding mothers are all too familiar with the experience of having their breasts begin to leak milk while they are at work, only to find out later that their baby had awakened from a nap at the same time and was crying for her. This kind of intuitive awareness is too common to be dismissed as coincidental and too valuable for us to dismiss as fallacious.

To reclaim women's wisdom is to put feminine modes of intuition and intelligence into respected places among the many options available to us for our health care. To reclaim women's wisdom, we have to proclaim that we are the true authorities about ourselves, and we have to reinstate traditionally feminine methods of healing as part of a sensible approach to medicine and wellness.

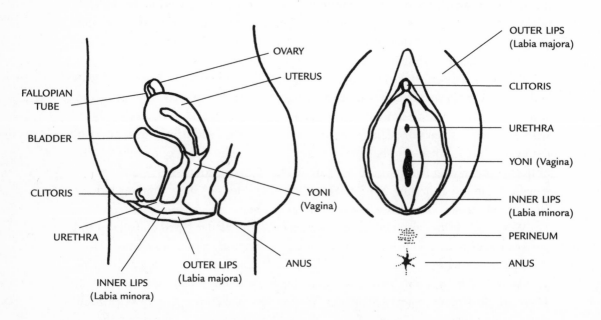

**Pelvic cross view**    **Pelvic front view**

One of the ways that I and other women have chosen to reclaim what is rightfully ours is to replace the word *vagina* with the word *yoni*. *Vagina* literally means a "sheath," and is obviously a reference to the idea that our sexual organs exist only in relationship to men's needs. The word *yoni*, however, is a Sanskrit word for the female genitalia, and refers to the sacredness of a woman's sexual self. In this book you will often see the word *yoni* used where you might commonly use the word *vagina*.

Learning to trust and recognize our intuition and body messages is particularly valuable for pregnant women. Pregnancy is a time when you and your baby are experiencing many increased nutritional demands as well as a greater need for nourishment in other areas, such as massage, exercise, rest, and relaxation. Our body awareness alerts us to our needs, and our intuition can help us to name exactly what we need to do to meet these. One example of using intuitive guidance occurred with a very young couple, with whom I worked long ago, who were having their first baby. The woman, actually still a teenager, had a very poor diet, consisting in large part of pizza and candy bars. I felt that she needed to recognize what her body told her she needed to eat. I taught her and her partner the following exercise: I had them sit facing each other, holding hands. I suggested they ask the baby what he or she needed right now for optimal nourishment. They were both completely silent for a few moments, waiting for a response from the baby. When they both became quite still, I told them to open their eyes and voice what they heard. Simultaneously, both the father and the mother said, "Carrots, the baby needs more carrots." So the mother ate more carrots, practiced this exercise more often, improved her diet greatly, and gave birth at home very easily (after a three-hour labor) to a healthy baby.

Today, as we try to ensure the healthy development of our babies during pregnancy, we can look beyond the conventional prenatal care offered by a typical obstetrician. Exploring your intuitive connection with your baby and trusting your inner wisdom can help you grow a healthy baby.

As you explore the various healing options available for supporting pregnancy health, I invite you to reacquaint yourself with your women's wisdom and discover the techniques that can best nourish you, your baby, and your family.

## Chapter 3

# The Baby inside You

For me conception rings a bell of immediate awareness in the center of my being. I know as soon as I conceive. Within days, my body tells me that I am no longer just myself but have a new companion. With each child, the experience is a bit different.

With my first, I could see an imaginary door open above me and light begin to pour through as my mate and I came together. With my second, I had vivid dreams of seeing a magnificent seashell in the ocean, too deep for me to reach, so my husband dove for it. The shell he handed me had a deep pink, shimmering lining that in waking consciousness reminded me of my womb's lining. At my third child's conception, my husband and I felt a breeze come over us, as if a door opened, and with my fourth baby, somehow I just knew she was with me. With the first couple of babies, I did home pregnancy tests (one of which was negative, though I was pregnant) to confirm what my body and spirit already knew, but after that I chose just to trust my gut feelings and my subtle physical sensations. This was part of my personal commitment to trust my body to tell me what I needed to know. As soon as I felt that I had conceived, I treated myself as if I was definitely pregnant, eating extra well, resting, and avoiding anything that might be harmful to my newly growing child. From the onset, this was my child, not an embryo or a fetus with potential defects or a pregnancy with potential complications, but my child. I truly believe that it is partially this attitude that has nurtured health in each child. But had one of my babies not been perfectly healthy, that baby would still have felt loved and accepted from the beginning.

Later in this book you will find a discussion of the various prenatal diagnostic tests that are commonly offered to pregnant women. There are times when these tests are medically warranted; however, routine use of such testing can prevent a woman from developing and trusting her connection with her baby. The real connection between a mother and her baby exists before the connection that is fostered by seeing the baby on a screen, knowing whether the baby is a boy or a girl, or hearing the baby's heartbeat by electronic amplification.

While it is true that you may feel more confident in your pregnancy after receiving some objective measure of your health or the baby's health via a prenatal diagnostic test (keeping in mind that many tests of fetal well-being are inaccurate), you will have to decide for yourself at what point you draw the line between a natural experience and a technological experience. Therefore it is up to you to be well informed as to the benefits, risks, and necessity of such testing, and to choose for yourself what you do and don't want done. Developing a strong prenatal connection with your baby, as well as trusting in your inner knowing, will enable you to make the most appropriate use of technology during birth, your child's early years, and possibly later.

While the intention of this chapter is to facilitate your inner awareness of your baby, having a clear visual idea of how babies generally develop can help make the conscious connection with your baby more tangible. As a midwife, I am so aware of feeling babies' arms, legs, little bottoms, and heads while still in their mamas' wombs, that a baby in the womb is almost as tangible to me as a baby in arms. However, pregnant women often sense that their baby is inside, kicking, rolling, and playing, yet the wholeness of this actually being a baby, a real person that will one day be in their arms, is often overlooked. The same goes for the dads. Therefore, at each prenatal visit, I show the parents or mother how to feel and massage her baby so that this awareness is strengthened. This chapter will be devoted to the development of the baby and the importance of the prenatal environment for your baby, as well as communicating with your baby prenatally.

> *It is my sincerest hope that those who read this book will be inspired to listen to and respect their bodies, and, in doing so, find a sense of well-being and confidence that will assist them throughout their lives.*
>
> *—A. J. R.*

# Your Growing Baby

The following discussion of a baby's development begins at conception, this being "week one." However, most health-care practitioners measure pregnancy from the first date of the last menstrual period, which is generally two weeks prior to conception. This comes out to ten lunar months—also the way that women in many traditional cultures counted their pregnancies and determined when they were due—ten lunar months from their last period. If you are trying to compare the following information with how far along you are in your pregnancy, count the weeks from conception, which is generally two weeks less than the number of weeks you are figured to be pregnant by your physician or midwife. This will also vary slightly according to the length of your menstrual cycles. For example, if your period occurs every five weeks you will likely be a week further behind. And of course, each baby has an individual growth rate. If you want a general idea of what stage of growth your baby is in, read about the development of a week before and a week after your week's gestation.

## Conception

Conception occurs and pregnancy begins when the sperm and ovum unite. This brings both parents' genetic potential into contact and creates the physical foundation of a new life—your baby. Fertilization generally occurs in the fallopian tube and then over the next five days, as the "zygote" divides into a cluster comprised of numerous cells, it makes its way toward the uterus, where by about the sixth day it attaches to the uterine lining. The process of implantation is complete by about the tenth or eleventh day after conception. By the end of the first two weeks, the placental formation has begun and the cells of the baby are beginning to differentiate. The first two weeks are known as the preembryonic phase.

## Weeks Three through Seven

From week three through week seven, the developing baby is referred to as an embryo. It is during this remarkable period of development that all of the baby's essential features and body parts will be formed. Because it is the most vulnerable phase of development for the baby, it is important for pregnant women to avoid all substances such as alcohol and drugs (including many prescription and over-the-counter medications), and environmental contaminants, such as pesticides, chemical fumes, and cigarette smoke, that could harm the baby.

By the fifteenth day after conception, when you might be expecting your period to start, you may notice breast tenderness and a feeling of fullness in your abdomen. You may find that your hair is hard to manage. This is the way you would normally feel before your period. If you tried to conceive, you may have already begun to take special care of yourself even before you missed your period. If your period is late, then it is sensible to treat yourself as if you were pregnant until it becomes evident that you are not. This will afford your baby optimal protection for healthy development.

During week three the shape of the baby begins to take form.

During week four the heart begins beating, and by the end of this week, the embryo has assumed the appearance of a salamander. There are arm and leg buds, facial and neck structures, and small pits that will later become the ears. By the end of this week, your baby is less than a quarter of an inch long.

The fifth week brings extensive growth of the brain and head and the beginning development of the eyes. Because a baby's growth occurs from top to bottom, the head is large in relation to the body.

During the sixth week since conception, the nose, mouth, and palate take shape, and the eyelids form. By this time, the arms and legs have developed rapidly so that by the seventh week the baby has clearly defined wrists, elbows, knees, fingers, toes, and so on. The baby is now about one-half inch long.

In the seventh week, the baby's urogenital system is developing, the neck area is established, and the external ears are visible. By the end of this week, the baby clearly looks like a human baby. The end of the seventh week is also the end of what is called the embryonic period.

At this point, all of the baby's essential structures, both internal and external, have been formed and require only further growth and development. By now, the baby can respond to touch: if it were possible to touch the baby's palm, the baby's hand would close. The baby can touch his or her own face, as well as make other gentle movements.

## Week Ten

At ten weeks, the baby will begin to have both hair and fingernails, and one can begin to differentiate boys from girls.

## Week Twelve

By twelve weeks, the baby is about three and three-quarters inches long and weighs about an ounce. The baby is able to make facial expressions, and the lips can make sucking motions. In fact, the baby can now swallow amniotic fluid and pee it out, too. The eyes are almost fully developed and the lids fused closed while the rest of this development occurs. By this time, your uterus is about the size of a large grapefruit and you are already entering the second trimester of your pregnancy. If you have been nauseated and uncomfortable, you will soon begin to feel much better.

## Week Fourteen

At fourteen weeks, the baby is covered with lanugo, downy hair that grows in whorls over the body, and the baby has fingerprints. Nipples appear, and the back, which has been curved, straightens. The bones are hardening, and the baby, who fills your womb, is now becoming more active. You may even notice movement, particularly when you are resting.

## Week Sixteen

By sixteen weeks, the baby measures seven or eight inches in length and weighs about four ounces.

## Month Five

At five months, the legs reach their full length and toenails form. By now, you are likely to notice some subtle fluttering movements or even some obvious "kicks and pokes." If you've not yet noticed movement, it is likely that you will soon. The baby also hiccups occasionally, which you will feel as a series of rhythmic "knocks" in your belly. Your baby can suck his or her thumb, can grasp the umbilical cord, and can even scratch his or her face. There is more hair on the head and eyebrows are formed. The eyes are still fused shut. The body is now covered with vernix (which literally translates as "cheese"), a creamy substance that protects the baby's skin while surrounded by water. The heartbeat may now be audible by fetoscope and will usually range between 120 and 160 beats per minute. The baby's ears are now fully functional, and because water conducts sound so well (when we are underwater sounds are muffled because we have air in our ears, but babies have no air in theirs while in the womb), the baby hears sounds all of the time—the rhythms of your heart and breath, the placenta, and your digestion, as well as all of your speaking, singing, crying, yelling, praying, and so on. The baby is able to hear and respond to music and will also respond to your emotions with more or less gentle movements. It is therefore optimal to surround yourself with beautiful and soothing music, as well as to make your own sounds as peaceful, joyous, and comforting as possible. Through sound, the baby begins to learn about the world. Your baby is now about ten or twelve inches long and weighs about eight ounces.

## Month Six

At six months, the skin is wrinkled, translucent, and appears red, due to the blood being visible through the skin. Permanent tooth buds are present and hair growth is obvious. The eyes are open again, and the baby can make both crying and sucking motions. Strong arm and leg muscles have developed, and if the foot is tickled, the baby will respond by planting the foot downward. You may notice that the baby responds to your touch with movements. The baby is twelve to fourteen inches long and weighs about one and a half pounds.

## Month Seven

At seven months, the lungs, though not fully mature, could function minimally outside the uterus. The baby would have a good chance of survival if born prematurely at this point. The baby now sees sunlight through your abdomen and will turn away from very bright light. He or she is about fifteen inches long and weighs three to four pounds. The baby will gain about a half pound a week.

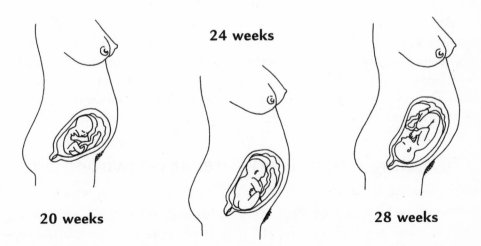

**24 weeks**

**20 weeks**

**28 weeks**

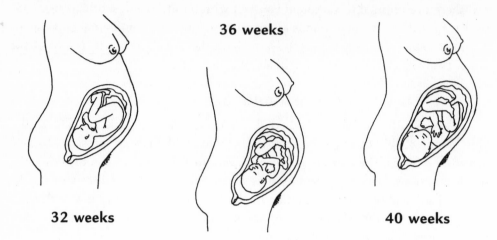

**36 weeks**

**32 weeks**

**40 weeks**

## Month Eight

During the eighth month, the baby begins to put on fat and the wrinkled skin begins to smooth out. Vernix and lanugo still cover the baby except for the face, but these will gradually lessen in quantity by birth. The eyes are open and the lungs are much stronger. The baby is between sixteen and eighteen inches long and may weigh between four and seven pounds.

## Month Nine

At nine months, the lanugo and vernix have begun to disappear, and the baby is reaching full maturity, ready for life outside of your womb. All of the sense organs are well formed and the rest of the organs are ready for extrauterine life. The wrinkles have disappeared and the baby's head will begin to settle into your pelvis, ready for birth. The baby is now nineteen to twenty-one inches long and on the average weighs between six and nine pounds.

# Creating a Nourishing Prenatal Environment

During pregnancy, you are quite literally your child's environment. So how can you create a home for your baby that is stable, nourishing, comfortable, and soothing? Well, in truth, you cannot do this 100 percent of the time, nor is this necessary. Every pregnant woman will experience some stress, whether it be a car that won't start or a toddler who spills things fifty times a day, or important deadlines that must be met, or clothing that doesn't fit. These stresses are temporary, and if you can deal with them without internalizing the stress to the point that you skip meals or lose sleep, your baby is unlikely to be affected. Even anxieties caused by financial issues, marital tensions, or housing problems, for example, can be resolved without upsetting your baby, provided that you take care of yourself responsibly and that you maintain communication with your baby, letting her or him know that yes, there is stress occurring right now in your life, but you still love and welcome the baby, and will in time resolve the stress. While the baby might not intellectually understand the exact reasons for the tension, she or he will have a sympathetic sense of your emotional state, as your state of mind influences the hormones, oxygen, and blood flow the baby receives. When you feel tense, the baby receives tension signals, and when you relax, so can the baby.

There are, however, situations that can cause both temporary and extended emotional impact to babies, and this may be of either a physical or psychological nature, or both. Some situations that occur are unpredictable and are part of the challenging experience of being human—for example, the death of someone you love, the loss of a job, an accident, or other misfortunes. Such experiences challenge the soul and, if they cause ongoing grief, they can cause the mother to withdraw from nourishing herself as well as providing the baby with emotional attention. It will take great will and strength of spirit to overcome such adversity and maintain the focus on creating a healthy environment for the baby.

> *We can nourish our babies so that they may enjoy prenatal wellness and be prepared to meet the inevitable challenges of the world.*
>
> *—A. J. R.*

Fortunately most of us do not experience traumas of such magnitude during pregnancy. Nonetheless, we can let the stresses of our lives consume and preoccupy us to such an extent that the results are similar—we withdraw our attention from physically and emotionally nourishing ourselves and our babies. In addition, our emotional reactions, such as depression, anger, or sadness, and the reactions and expressions of others, especially our mates, can have a profound effect on the baby's well-being. The hormones you produce during such stressful times can reduce the flow of oxygen and nutrients to the baby; babies will react to intense and unpleasant emotional outbursts with vigorous kicking. Extended stress can result in emotional insecurity and failure to thrive. Such behavioral patterns that are established in the womb, depending on the intensity of the situation, can persist as lifelong patterns of physical and emotional illness to varying degrees.

Furthermore, habits of the mother—such as smoking cigarettes and drinking alcohol or using other drugs, all of which have notably harmful physical effects—may also have adverse psychological effects on the baby. The baby lives in a constant state of negative expectancy, never knowing when the mother will again engage in the behavior that causes the baby to be poisoned or asphyxiated or have other harmful physiological responses. Listening to rock music has also been shown to cause an adverse reaction in the baby, leading to violent kicking. Even rushing around all day, day after day, can cause a baby to become overstimulated and affect his or her development.

Of course, all of this places a great responsibility on the woman to act wisely. This responsibility should not be shouldered by mothers alone but shared by fathers and the culture in general. Women should be supported in appropriate ways so that they have the time to eat well, rest, exercise, and engage in activities that nourish body and spirit. No woman should have to worry about an abusive husband, how she will feed herself or her children, or whether she will be fired from her job for taking days off to care for herself. Unfortunately, the needed support does not always exist in our homes or in society. As mothers, we must work together to create such changes. The choice is ours: we can nourish our babies so that they may enjoy prenatal wellness and be prepared to meet the inevitable challenges of the world, or we can start them with emotional and physical difficulties that leave them less prepared to succeed in this complex world.

How we respond to stress is up to us. None of us has to have a drink or a cigarette—these are personal choices. When you fully grasp the importance of the connection between you and your baby, the choices become more apparent—you'd never give your baby a beer or a cigarette. Similarly, when your awareness extends to the effects of your emotional state on your baby and how these can adversely or beneficially influence your child's sense of security, belonging, confidence, and emotional health, it becomes most important to surround your child with a sense of well-being, even in the midst of a struggle. As many mothers of young babies have experienced, if the mother can stay calm even in the midst of chaos, the baby is more likely to do so, and if you are very upset, the baby will likewise become fussy and irritable. The next section explores how to communicate well-being to your baby throughout your pregnancy. Learning these skills now will help you deal with stresses that sometimes arise during parenting while still letting your daughter or son know that she or he is loved, safe, and a welcome member of your family. In turn, your child will also learn to make use of these skills.

# Communicating with Your Baby

Communicating with your baby, as with anyone, is a two-way exchange—that is, you can communicate with your baby and he or she can communicate with you. It is quite possible for this communication to begin even before pregnancy occurs through dreams and extrasensory awareness. For example, before I conceived my second child, I had a vivid dream, which I recorded in my journal, of being in a snowstorm with a close woman friend. In the dream, she went into a room and I assisted her at the birth of her child, a girl, and then I went into an adjacent room and birthed my own baby, also a girl. Several months after this dream, my friend conceived a baby, and in the following month I too conceived. Later I assisted her—in the midst of a snowstorm—at the birth of her daughter, and weeks later I birthed my baby, also a daughter.

It has been my experience as a woman, a mother, and a midwife, that babies require our love for their health as much as they require food. They have a genetic and biological need to be loved and touched, talked to and soothed, long before birth. And loving our babies prenatally not only nourishes them, it feeds us in return, for all of the spiritual forces that help to grow our babies return the gift of love to us. We become infused with grace and light. The connection we build is one that can never be severed. Unlike the tangible, physical umbilical cord that becomes detached after birth, the deep connection we build deliberately with our babies will prevail, preventing detachment from ever developing. Many mothers feel this even though they didn't build a prenatal bond with their babies. We are even more blessed with empathy for our children when we open our hearts to them from the beginning. Fathers, too, can develop and benefit from such prenatal bonding.

## *Talking to Your Baby*

It is not hard to speak to your baby. Talk to the child inside of you throughout your day, sharing even mundane tasks, the music you love, your musings about the beauty of the world around you. When you feel sadness or anger, talk to your baby about it. Although the child may not intellectually understand your concerns, he or she will feel the calm and soothing nature of your voice, which will reassure the child that you are both okay. Massage your baby during the day by rubbing and patting your belly, and also each morning when you rise or each evening before you sleep. During these relaxed times, put a little oil on your hands and rub deeply, actually massaging the parts of the baby's body that you feel. This cannot hurt your baby, and babies respond positively to such caring during the pregnancy with excellent growth as well as after birth. Babies that have been regularly massaged prenatally will love to be massaged throughout childhood. This is an excellent technique for the prevention of illness as well as a remedial treatment. Talk to your baby as you massage her or his body, or sing a special, beautiful song. Chances are the baby will continue to be soothed by this song after birth and will quickly learn to sing it once she or he learns to speak.

Some mothers enjoy reading verses of poetry or children's books to their babies even before birth. These books will probably become your child's all-time favorites, as babies definitely have exhibited preferences from their prenatal time.

Speaking affirmations to your child can foster your confidence as well as nourish the baby's growth with ideas that reinforce his or her well-being. For example, as you massage your baby, you can repeat a few times, rhythmically, "You are so welcome and wanted here, we love you so," or "You are a strong and healthy baby," or "I welcome you for whoever you are." These positive statements can also be used to help you dispel anxieties that may creep into your mind about the baby's health or normal development. As you get closer to the birth, you can say things like: "We are so ready for you to be born, we welcome you into our open arms" or "It is safe to be born, and we look forward to holding and caring for you, dear baby."

> *If you listen to your baby and be very quiet, you may "hear" your baby telling you something important.*
>
> *—A. J. R.*

## Listening to Your Baby

Listening to your baby takes inner trust and quiet. Each day when you take time to quietly rub your baby, become silent and ask your baby, either in your mind or aloud, what he or she needs, and how you can best serve your child's needs. Ask if there is anything the baby wants you to know. Then just listen very quietly and you may be surprised at what you hear. You may not hear a baby's "voice," but in time you may feel a message coming through to you.

Many women find themselves experiencing an intense need to be near their mates during pregnancy, odd desires for foods, and even yearnings to be in certain environments, such as at the beach or in a forest. While we cannot assume that all of our emotions and desires stem from the baby, the baby does make his or her will and desires known through the mother. If you find yourself having feelings, thoughts, or desires that are unfamiliar, you may want to open yourself to the possibility that the baby may be trying to communicate with you.

Dreams are another vehicle for your baby to communicate with you. Many women dream that their baby is already born and is a child of three years old or so. When you dream of your baby, try to talk and listen. However, it is not necessary to take all birth dreams literally. Many women will have disturbing dreams of a deformed baby or other problems, yet these dreams are most often not really premonitions. They frequently are simply a landscape in which women can safely explore their anxieties. Women who work out these anxieties prenatally often experience smooth births and have healthy babies. If you have particularly disturbing dreams, discuss this with your midwife or a trusted friend.

## Creative Insights

Keeping a journal of your insights about your baby or dreams can be a delightful way to preserve these experiences for both of you to cherish for decades to come. Make a note of the words to the songs you sing, stories you read to the baby, or particularly magical places you visit during your pregnancy.

One of my favorite forms of receiving insight about my baby is through artwork. I am not a professional artist, nor am I artistically gifted. I just enjoy the experience of creating, so I'll sit down with blank paper and supplies and let my body talk through whatever medium I am using. I find that colored chalks and oil pastels reflect the subtle energy of pregnancy since the lines and colors can be blended to create a smooth, soft image. Many supplies are available inexpensively at an art supply store; you can therefore enjoy yourself without spending a fortune. It is best to avoid art supplies that contain toxic metals (as do many oil paints) and those with strong fumes. Acrylic paints, most watercolor paints, pastels, colored pencils, and chalks are safe for use during pregnancy.

I've found myself creating images of angels' wings surrounding babies, mothers holding babies, buds opening, and so on. Let your body speak to you. Go deep within yourself to find the reservoir of creativity that resides in your womanplace, and express yourself from there. Artwork can open and release blocked creative energy and be highly therapeutic, but only if you do it for enjoyment and don't judge your results.

The joyous welcoming of your child into your life sends messages to your child that will help him or her to thrive and develop a sense of self-esteem long before birth. None of us can be happy 100 percent of the time, but we can choose to stay in close touch with the messages we are sending our babies. How we treat them prenatally can set the tone for how they will treat themselves and expect others to treat them for much of their lives. While prenatal influences are not the only influences that emboss patterns on our psyches and emotions, they do hold great sway over us. We can help a whole generation of children to feel loved. This will sow the seeds of loving each other and creating a just world coming from our most evolved awareness.

## Chapter 4

# Prenatal Care

The most significant prenatal care a woman receives is the care a woman gives herself. Ultimately, it is this care that all other forms of prenatal care should nurture.

When most people refer to prenatal care, they mean prenatal medical monitoring. Focused on detecting and reducing problems such as premature delivery, birth defects, and infant mortality, conventional prenatal care neglects to place adequate emphasis on nutrition, exercise, and emotional, social, and psychological health, all of which are essential to mothers and babies. The key to excellent prenatal care is individual care rather than routine procedures that ignore the unique needs of mother and baby. To restore a healthy balance to prenatal care in this country, we need to place more emphasis on projects that give all women access to healthy foods, reduced stress, and other necessities of prenatal health, rather than narrowly directing our resources to the research and development of sophisticated methods of prenatal testing. An ultrasound cannot help a baby grow—food does!

Prenatal care also includes the care a pregnant woman receives from others besides her health-care provider—be it her mate, children, mother, friends, or childbirth educator. A back rub, some help with older kids, a kind word, or nurturing and informative classes with a knowledgeable childbirth educator can enhance the care you are able to give yourself.

Again, none of this can replace the need for you to take care of yourself optimally, but it can contribute to your wellness by creating a very effective support network for you.

## Choosing Your Prenatal Care Provider

The purpose of prenatal care is to support the mother, her baby, and her family so that a healthy pregnancy can ensue, followed by a healthy birth, baby, postpartum, and integration of the baby into the family. This means working with a care provider who is sensitive to women and their families and knowledgeable about their needs, including optimal nutrition, exercise, mental and emotional well-being, and spiritual growth. In addition, this care provider should understand what compromises a healthy pregnancy for both the woman and baby, and have the ability to identify both health and health problems. The care provider must be sensitive, considerate, responsible, and professional yet warm. She must help the mother to become educated, well-informed, and confident about her body. She must also maintain an excellent relationship with other health-care practitioners so that she can help the mother to receive the care she requires.

I generally refer to prenatal care providers as women throughout this book. I believe that women are the most appropriate care providers for pregnant women. While there are sensitive male obstetricians and male nurse-midwives, I strongly believe that it is women's rightful place to provide prenatal and birth care. This is how it has been throughout history until the recent past, and this is how I believe it should be again. However, many women still take comfort in a male physician. If you do choose a male care provider, choose one who truly respects women.

Most practitioners (obstetricians, certified nurse-midwives, or traditional midwives, certified or not) see pregnant women on generally the same prenatal schedule, once a month until thirty-two weeks of pregnancy, then bimonthly until thirty-six weeks, then weekly until the birth. Many of the same procedures are done—for example, checking urine, determining the position of the baby, checking the blood pressure, and so on (see "Prenatal Visits" later in this chapter). However, the way a practitioner has been trained greatly affects her or his philosophies and perspectives, and thus, your care. This section provides an overview of the main types of care providers currently in the United States. Of course, these descriptions are generalizations, and any practitioner may be more or less holistically or medically oriented. You will have to decide which approach you are looking for and then choose an appropriate care provider. Many practitioners offer a free consultation.

When choosing a health-care practitioner, always ask questions that are important to you that will help you choose the most appropriate practitioner for you. Here are several essential questions to ask midwives:

- What training and experience do you have? Are you involved in continuing education?

- Can you handle both complications and emergencies?

- Do you have medical backup or a contingency plan for emergencies? What will be your role in an emergency? Will you continue to be with me during the emergency?

- What kind of equipment do you carry? Do you know how to use this equipment?

- Do you intend to see me with an assistant or by yourself? What about births?

- Is there a backup care provider should you be ill or otherwise unavailable at any point during the pregnancy or the birth?

- Do you have clear protocols and, if so, are these protocols rigid or flexible? For example, what happens if I go into labor prematurely or if I go past my due date? What if my baby is breech, and so on?

- What are your fees and what do they cover? Are any expenses covered by medical insurance? Am I entitled to any reimbursement in the event that I need to transfer out of your practice, for instance, if there is an emergency and a planned home birth becomes unreasonable?

- What are your philosophies about birth? Are they consistent and harmonious with my own?

If you are interviewing an obstetrician, you will want to ask:

- What are your credentials?

- What is your cesarean rate?

- What is your episiotomy rate?

- What is the rate of medicated births in your practice?

- How many women in your practice request rooming-in with their babies?

- How many women in your practice breastfeed their babies?

- What are your feelings about natural birth?

- How much time do you spend with women at prenatal visits?

> *"It's like growing food—if you take care of the soil, the food will grow. Cluck over the mother, nurture her."*
>
> —Candace Fields-Whitridge, CNM

> *"Care that is provided by another woman can be special. A midwife is a birthing woman's equal, not her authority. She is a confidante. She understands the importance of being respectful and gentle with another person's most intimate parts of herself. She knows that safety in childbirth is more a matter of prevention than treatment, of listening closely, helping a woman have a healthy attitude, and promoting normalcy. She protects both the privacy of the woman and the integrity of the family."*
>
> —Elizabeth Davis, *Heart and Hands: A Midwife's Guide to Pregnancy and Birth*

- Will you be at my birth or will another physician attend (and if so, who will that be)?

- What are your policies for women who go past-due, who have had previous cesarean sections, for permitted length of labor and pushing (or any other concerns or questions you might have)?

- Do you encourage women to participate actively in prenatal care and the birth?

You must be honest and comfortable with your care providers if you are really to meet your needs. It is of utmost importance that you work with someone you trust, whether this be a practitioner with an unconventional training, or a formally trained physician. If you aren't comfortable, seek another practitioner. This is your pregnancy and your decision to make. Ideally, your mate should feel comfortable with this person as well. The practitioner should respect you as an equal and talk to you with respect, answer your questions directly, and never treat you in a condescending way. If you feel that you are being treated in a way that makes you uncomfortable, find another practitioner with whom you do feel comfortable. In birthing, it is essential that you can be open, both literally and figuratively, and that your confidence in yourself be nurtured and reinforced.

## Direct-Entry and Certified Professional Midwives

Midwives come from a philosophy that honors the importance of the pregnant woman in the entire childbearing experience. At all times, the woman is treated with respect and sensitivity for the intelligent adult that she is. Midwives also maintain respect and sensitivity for the needs of the baby. Perhaps the central belief that unites midwives is that pregnancy and birth are natural processes for which women are inherently and biologically capable, and that with the participation of the woman in caring for herself and with the assistance and guidance of the midwife, the woman will enjoy a healthy experience. Midwives honor childbearing as a rite of passage and therefore encourage full participation by the mother during pregnancy and birth, and support her in this transition, helping her to grow in confidence and ability to nurture herself and her baby both before and after birth.

Direct-entry and certified professional midwives (CPM) primarily attend home births. However, many presently have birthing centers or clinics where they provide prenatal care and birthing services. Midwives (with occasional assistance from a physician or nurse-midwife) have been fighting the battle to keep alive the right to birth at home with a skilled attendant. This right to birth at home has been challenged in most states, to the point that many midwives have been arrested or harassed. While I cannot discuss this issue at length in this book, I encourage you to read books such *The American Way of Birth* by Jessica Mitford and *Immaculate Deception* by Suzanne Arms, as well as other titles found in the bibliography. For a complete discussion of the statistics on midwifery and homebirth safety, as well as choosing a care provider and birth setting, you might wish to consult my book *A Pocket Guide to Midwifery Care.*

Midwives, who are variously referred to as traditional midwives, lay midwives, or direct-entry midwives, maintain advanced levels of knowledge and understanding about the normal physiological processes of childbearing, as well as variations and deviations from normal. They are also knowledgeable about both preventing and treating problems that can arise during pregnancy, birth, and the postpartum period. Midwives have incorporated conventional knowledge, skills, and techniques for assessing both pregnancy health and complications, and complementary healing modalities such as dietary awareness, herbalism, and massage. Many of the innovations and progressive changes that have occurred in hospitals in recent years have been inspired by the kind of intimate, professional care provided by midwives.

Most midwives train as apprentices under the tutelage of other experienced midwives, gaining extensive clinical experience by attending numerous women throughout pregnancy, birth, and afterward. Midwives also engage in extensive independent academic study, familiarizing themselves with both conventional and traditional theories, techniques, and procedures for providing women with optimal health care. There are also several schools in the United States that provide formal midwifery training. The national midwifery organizations—the Midwives Alliance of North America (MANA) and the North American Registry of Midwives (NARM)—have developed a national certification process for those midwives who demonstrate their proficiency by passing an eight-hour written examination and an equally lengthy clinical examination. This certification (which confers the title of Certified Professional Midwife, or CPM) has been fostered in order to gain validity in state governments so that midwifery care can be made accessible to a broader range of women. The primary disadvantage of the certification and legalization processes is that they make midwives subject to external protocols that might be more limited in scope than those adopted by strictly independent midwives.

Studies indicate that in midwife-assisted births, even in high-risk women, there is a reduction of maternal and infant morbidity and infant mortality. Other countries that rely primarily on midwifery care have the lowest infant mortality rates in the world. (The United States ranks twenty-fifth in international infant mortality ratings; many other developed countries have a lower infant mortality rate.) At present, in many states midwives are illegal. Midwives can generally be found, however, with a bit of effort, by contacting local childbirth educators and La Leche League leaders, natural food stores, or by contacting MANA or other organizations found in the resources section of this book.

As with all professions, midwives vary in their skills and integrity. It is therefore up to you to determine the level of skill you want your midwife to possess (including the type of equipment she carries to births) and to explore her references and documentation of her training. To some women seeking a midwife, a midwife's skills at handling complications may be less significant than their personal relationship with her. It is your birth and if you choose a midwife with minimal experience because you feel that your relationship with her is the most important factor, that is your right; however, this choice must be based on honest information provided by your midwife, and it is your responsibility to arrange access to a practitioner or facility capable of handling an emergency should one arise beyond the capability of you or your practitioner. It is unfair to you and your baby, as well as your midwife, to expect her to be able to help you should an unexpected complication arise for which she lacks the necessary skills.

Midwives, because they are independent professionals, are able to provide mothers and their families with individual care. They are not bound by the regulations of hospitals or the time limitations of a medical office. In addition, most midwives have borne children and loved the experience. As women and mothers, they are uniquely capable of understanding pregnant women. They have firsthand knowledge of what they teach and do. Because midwives consider themselves your partner in your health care rather than in charge of your health care, you will usually find that you will be comfortable expressing your needs and desires, and they can help you achieve these. Most independent midwives provide prenatal care in their own homes,

> *"Pregnancy is a great time to have sex—you can't get pregnant!"*
>
> —*Ina May Gaskin*

providing you with a comfortable and informal atmosphere. They will also do at least one prenatal visit at your home prior to the birth.

Because most midwives rely on low-tech diagnostic techniques using their common sense, intuition, and sensitivity, many midwives are uniquely able to detect and avert pregnancy problems without the use of invasive (and expensive) procedures. Because midwives tend to choose their profession out of their deep caring for mothers and babies, they will provide you with excellent continuous care, seeing you from the time you initially contact them to the first months after your baby is born. Unlike other practitioners, most midwives make themselves readily available to their clients by phone for questions and concerns, in addition to being on call by pager for urgent situations. However, because midwives are not recognized as members of the medical profession in most states, nor are they trained to perform certain emergency medical procedures, your midwife is unlikely to be able to continue to provide you with treatment should an emergency arise and transport to the hospital become necessary. Most midwives will, however, accompany you to the hospital and continue to serve as a support person and advocate for you and the baby.

In the states where midwives are treated with hostility, your midwife might not be able to accompany you to the hospital, or, if she does, may prefer to accompany you provided you do not refer to her as a midwife. In states where midwifery is legal, or where there are supportive obstetricians willing to serve as a medical liaison to the hospital in case of emergency, a backup physician can be obtained before the birth. It is important that you discuss the issue of an emergency at some point during the pregnancy, and decide upon a clear course of action. Most midwives will have clear protocols that they can explain to you.

If you are working with either a direct-entry midwife or a nurse-midwife (see below), she should be able to provide you with the name of an obstetrician should you not be a candidate for a home birth or a birthing center birth, or should medical problems arise during your pregnancy. If you are at risk or have developed problems, you may need to work with an obstetrician, but you may in addition want to work with a midwife as a consultant, as problems of pregnancy and birth can often be reduced. In such cases, a team of health-care providers can be ideal.

## Nurse-Midwives

Nurse-midwives have completed the same training as registered nurses, then specialized in midwifery care. They first attend academic classes and gain clinical experience in caring for childbearing women and general gynecological care. They then begin midwifery training. Their ability to practice is limited by the fact that they can practice only if they have the consent of a supervisory obstetrician.

In general, nurse-midwives are more woman-centered than obstetricians and are likely to respect birth as a natural process. Nurse-midwives are very dedicated to their professions and are a great alternative for women who are seeking woman-centered medical care. However, their decisions regarding care are subject to the protocols of both their supervisory obstetrician and the hospital or birthing center in which they practice. Nurse-midwives may or may not be aware of complementary therapies that can facilitate health during pregnancy and birth. Instead, they are trained to rely on technology for information and may feel more secure by so doing. Few nurse-midwives attend home births compared to independent midwives, though there are some who do so.

## Obstetricians

Obstetricians are physicians who, in addition to their four years of medical training, have trained four additional years in obstetrics and gynecology, preparing them to assist women through both normal and complicated pregnancies and births. They are trained to provide women with gynecological care from puberty through old age.

Unfortunately, obstetricians are trained to manage pregnancy and birth as medical events. Few obstetricians are trained to let the mother be the orchestrator of her own health care and, because of their training, may come to see all pregnant women as emergencies waiting to happen. Additionally, because they often feel it necessary to protect themselves from lawsuits, they may use routine protocols with all patients. Overwhelmingly, obstetricians require that patients give birth in a hospital setting. However, some obstetricians will help women achieve natural births in the hospital. A few courageous obstetricians do have home-birth practices. These obstetricians may be ostracized by their colleagues, and some have had their licenses suspended.

Because of their training, which encourages obstetricians to rely on technology, few are comfortable with personal care, opting instead for routine tests and procedures to determine the well-being of the mother and baby. Similarly, few receive training in preventive health care. If you choose an obstetrician, you'll need to get input from other sources.

Most obstetricians are men (though the rate of female medical residents is now nearing 50 percent) and may therefore carry with them, consciously or not, culturally conditioned, condescending attitudes toward women. This can greatly affect the care you receive and the way you are treated. So please take care in choosing your doctor. Please insist upon natural, woman-centered, and family-centered childbirth. This will cause changes in obstetrical practice and lead to greater choice in hospital birth experiences in the future.

Obstetrical care is the best choice for those women with a high likelihood of developing complications during pregnancy or birth, such as those with diabetes, kidney or heart disease, toxemia, hypertension, or any problem that is likely to require medical intervention or emergency care.

## Osteopathic Obstetricians

Osteopathic physicians trained with a specialty in obstetrics go through medical training and a residency program nearly identical to other obstetricians, and have exactly the same privileges and rights, including permission to do cesarean sections and other surgery. Many osteopathic obstetricians hold positions on hospital staffs. Osteopathic training integrates an acceptance of holistic healing with organized medicine, making many osteopaths open to a natural approach to childbirth. You may want to consult with an osteopathic obstetrician if you prefer to have an obstetrician for your prenatal care and birth.

## Self-Care

I present this option as the last in this list because it is the least likely choice for most American women. However, a small percentage of couples and single mothers choose to provide their own prenatal care, paying close attention to a lifestyle that supports a healthy pregnancy and prevents problems. These women recognize that excellent self-care and intuitive awareness can guide them through pregnancy and birth safely, joyously, and in optimal health. This is a very empowering experience and creates a deeply intimate atmosphere in the family. In my own family, we've had three such pregnancy experiences in which my husband and I have independently cared for myself and the baby. It is important to say that I have spent nearly fifteen years as a midwife, and also have an excellent support network of other midwives and physicians upon whom I can call for support in the event of an emergency. Nonetheless, I have found that by looking inward for the information about my wellness and my baby's health, I have developed an enduring confidence in my body as well as deep connections with my children. One need not be a midwife to achieve this level of awareness.

If you choose to provide your own prenatal care, it is essential that you possess the humility that allows you to be able to ask for help, support, advice, or information at any time you want or suspect you need these, and that you be uncompromisingly committed to your well-being during pregnancy. I have seen couples so stuck on the idea of doing everything themselves that they endure unnecessary health problems that might have been easily resolved had they been willing to see a practitioner. It is important to be realistic and establish some sort of contingency plan for yourself in case a problem or emergency develops.

You may feel that you want a midwife or other experienced practitioner to support you on your independent path, but you should realize that in choosing the do-it-yourself route, you may be limiting your ability to consult with practitioners, because most practitioners, including midwives, will not want to be held responsible for you if you have not seen them regularly for prenatal care as a client, or if you have made choices with which they do not agree.

## Prenatal Visits

Prenatal visits ideally provide the opportunity for you (and your family) to have personalized and intimate time with someone who is knowledgeable about pregnancy and birth, who can answer your questions and give you information, support, encouragement, and confirmation of the baby's growth and health, as well as your own. It is also a time when a basic prenatal examination can indicate if there are any problems developing that require further assessment, treatment, or just watching. Prenatal visits should provide a chance for you and your care provider to get to know each other, developing a comfortable relationship that you can call upon for support during your pregnancy, birth, and transition to motherhood. During these visits, your care provider should also help Dad and siblings to feel the baby, listen to the baby's heartbeat, and so on. This helps all members of the family develop a deep prenatal bond with the baby and also lessens the difficulty of introducing a new baby to older siblings. In my experience, children who have been well integrated into the prenatal care readily accept their siblings and often participate in their care. A wise practitioner will always honor the primary relationship of the parents and do what she can to foster communication between them, helping the father accept his role as an active participant.

Prenatal care can vary greatly depending upon the type of practitioner you are seeing and her personal philosophy. The setting in which your prenatal visits occur, the regulations to which your practitioner is subjected, and the extent to which you help to shape your own care also matter.

## Midwife Visits

As discussed above, a direct-entry midwife is likely to be steeped in a philosophy that is woman-centered, based on the belief that pregnancy is a natural process. Most traditional midwives, while utilizing noninvasive methods for prenatal testing, will tailor their actions to the individual needs of the pregnant woman. Not only will she provide the same standards of pregnancy care provided by other practitioners, but she will also try to see how the pregnancy affects the woman's life and vice versa. Midwives, therefore, have to develop personal relationships with their clients. Most traditional midwives spend at least an hour per prenatal visit with their clients, often more than this. This depth of relationship is beneficial to a pregnant woman as well as her family. It can raise your sense of comfort, enabling you to relax your inhibitions and discuss personal issues that might affect your health, such as marital stress, herpes outbreaks, or parenting concerns. It can also reduce your anxiety about entering labor. You, as a woman, will be willing to discuss intimate physical discomforts or concerns with your midwife that you might be reluctant to discuss with a male practitioner.

The setting for prenatal care is generally the midwife's home or your own home. This environment, in my opinion, also increases a pregnant woman's sense that pregnancy is a normal, everyday event—that she is a client, not a patient—and that her birth can also occur in a relaxed, comfortable, and nonmedical environment. In addition, a traditional midwife is likely to include you in all procedures, teaching you if you're interested, and encouraging you if you're not, to be an active participant in your prenatal care—earning how to perform your own prenatal tests, understanding the significance of these, and learning how to care for yourself. As most midwives are very glad to share information openly with pregnant mothers (and families), your prenatal care is a perfect chance for you to learn about how your body works, the process of pregnancy, and your anatomy and physiology—in other words, how to be closely in touch with your body and baby.

> *When you are pregnant is a perfect time to get information about how your body works.*
>
> *—A. J. R.*

## Nurse-Midwife Visits

Nurse-midwives most often provide prenatal care within the context of an obstetrician's office, and though many try to establish personal relationships with their clients—and succeed at this—they are still subject to the limitations of time allowed for visits. Frequently nurse-midwives will meet with clients for only fifteen to thirty minutes. Additionally, you may not have the choice of which midwife you see prenatally (or which midwife attends your birth) if you are working with a group practice. Nurse-midwives have access to technology and medications, so if you want or need to employ tests or medications that require a prescription, you will have someone who can prescribe these, whereas most direct-entry midwives will have to refer you to a physician or lab. (If any situations arise that are beyond her scope, the nurse-midwife is obligated to refer you to an obstetrician.) The disadvantage of this is that the use of medications and procedures increases when they are easily available. You might find yourself subjected to greater levels of intervention if you work with a nurse-midwife rather than a traditional midwife. For example, if your urine sample reveals the presence of sugar, a traditional midwife is likely to first try to rule out diabetes using other noninvasive physical tests such as assessing your history, diet, and other symptoms, before recommending blood sugar testing. A nurse-midwife might be obligated to verify that there is no diabetes by requiring you to undergo blood sugar tests that require fasting or blood sugar loading, neither of which are healthy for you or your baby. Nurse-midwives who practice independently (often found in rural areas) or who practice in their homes are often more natural in their approach to prenatal care than those working in clinics, hospitals, and most obstetrician's offices.

## Obstetrician Visits

When you see an obstetrician, you will first be seen by the nurse who will weigh you and check your pulse, blood pressure, and urine. She will then take you to an office where you will wait for a period of time until the obstetrician comes to examine you. While there are some excellent obstetricians who provide holistic medical care and spend time familiarizing themselves with their patients' needs, most of these office visits will be brief, with the pregnant woman sometimes seeing the doctor for only fifteen minutes. The advantage of working with an obstetrician is that she or he can provide you with continuity of care in situations ranging from a normal vaginal birth to a complicated cesarean section. Neither traditional midwives nor nurse-midwives can offer this. Obstetricians are also much more likely to see birth as a medical event (you are a patient, not a client). This view of birth has its advantages and disadvantages. Moreover, since at least half of all obstetricians are men, you may find yourself inhibited in some discussions, even to the point of enduring certain physical discomforts, such as a symptomatic yeast infection, because you are too embarrassed to discuss the vaginal itching and discharge. You may also hesitate to discuss difficulty in your sexual relationship for similar reasons of embarrassment.

When working with most obstetricians, you are not likely to be involved in the medical aspects of your care, such as understanding routine tests and procedures. While some women may prefer not to take this responsibility, I believe that participating in your pregnancy empowers you as a woman. Your care provider should not be more knowledgeable about your body than you are.

# Prenatal Testing

In my practice as well as during my own pregnancies, medical technology has not been my focus. Rather, emphasis has been and is placed on nutritional awareness and other aspects of physical wellness, such as exercise and rest, and emotional and psychological health. Personal and social issues (such as financial stress or relationship tensions) may be disturbing the mother and may interfere with her taking care of herself. I also explore what the pregnancy means to a woman and how she is feeling. In addition, I physically assess the pregnant women with tests that are noninvasive and harmless, yet can confirm the mother's feelings of wellness or discomfort, or may reveal the development of a problem. These basic tests, the same as those that are performed by obstetricians and nurse-midwives, include testing the urine with coated test strips (the mother does this herself), checking the mother's pulse, blood pressure, and weight, measuring the growth of the uterus abdominally using a tape measure, feeling the baby for growth, listening to the baby's heart rate, and feeling the baby's position. Midwives, as well as other practitioners, may also perform a few more tests such as checking for kidney tenderness if a urinary tract infection is suspected, or checking the hemoglobin if anemia is thought to be a problem. The pregnant woman will also be asked whether she has had any problems such as nausea, headaches, dizziness, visual disturbances, heartburn, unusual urinary frequency, and other signs that may indicate the need for further attention.

Most practitioners also require pregnant mothers to obtain complete prenatal lab tests, which usually check blood type and Rh factor, hemoglobin, and an analysis of red and white blood cells, as well as ascertaining whether there is an immunity to rubella (German measles) and toxoplasmosis (contracted from handling infected cat feces and ingesting raw meat, both of which should be avoided by all pregnant women). You will also be tested for sexually transmitted diseases. It is also common for practitioners to require vaginal cultures to rule out the presence of gonorrhea and chlamydia.

More than ever, invasive—and sometimes unreliable—procedures have become routine components of prenatal care. A mere twenty years ago, many tests such as amniocentesis were performed only if problems were suspected or there were significant risk factors. Other tests, such as chorionic villi sampling, were not yet developed. The increase in such tests' availability has led to them becoming entirely routine in the obstetrician's office.

Fear of litigation should an obstetrician not detect a problem further leads practitioners to employ tests, protecting their own professional and personal interests and offsetting legal claims against them.

Every obstetric test has advantages and disadvantages. For example, knowing that she will give birth to a child with Down's syndrome, as revealed by an amniocentesis, may enable a woman and her partner to prepare for this, emotionally, psychologically, and materially, and find resources, organizations, and special supplies that they will need for caring for their child. Or if they choose to abort the child, they will avoid the stress that they perceive will accompany both raising a Down's syndrome child and the stress for the child in a society that is often discriminatory. However, the amniocentesis procedure can also cause damage to an otherwise perfectly healthy fetus, or even cause the miscarriage of a normal baby. It is up to each woman to become educated about the risks and benefits of the tests available to her prenatally, and to develop the confidence to agree to tests that she does want done, and to refuse the rest. It is essential that we examine our routine reliance on such equipment and tests as the doppler and diagnostic ultrasound, alpha-fetoprotein, chorionic villi sampling, and amniocentesis during pregnancy. In addition to their potential harm to the baby—about which much is still unknown—these tests externalize the mother's authority and body wisdom, keeping her distanced from the trust she might otherwise learn to develop in herself. This is not to say that testing is always unnecessary; it can be a great relief to a concerned mother to know that her baby appears to be healthy and growing well; it can also provide invaluable life-saving information when a problem is suspected.

Following are explanations of the purpose, procedure, risks, and benefits of several of the most common prenatal tests that might be considered invasive. I use the term invasive to mean that these tests require penetrating the body, either directly or by sound waves, or that they have the potential for harmful effects. Prenatal testing

> *It is up to each woman to become educated about the risks and benefits of the tests available to her prenatally, and to develop the confidence to agree to tests that she does want done, and to refuse the rest.*
>
> *—A. J. R.*

is an important issue in prenatal care, particularly if you are working with a medical practitioner, and I therefore encourage you to read *Pursuing the Birth Machine* by Marsden Wagner, *The Encyclopedia of Childbearing* by Barbara Katz-Rothman, *Obstetric Myths versus Research Realities* by Henci Goer, and *Immaculate Deception* by Suzanne Arms (see bibliography).

## Doppler Ultrasound

The doppler is an electronic device used routinely at a prenatal examination by both doctors and nurse-midwives, and occasionally by midwives, to hear the fetal heartbeat. It can detect the fetal heartbeat as early as eight weeks into the pregnancy. The doppler works by directing a continuous sound wave at the baby, which is then received by the amplification device and makes the heartbeat audible to those in the room. Many women enjoy hearing their baby's heartbeat amplified, but do not question the safety of the doppler. In fact, the doppler has not been conclusively proven safe for use in pregnancy; not enough long-term evidence is available. Nor has the doppler been proven more effective or accurate in assessing fetal heart tones than the completely benign use of the fetoscope, a fetal stethoscope. One minute of exposure to doppler has been estimated as equivalent to thirty-five minutes of imaging ultrasound exposure. The doppler is very useful for hearing the fetal heartbeat when it is difficult to hear it manually. You may want to request that your care provider use the fetoscope in place of routine use of the doppler, reserving its use for medical necessity, such as when the safety of the fetus is of concern and the heartbeat is inaudible with a fetoscope (for example, threatened miscarriage or lack of normal fetal movement).

## Diagnostic Ultrasound (Ultrasonography, Sonography)

Imaging ultrasound employs a similar technology to the doppler ultrasound but produces a screen image of the fetus and the placenta, which can be evaluated diagnostically. It is used routinely—most pregnant American women can expect to have at least one, and frequently several, ultrasounds. It too has not been proven safe for use in pregnancy.

While pregnant women find it exciting or reassuring to see a picture of their baby, imaging ultrasound is more appropriately reserved for use when there are medical indications such as suspected fetal demise, suspected placenta previa, a significant size/dates discrepancy, and determination of fetal position if it is difficult to determine it with palpation alone. If you do require an ultrasound, you can request that it be done by a technician with a lot of experience in order to reduce the amount of time that you are exposed.

## Maternal Serum Alpha-Fetoprotein Testing (MSAFP)

Alpha-fetoprotein (AFP) is a substance produced by the liver of the fetus, minute quantities of which appear in your bloodstream. The level of AFP rises progressively throughout pregnancy. Maternal blood levels are assessed for the amount of AFP present; an abnormally low or high level may indicate the presence of fetal anomalies. This test may be performed routinely without your knowledge at the time of your initial prenatal lab screening.

MSAFP is not a harmful test; however, it has a high rate of false positives. When a woman is determined to have abnormal AFP levels, she is then referred for further testing, usually an amniocentesis. Frequently, then, the woman will be anxious until the amniocentesis is performed. She will then be exposed to tests with higher risks for the mother and baby. The optimal time to have the MSAFP test performed is between fifteen and eighteen weeks' gestation, as the test is thought to be the most accurate when done during this time.

When a fetus is determined without a doubt to have anomalies, the only choices are to have the baby or abort.

## Amniocentesis

To perform an amniocentesis, a doctor inserts a long, sterile needle through your abdominal and uterine walls into the amniotic fluid. This test is done with an ultrasound in order to view the fetus and placenta. The amniotic fluid that is collected contains fetal cells that will provide information on fetal well-being and can indicate whether the fetus has certain birth defects (such as Down's syndrome), hemolytic anemia (destruction of the red blood cells that occurs from Rh disease), and many diseases, including carbohydrate, fat, and amino acid metabolism disorders, and cystic fibrosis. It can be used to determine lung maturity when a premature labor is occurring or if a preterm cesarean section is necessary.

Risks include puncturing the umbilical cord, placenta, or uterus, or causing infection or miscarriage. In addition, if an insufficient amount of fluid is collected, or if the culture of the fetal cells doesn't grow, the test will need to repeated.

If the baby is determined to have a disorder, you must then choose whether to keep the baby or abort. Amniocentesis cannot screen for all possible fetal disorders, and it can potentially damage a normal fetus. You must weigh the risks and benefits of having this test done, especially if you plan to keep the baby no matter what the problem is.

## Chorionic Villi Sampling (CVS)

To perform this test (at between nine and eleven weeks' gestation), tissues are removed from what will develop into the placenta. The tissue is obtained by going through either the abdomen or cervix, and using an instrument to remove the tissue while directly looking at the area. This test can check for chromosomal abnormalities, but cannot detect all of the problems that can be picked up by amniocentesis.

Risks of this test include damaging the embryo (damage can be as severe as the loss of a limb), damage to the cervix and uterus, infection, hemorrhage, and miscarriage. This test should not be done in the presence of a vaginal infection, Rh sensitization, or multiple gestation. I seriously suspect other potential problems we've not yet discovered, as disrupting the placenta is a significant interruption of what nature intended.

As with other diagnostic tests, you must evaluate the risk to benefit ratio. If you plan to abort the baby if there is a problem, CVS can provide you with quick and early diagnosis. (Results are usually available in twenty-four hours.) If you plan to keep the baby if there is a problem, you must keep in mind that an otherwise healthy baby can suffer severe damage as a result of this procedure.

> *We have become so highly acculturated to accepting birth as a technological and medical event that we must unlearn the cultural conditioning.*
>
> *—A. J. R.*

## Childbirth Education Classes

Ultimately, our bodies know how to birth and need very little instruction. However, there are three main aspects of childbearing in our modern culture that make childbirth education classes useful. First, we have become so highly acculturated to accepting birth as a technological and medical event that we must unlearn the cultural conditioning that can undermine our efforts to birth naturally. Second, we have lost our connection to the elders of our communities who share with us the information and wisdom that facilitates these transitions that we must make in becoming mothers, fathers, and families. We must learn on our own by trial and error, a task that is both difficult and fraught with stress. Third, we have become isolated in nuclear units, thinking that our problems are unique, unusual, or worse than those of other families. This can lead to unnecessary stress, shame, confusion, and in the long run, if not addressed, depression, exhaustion, and divorce. For example, many couples experience sexual tension during pregnancy (one partner may want more physical intimacy than the other), or confusion and anger over unmet expectations (pregnant women may want their mates to be more involved in touching the baby or buying baby clothes than the partner cares to be). Many pregnant women experience similar physical and emotional challenges, and many men feel unsure in their new role.

Childbirth education classes provide a forum for parents to explore such issues under the guidance of a childbirth educator, usually a woman (or a couple) who has knowledge about pregnancy and birth through both study and personal experience. While midwives can provide excellent prenatal education that can often substitute for prenatal classes, the opportunity to share and learn with other couples is very valuable, particularly for first-time parents. In an obstetrician's office, rarely is there time allocated for prenatal education. Classes in this case are also necessary if you are to have any understanding of the birth process, or of hospital procedures and protocols.

There are numerous childbirth education organizations offering their own philosophies, material, and educational styles. Classes offered in hospitals are nearly always geared toward a hospital birth. While natural childbirth might be a term that regularly pops up in the discussion, you are also likely to receive complete information on the drugs of choice for pain relief, full preparation for a cesarean section, and minimal information that would truly support you in achieving either a natural pregnancy or birth. If a truly positive and natural experience is your goal, you will want to seek a childbirth teacher who is well versed in positive, natural birth and who orients classes toward home birth or home and hospital birth. Whether you are planning a home or hospital birth, it is imperative that the classes educate you about medical procedures commonly used during birth so that you can discriminate between necessary procedures and hospital policies, protocols that might expose you to unnecessary testing, and intervention that the hospital requires in order to reduce its insurance liabilities. It is your right to exercise authority over your own body.

Ideally, classes should begin in early pregnancy in order to address the needs of pregnant mothers, couples, and families. For example, there should be discussion of nutrition and common discomforts during each trimester, there should be discussion of emotional issues that are likely to arise, and there should be preparation for the experience of pregnancy and parenting, of which birth is just a part (albeit a very profound part). Classes that encourage you to focus mainly on breathing techniques will distract you from finding your own strength, and in a subtle way promote a fear of birth. Such classes may stress the necessity of avoiding the pain or intensity of labor. You will know what to do. A good class will help you identify your inner resources for birth and prepare you for parenting and breastfeeding. A good class will help you find confidence in your abilities, while welcoming the intensity of birth and parenting.

In the resources section, you will find organizations that offer childbirth education services with trained teachers around the United States, Canada, and Europe. Midwives often offer classes to their clients, and so do hospitals. If not, they can recommend childbirth educators in your area.

There is much literature available on pregnancy, birth, and parenting. You can learn a lot by reading either on your own or with your mate (some men are very reluctant to read pregnancy and birth books, so you might have to be persistent), or by joining a study group with other pregnant moms. Cascade Health Care Products's *Birth and Life* catalog (see resources) offers a comprehensive selection of titles, and is well worth receiving. Local women's bookstores and even many large bookstores carry a selection of such books. Libraries often have limited book selections but may be convinced to expand their resources if enough women request that they do so.

## Chapter 5

# Nutrition during Pregnancy

The words *nutrition* and *nourishment* both have as their root the word *nourir,* which literally means "to suckle." A similar word, *nurturance,* means affectionate care and attention. *Nurture* is also defined as "the sum of the influences modifying the expression of the genetic potentialities of an organism." From this etymological and defined perspective, it is apparent that nutrition is much more than obtaining a certain amount of vitamins and minerals. Optimal nutrition is a way of loving and caring for ourselves and others that allows us and those we serve to reach our (or their) fullest potential. Indeed this is obvious when a close relative or friend serves us a bowl of warm soup and we feel that we are being fed much more than the food itself. Excellent nutrition is more than just taking in a certain number of recommended daily allowances, it is also an awareness of how we prepare, eat, and digest our food, of how we feel about our bodies as well as our emotional, mental, and spiritual selves, of what chemicals are in the foods we eat and how these affect not only our own health but also our baby's health and the health of our environment. Nourishment is a holistic experience that goes far beyond simply eating.

Because we live in a fast-paced and highly industrialized culture, one that places material gain and external approval over an intrinsic sense of wellness and satisfaction, many women do not take the time to nourish themselves—nor do many women truly know how. Many women entering pregnancy, for example, know very little about eating well. I've worked with highly educated women, including health-care professionals, whose idea of a nutritious vegetable is canned green beans, and whose idea of a high-calcium food is ice cream. Similarly, most women do not know how to relax deeply, do not know how to exercise to improve the health of their pelvic muscles, do not know how to use their Earth-given gifts of herbs to support pregnancy health, do not know how to supplement their diets with essential nutrients, nor how to prevent or reduce many common pregnancy discomforts. But many pregnancy problems, including serious complications, can be prevented with optimal pregnancy nourishment, precluding the need for testing and interventions during pregnancy and birth, and also for their newborns. An optimally healthy woman will usually feel well for most of her pregnancy, and therefore have a greater chance of enjoying the experience and looking forward to her baby's birth with joy. So many women consider the common complaints of pregnancy to be "natural." To some degree, it is likely that the changes that occur during pregnancy will cause periodic discomfort, but many common problems are a reflection of a lifestyle that did not prepare us to be healthy pregnant women. While some nausea may be unavoidable, such problems as persistent constipation, headaches, leg cramps, and exhaustion can be prevented or relieved with good nutrition.

Optimal pregnancy health not only helps to ensure that your baby is healthy, intelligent, and resistant to infections, but will ensure that you are healthy during the pregnancy and birth. This will lay a foundation of health that can support you when you are breastfeeding during the precious first few years of your child's life. It will also help you meet the demands every parent of young children must face. A well-nourished person is better able to cope with stress than one who is inadequately nourished.

In my work with pregnant women, from the earliest prenatal visit, I place a great emphasis on nutrition. The reason is simple: there is overwhelming evidence that excellent maternal nutrition almost always results in healthy mothers and babies, while a poorly nourished mother is likely to experience complications during the pregnancy and birth, and her baby is also likely to have problems. This evidence ranges from scientific studies of many types to the personal experience of mothers and midwives who time and time again see the effects of excellent and poor nutrition.

But what is excellent nutrition? So many of us, raised on sugared cereals, canned vegetables, pizza, and TV dinners, have no clue as to what constitutes good nutrition beyond what we see and hear on television or in popular magazines or newspapers. Some shoppers may be familiar with the labels on packaged foods, which tell us what the recommended daily allowances (RDA) of certain nutrients are. However, do we question where these standards come from, or how they relate to us? Do we even know what the nutrients are, what they do in our bodies, why we need them, and where we can get them? Many people remember the four basic food groups from elementary school or are familiar with the more recent food pyramid. However, we really have no idea what whole foods are or what variety of foods we should eat to ensure optimal nutrition. We can prepare our food in more wholesome ways, we can eliminate junk foods, and we can eat more fresh fruits and vegetables. I can recall my own first pregnancy when I put ketchup on the freshly picked organic kale and collard greens that my mate had lovingly harvested for me, in order to make them palatable. Before pregnancy, I'd never eaten these highly nutritious greens that he, as a Southerner, had known since childhood. Now I devour these vegetables daily, as do my children, frequently with no more garnish than a dash of tamari.

In a culture that equates thinness with success, beauty, and health, women are afraid to eat for fear of becoming overweight. So we have a substantial population of women in our society with eating disorders (an estimated one in five women), many of whom are of childbearing age. Many women are so out of touch with their bodies that they don't even know when they are hungry, a result of suppressing their instinctual, life-preserving urge to eat. What often happens is that women try to get by on as little food as possible, living in a state of hypoglycemia, frequently overloading on sugar and carbohydrates to restore their low blood sugar level to a semblance of normality. This, combined with the fact that the few foods women permit themselves to eat are junk foods, it is no wonder that our country has a high rate of premature, underweight babies, and a high rate of pregnancies fraught with discomforts and problems. When you add to these issues the poor women whose access to healthy foods is difficult, and the omnipresent factor of stress, which adds to our caloric and nutrient needs, we have a prenatal nutritional mess.

Yet all women can learn to eat well and to be informed about their unique nutritional needs. We can learn to be wise shoppers and to recognize that we pay more for packaged foods than for fresh foods, that buying junk food instead of nutritious food is throwing away our nutrition, money, and health, and that preparing our own foods, to whatever extent we can, is less expensive than eating out. Even women who are in high-risk categories for

> "For each of us as women, there is a deep place within, where hidden and growing our true spirit rises. . . . Within these deep places, each one holds an incredible reserve of creativity and power, of unexamined and unrecorded emotion and feeling."
>
> —*Audre Lorde*

pregnancy complications due to the problems associated with poverty can bear healthy children when their diet is improved. Poor women of color have significantly higher mortality, morbidity, and congenital problems than white women. It is essential that individual communities find ways to support those women who are at greater risk, such as providing free prenatal classes, promoting social services that provide prenatal care, and starting community gardens to provide seasonal fresh vegetables to pregnant women.

## Committing Yourself to Eating Well

The first step that a pregnant woman can take toward becoming well-nourished is to make the commitment to do so, knowing that she and her baby deserve it. Ideally, the father or partner should also make the commitment to support the pregnant mother in shopping, cooking, and so on. There will be days when a pregnant woman just doesn't feel like cooking but still really needs to eat well. Without some form of support, meals are likely to be missed or skimped, and mother and baby may go without adequate nourishment.

In order to be able to nourish yourself, you must reconnect with your instinctual sense of hunger, which is inherent in human beings. You will have to learn to eat when you are hungry, not for reasons such as frustration, anger, depression, or boredom. Likewise, you will have to learn not to skip meals due to emotional upset or stress. You must learn to love and appreciate your growing body, and eat without worrying about your weight (see "Weight Gain" later in this chapter). And you must learn what foods are necessary for optimal health, first by studying, then by recognizing how different foods cause you to feel, and what you intuit you and your baby need. (See chapter 3 for more information on using inner guidance during pregnancy.)

## Every Woman Is Unique

Every pregnant woman is going to have a unique appetite. She will come from a different ethnic background and seek different comfort foods. The best place to start to plan your diet is to list what you eat presently. From there, you can add foods that may provide you with the extra nutrients that pregnancy requires, and perhaps you'll be open to acquiring a few new tastes. The most effective way to begin is to write down what midwives refer to as a "diet diary." This is a record of all that passes your lips (such as food, pills, and cigarettes). Five to seven days will give the broadest, clearest picture of your eating habits. A three-day diary is the absolute minimum. See the accompanying diet diary form that I give a pregnant mother, which outlines the ideal of three meals and three snacks daily. You can use any notebook to write in.

By glancing at this chart, you can see that a pregnant woman will ideally be eating quite often. This does not mean that you need to gorge each time you eat. It does mean that you eat something nutritious every few hours. Ideally, every time you eat you should be meeting your daily needs. By eating a wide variety of foods from the "Essential Nutrients" section below, you will be doing just this.

Another excellent idea, taught to me by midwife Sarahn Henderson, is to create the ideal pregnancy diet diary. Using the same form, create a diet diary of what you would be eating for five days if you had an ideal prenatal diet. You can use nutritional guidelines from this book and others (see bibliography). You will learn a great deal from this exercise, and might even come up with a few new ideas and recipes in the process.

# Diet Diaries

When I have a woman write down a diet diary, I have her keep a record of the intake of all substances over the course of five to seven days. The following samples represent a day from the diet diaries of several different women. All of the women are in mid- to late pregnancy, as diet diaries done during the first trimester may reflect inability to eat optimally due to prenatal nausea. (Of course, it is still important to eat well when you are nauseated, and, in fact, a healthy diet can often reduce nausea.) Diet diaries are brought to an initial prenatal visit and are reviewed as a part of the medical and personal history. The women in these samples began prenatal care with a midwife at the weeks' gestation noted near the mother's name. (All names were changed for the purpose of confidentiality.)

Diet diaries are assessed on the basis of general food groups as discussed later in this section, with the idea that a woman should ideally be eating a certain number of servings from each group. It would be impractical for a woman to record her food intake on the basis of grams, milligrams, international units, and so on, and impossible for a midwife to evaluate her diet in this way without knowing the exact sizes of individual servings and specific nutrient contents of various brands of foods that might be used. For example, did the woman drink six ounces of soy milk or ten ounces, and how much protein per ounce does that soy milk brand claim to have?

It is important to remember that there might be days that you don't eat optimally, but that the goal is to try to eat optimally as often as possible.

# Diet Diary

*From*_____ *to*_____

| | Day 1 | Day 2 | Day 3 | Day 4 | Day 5 |
|---|---|---|---|---|---|
| **Breakfast** | | | | | |
| **Snack** | | | | | |
| **Lunch** | | | | | |
| **Snack** | | | | | |
| **Dinner** | | | | | |
| **Snack** | | | | | |
| **Drinks (specify)** | | | | | |
| **Supplements** | | | | | |
| **Other** | | | | | |

## Stephanie's Diet Diary

*23 weeks pregnant with her third baby*

**BREAKFAST**
2 scrambled eggs
$^1/_2$ bagel
Water
Peppermint tea with milk and sugar

**LUNCH**
Manicotti with cheese and sauce
Green salad with alfalfa sprouts
Water
Milk

**SNACK**
Water
Apple

**DINNER**
Potato omelette
Rice, peas, and beans
Broccoli, green beans, and carrots
Orange
Milk

**EVENING**
Water

Overall, this mother ate a very healthy diet this day. If you compare it to the recommended amounts, she received many of the servings needed for optimal wellness. Improvements might be in getting her complex carbohydrates from a whole-grain source such as brown rice and a whole-wheat bagel, rather than the white-flour variety. Her overall food choices reflect a wide variety of foods, and no reliance on sweets, empty calories, or junk foods.

## Jenny's Diet Diary

*27 weeks pregnant with her first baby*

**BREAKFAST**
Cheerios with blueberries and soymilk
1 piece whole-wheat toast with
    strawberry jam
Prenatal vitamin

**LUNCH**
$3^1/_4$ ounces tuna
Wheat Thins
Water
Raisins

**SNACK**
Apple juice
Iron supplement
Vitamin C

**DINNER**
Spaghetti with tomato sauce
Mozzarella cheese
2 pieces whole-wheat garlic toast
Cucumber
Mineral water
Chocolate nonfat frozen yogurt

Jenny's diet contains few fresh vegetables, little protein, few calcium sources, and very few fluids. She shows a reliance on sweets for energy, which she probably craves due to the lack of whole grains and protein. She often had sugar in her urine, which would disappear after several days of moderating her sugar intake. She could add a salad to her lunch, a leafy green to her dinner, and a serving of squash, steamed carrots, or a slice of cantaloupe to one of her meals. To her spaghetti sauce, she might add texturized vegetable protein, ground tofu, or ground beef for protein. At breakfast, she might replace the Cheerios with a whole-grain cereal. She could have a more substantial grain with her lunch, and perhaps some cottage cheese with the apple for her snack. She should increase her fluid intake.

## *Nita's Diet Diary*

*32 weeks pregnant with her second baby*

**BREAKFAST**
2 whole-wheat waffles
1 fried egg
Grapefruit juice

**SNACK**
Milk with Ovaltine

**LUNCH**
Peanut butter and banana
Noodles and cheese
Green beans and red pepper

**SNACK**
Banana

**DINNER**
Artichoke with mayonnaise sauce
Large green salad with carrots, garbanzo
    beans, and sunflower seeds, oil and
    vinegar dressing

**OTHER**
2¹/₂ quarts of water
Prenatal vitamins
Fresh carrot-apple juice

Nita has an excellent diet in general and is conscientious in eating protein, vegetables, and fresh, wholesome foods. I might suggest a more natural alternative to Ovaltine, as it contains a fair amount of sugar. Also, Nita might incorporate whole grains into her dinner meal, or as part of her snacks.

## *Michelle's Diet Diary*

*25 weeks pregnant with her first baby, working full-time as a health-care provider in a busy practice*

**BREAKFAST**
1 cup of decaffeinated coffee
Banana

**SNACK**
Crackers

**LUNCH**
Turkey with cheese sandwich

**SNACK**
5 pieces of chocolate

**DINNER**
Tuna with pasta and cream sauce

**OTHER**
2 quarts of water
2 prenatal vitamins

Michelle's diet, even to the untrained eye, is obviously devoid of almost all nutritional value, short of two protein servings and plenty of fluids. In fact, she has far fewer nutrients than she requires and is actually further depleting her nutrients by drinking coffee and eating chocolate, which rob minerals from the body. Michelle improved her diet somewhat by learning about foods that she could carry along with her to work, having prepared them in advance. Even with those changes, her baby weighed only just over five pounds at birth, compared with all of the other babies in these samples, which weighed at least seven and a half pounds. She also had a very difficult time establishing breastfeeding. Michelle needed a full education in nutrition for pregnancy health.

## *Amina's Diet Diary*

*33 weeks pregnant with her second baby*

**BREAKFAST**
Prune/bran drink
2 pieces of whole-wheat bread with peanut
butter

**LUNCH**
Carrot and celery sticks
Cottage cheese
Raisins
Apple
Crackers with cheese

**DINNER**
Roast beef
Potatoes
Green beans
Corn

**EVENING**
Prune/bran drink

**OTHER**
$\frac{1}{2}$ gallon water
Floradix (2 times daily)
Spirulina (2 tablets, 3 times daily)

Amina has a good basic diet, but might add a calcium-rich snack and a calcium serving to one of her meals. In addition, she rarely eats leafy green vegetables and consequently suffers from constipation. Leafy greens are also rich in calcium. A bed of lettuce for her cottage cheese and a serving of collard greens with dinner might round out her diet nicely.

## *Diane's Diet Diary*

*30 weeks pregnant with her second baby*

**BREAKFAST**
Orange juice
Oatmeal with raisins

**LUNCH**
Salad
Cheese toast
Cookie

**SNACK**
Bagel with cream cheese

**DINNER**
Potato
Broccoli

**OTHER**
Prenatal vitamins
Calcium supplement
1000 mg vitamin C

Diane's diet diary is severely lacking in essential nutrients. Throughout her pregnancy she had recurrent bladder infections, sugar in her urine, and depression. She bled heavily at birth and was depressed afterward as well. Her diet is lacking in protein and calcium, contains no yellow or orange vegetables, and is heavy in sweets, including fruit juice, raisins, and cookies. She needs to add protein, calcium, and vegetables at each meal and snack, and try to find foods that are filling and nonsweet. In fact, when she tried this approach, the sugar did not show up in her urine samples.

The diet diaries in these samples come from women ranging from eighteen years old to the midthirties. These women's professions are stay-at-home mother, artist, musician, schoolteacher, chiropractor, and medical doctor (not in that order).

To understand the evaluation of these diet diaries, you will need to refer to the following information on specific nutrients so that you will know which foods provide which nutrients.

# Essential Nutrients

Because it is ideal to get your nutrients from foods rather than relying on supplements, I am including a wide variety of food sources from which various nutrients are available. The best way to ensure that you are eating well is to include a wide variety of healthy, natural foods. Your best bets are foods that are as close to a natural state as possible—minimally processed with no additives or preservatives. The core of a healthy diet will be made up of whole grains, beans, fresh vegetables, fresh fruits, nuts, seeds, and smaller amounts of dairy products, and complementary amounts of meats, particularly fish and poultry. If you are unaccustomed to natural foods, try to find a few interesting cookbooks and begin to add healthy foods slowly to your diet. If you already are eating a very healthy diet, then make sure you are eating adequate amounts, which are needed by your growing body and baby.

Let your intuition guide you in your food choices. Suspend your conscious mind for a few minutes each day to allow messages to arise from your right brain or intuitive mode of thinking. If your intuition tells you to eat a piece of salmon though you are an ardent vegetarian, you may choose your intuited needs over your ideals. Similarly, if you dislike collard greens but your body says "greens," you may have to develop a taste for collards

### Recommended Dietary Allowances of Nutrients for Pregnant and Nursing Women

| NUTRIENT | PREGNANCY | NURSING |
|---|---|---|
| Protein | 74 g | 64 g |
| Calories | 2300 | 2500 |
| Vitamin A | 5000 IU | 6000 IU |
| Vitamin D | 400 IU | 400 IU |
| Vitamin C | 80 mg | 100 mg |
| Vitamin E | 15 IU | 16 IU |
| $B_1$ | 1.4 mg | 1.5 mg |
| $B_2$ | 1.5 mg | 1.7 mg |
| Niacin | 15 mg | 18 mg |
| $B_6$ | 2.6 mg | 2.5 mg |
| Folic Acid | 800 mcg | 500 mcg |
| $B_{12}$ | 4 mcg | 4 mcg |
| Calcium | 1200 mg | 1200 mg |
| Phosphorus | 1200 mg | 1200 mg |
| Magnesium | 450 mg | 450 mg |
| Iron | 30 to 60 mg | 30 to 60 mg |
| Zinc | 20 mg | 25 mg |
| Iodine | 175 mcg | 200 mcg |

(from the Food and Nutrition Board of the National Academy of Sciences, 1980)

and find a few delicious recipes! To develop this intuition, allow yourself to be very still and quiet for a few minutes, and then simply ask yourself or the baby what you need. Make a note of what you imagine the answer to be. Try this each day for a week and follow through on the messages that you receive.

Eat for nutrition and pleasure, and you will meet your needs. Enjoyment of food is one of the most important keys to good digestion, which must also occur if you are going to absorb and utilize the foods you do eat.

Here's a general guideline to the food servings you need to eat daily:

- Calories: eat plentifully of healthy foods to ensure adequate calories daily—pregnancy is not a time to try to minimize calories.

- Protein: 4 servings.

- Vitamin C foods: 2 servings.

- Calcium foods: 4 servings.

- Green leafy vegetables and yellow fruits and vegetables: 3 servings.

- Other veggies and fruits: 1 to 2 servings.

- Whole grains and other complex carbohydrates: 4 to 6 servings.

- Iron-rich foods: some daily.

- High-fat foods: 2 servings.

- Salt: daily in moderation to taste.

- Fluids: at least 6 to 8 glasses a day.

- Supplements: nutritious herbs, highly concentrated food supplements such as spirulina, and, when necessary, a vitamin/mineral supplement.

These daily serving amounts are known as "the daily dozen" in *What to Eat When You're Expecting* (Eisenberg, Murkoff, and Hathaway). They will provide you with a good framework to which you can add healthy foods of your own choosing. Note that all of these requirements increase when you are carrying two or more babies. Remember, this is an ideal that you should try to achieve as closely as possible. You will have better days and skimpier days, depending on how you feel and what is going on in your life. I also suggest that you pay attention to how you feel when you eat or miss a meal, or when you eat a healthy meal compared to a sweet snack. In time, your body will come to crave the healthy meals over the empty foods.

The National Academy of Sciences has published recommended dietary allowances of nutrients for pregnant and nursing women (see chart on page 61). These numbers reflect the actual amounts of nutrients that pregnant and nursing women need in order to maintain a healthy pregnancy. When referring to this chart, it is important to keep a few things in mind:

- We are all unique—so are our needs.
- The numbers in this chart reflect dietary needs to the best of present scientific knowledge. As knowledge changes and grows, so do charts such as this one.
- Following a chart of nutrients is less important than eating amply of a wide variety of whole, natural foods daily.
- A healthy diet comes from an open mind and a commitment to paying attention to your personal needs.

Following are descriptions of the common essential nutrients, along with their functions and the sources from which you can obtain them.

## Protein

Protein is one of the most abundant substances in the body, second only to water. It provides the structural framework upon which all body tissues depend for healthy growth. Bones, muscles, skin, blood, hair, nails, organs, and connective tissue are all made from proteins. The baby's hormones, growth, metabolism, and sexual development are made possible with protein. Protein is necessary for basic chemical reactions, including the maintenance of fluid and pH balance. Protein encourages and contributes to the formation of antibodies necessary for fighting infection. If we have an adequate protein and carbohydrate ratio, our blood sugar level remains stable and we are provided with energy as we need it.

Protein provides the raw material for making the baby, placenta, and a strong uterus. It contributes to the formation of breast milk and is essential for healthy blood clotting. There are about twenty-two amino acids—the structural components of protein and the end products of protein digestion—needed by the body. All but eight of these can be produced in the body or converted into another kind should a shortage of any occur. The eight that must be obtained dietarily are called the "essential amino acids." These eight amino acids are available in many foods in varying proportions. However, for the protein to be used optimally by the body, they need to be present in specific amounts. Foods in which the amino acids are always present in these specific quantities are known as "complete proteins" and include such foods as meats, dairy products, and soybean products. When eating meat as a protein source, organic is preferable. Though it may be slightly more expensive than inorganic meat, avoiding the many chemical contaminants found in meat (antibiotics, growth hormones, and other chemicals given to the animals during growth) is preferable for the health of both the mother and the baby. Foods such as grains, seeds, nuts, and legumes are known as "incomplete proteins" as they are either missing or low in specific amino acids. When eaten in various combinations, grains and legumes form complete proteins that are highly nutritious and assimilable by the body. Vegetables also contain usable proteins, but in smaller amounts than the foods already mentioned. See below for a discussion of protein combining.

Protein is not well stored in the body and a continual supply is necessary for the healthy functioning of all of our cells. Protein deficiency may manifest itself as follows: abnormal growth and development, loss of muscle tone, lack of vigor and stamina, mental depression, increased susceptibility to infection, poor wound healing, and slow recovery from illness. Protein loss occurs through stresses such as injury and illness. During such times, extra protein is required to replace or repair tissues. Childbearing, due to the increased size and amount of the mother's tissues, the baby's needs, labor, birth, postpartum healing, and lactation, requires a great increase in protein consumption. While protein requirements are influenced by a woman's size, nutritional status, and activity levels, it is generally thought that 75 to 100 grams of protein daily will fulfill the protein requirement for pregnancy. Eating at least four servings of protein-rich foods as part of meals, with complementary high-protein snacks (such as yogurt, cheese and crackers, or hummus dip) daily will provide you with adequate protein. I personally have found that the lower end of this range is optimal, the upper end producing very large babies and difficult digestion. Inadequate protein intake during pregnancy is associated with toxemia.

An exhaustive list of protein quantities in different foods is beyond the scope of this book, but I direct you to *What to Eat When You're Expecting* (Eisenberg, Murkoff, and Hathaway). *Holistic Midwifery* by Anne Frye, written for health-care professionals, also offers many pages of food servings and their nutrient quantities. The book is clear enough that you don't have to be a midwife to understand and make use of the information. By learning to recognize what foods are rich in different nutrients, you will be able to construct a good diet for yourself.

# *Carbohydrates*

Carbohydrates are the main source of energy for all body functions including digestion and assimilation of food and all muscular activity. Carbohydrates provide immediately available energy for producing heat in the body. Broken down into glucose, carbohydrates provide fuel for the brain, nervous system, and muscle tissues; in the form of glycogen, carbohydrates can be stored by the liver and muscles. Carbohydrates, when available in excess, can also be stored throughout the body in the form of fat and used as reserve energy when needed. (The utilization of fat results in weight loss.)

Carbohydrates are needed in the largest quantity of all the nutrients required by the body. They make up the bulk of our diet. They are available in three main forms: simple sugars, starches (complex carbohydrates), and cellulose (the indigestible parts of fruits and vegetables that provide us with the fiber needed for healthy bowel functioning).

Simple sugars can be found in both refined foods (sugar, candy, soft drinks, chocolate, and so on) and unrefined foods (honey, maple syrup, and other natural sweeteners as well as fruits). In these forms they are almost immediately digested, quickly raising blood sugar levels and eliminating feelings of hunger. It is important to realize that the feeling of hunger, although triggered somewhat by falling blood sugar levels, is more than a signal to put more sugar in the body. It is also a call for vital nutrients. Both refined and unrefined sugars have the ability to satisfy hunger with quick fuel. This can lead us to forgo eating nutritious foods that will provide us with longer-lasting energy. This is true for fruits as well, though they do provide essential vitamins and minerals. Since excess carbohydrates are stored in the body as fat, you can actually become overweight at the same time you are becoming malnourished. Simple sugars are short-lived in the bloodstream, leaving us with sudden feelings of fatigue, depression, irritability, headache, and the need for another boost of energy. Persistent overconsumption of simple sugars can also lead to an overly large baby and maternal diabetes (with complications for both mom and baby).

Starches are complex chains of sugar units. When carbohydrates are eaten in this form, the sugar units are separated and digested slowly, thus taking longer to reach the bloodstream and satiate hunger. This slow digestion allows the body adequate time to absorb the range of nutrients in these unprocessed starchy foods. With complex carbohydrates, blood sugar levels remain steady for a longer time than with simple sugars, so hunger is sated for a considerably greater length of time.

If carbohydrate intake is insufficient, the body will use protein and fat for energy. This leads to a harmful chemical residue in the body known as "ketones," which if present consistently or in high amounts can be dangerous for both the mother and the baby. It is therefore essential that pregnant mothers base their diets around complex carbohydrates as their source of energy (four to six servings daily), getting these from whole grains (brown rice, whole wheat, millet, oats, rye, barley, amaranth, and so on), seeds, and a variety of starchy vegetables such as potatoes (both white and sweet), squashes, and beets.

## Fats

Fats, or lipids, are the most concentrated form of energy in the diet, providing twice as many calories per gram as carbohydrates and protein. Fats act as carriers of the fat-soluble vitamins—A, D, E, and K. By aiding in the absorption of vitamin D, fats make calcium available to body tissues. Also, fats are important in converting carotene to vitamin A. Fat deposits surround, hold in place, and protect major organs. A layer of body fat helps the body deal with temperature changes in a room or outdoors and preserves body heat. There are three essential fatty acids (substances that give fats their different properties such as melting point, flavor, and texture). They are synthesized by the body if one of them, linoleic acid, is present in the diet. These unsaturated fatty acids are necessary for healthy blood, arteries, nerves, skin, and other tissues. They aid in the digestion of cholesterol.

Cholesterol is a fat-related substance and is needed to form sex and adrenal hormones, vitamin D, healthy blood, skin, the nervous system, brain and liver tissue, and the bile that is necessary for the digestion of fats.

Although rare, a deficiency of fats will lead to a deficiency of fat-soluble vitamins and related disorders. Excessive intake of fats could also lead to digestive and other health problems. An acceptable intake is one tablespoon of fat daily in the form of a pure vegetable oil (unrefined, cold-pressed oil), as well as foods rich in this nutrient. Significant sources of fats are nuts, seeds, vegetable oils, butter, margarine, dairy products, and fats in meat. Salmon, mackerel, and herring are excellent sources of essential fatty acids and can be eaten a couple of times a week. Essential fatty acids are also found in the oils derived from evening primrose, walnuts, black currants, flax seeds, and borage. Raw walnut oil or flaxseed oil can be added to salads and other dishes after cooking, or a supplement of 500 mg of any of these oils, with the exception of the walnut oil (do not exceed this dosage unless there is a specific reason for doing so), can be taken daily throughout pregnancy to ensure adequate intake.

## Vitamins

### VITAMIN A

Vitamin A is most noted for its role in preventing and fighting infections. It promotes healthy skin and mucous membranes, strong bones, rich blood, and keen eyesight. Proper digestion of proteins requires the presence of vitamin A. Requirements may vary greatly from person to person, and both deficiency and excess of this vitamin can be harmful. Therefore it is important to eat foods rich in vitamin A, but to avoid supplementation of this individual vitamin during pregnancy (other than what is in your prenatal vitamin, if you are taking one).

Acute vitamin A poisoning can be recognized by nausea, vomiting, dry skin, diarrhea, hair loss, sore lips, and flaky, itchy skin. This usually only occurs as a result of excessive supplementation and, unless caused by chronic excess, will disappear soon after the vitamin supplement is withdrawn. In early pregnancy, however, excessive supplementation can result in permanent fetal malformations.

Symptoms of vitamin A deficiency include frequent colds and respiratory problems, sinus trouble, rough skin, acne, dandruff, and night blindness.

Vitamin A is destroyed by light, staleness, drying of foods, and chemical fertilizers. It is leached out of the body by ingesting mineral oil. The body accepts vitamin A more easily in foods that are cooked, mashed, or puréed.

Rich sources of this vitamin include yellow and orange fruits, yellow vegetables, dark green vegetables, orange vegetables such as carrots and sweet potatoes, dairy products, eggs (especially the yolk), and liver.

Herbal sources include alfalfa, watercress, nettle, red raspberry leaves, dandelion, comfrey, nori, yellow dock, and lamb's quarters.

### VITAMIN B-COMPLEX

The B-complex vitamins are grouped because they have similar functions and tend to occur together in nature. Similarly, a deficiency of a single B vitamin is less likely than a general B vitamin deficiency. B vitamins are essential for a healthy nervous system, as well as for the metabolism of carbohydrates, fats, and proteins. They also help maintain muscle tone in the gastrointestinal tract and health of the skin, hair, eyes, mouth, and liver. Since they are water-soluble vitamins, they are not stored in the body and must be ingested through the diet on a regular basis. Some of the B vitamins are produced naturally in healthy intestines.

There are quite a few B-complex vitamins. The following are considered especially important for health during pregnancy:

*B1 (thiamin)* is necessary for children's consistent growth, a healthy nervous system, and good muscle tone in the stomach, intestines, and heart. B1 aids in the conversion of glucose into energy and helps stabilize the appetite and blood sugar by the assimilation of starches and sugars. Signs of deficiency include constipation, loss of appetite, digestive problems, fatigue, apathy, uncertainty of memory, and nervousness. B1 is stored in the body only in very small amounts, so daily intake is necessary. Found in the outer layers of grains, it is usually lost in the refining process. It is destroyed by heat, oxidation, and alkaline substances such as baking soda. Sources include whole grains (especially wheat germ), nuts and seeds, legumes, potatoes, peas, nutritional yeast, bananas, and avocados.

Herbal sources include dandelion, alfalfa, red clover, red raspberry leaves, nori, kelp, catnip, and watercress.

*B2 (riboflavin)* is necessary for the assimilation and digestion of carbohydrates, fats, and proteins. It aids in cell respiration. Maintenance of healthy skin, nails, hair, and good vision depends on vitamin B2.

This nutrient is found in nutritional yeast, whole grains (especially wheat), dried beans and peas, seeds (especially sunflower), leafy green vegetables, cottage cheese, milk, and organ meats.

Signs of deficiency in B2 include digestive troubles, skin and eye problems, cracking at the corners of the mouth, hair loss, poor lactation, sluggishness, retarded growth, dizziness, trembling, urinary difficulty, vaginal itching, and bloating of the body.

Herbal sources include rose hips, dandelion, dulse, kelp, and fenugreek.

*B6 (pyridoxine)* is required for a healthy nervous system and utilization of carbohydrates, fats, and proteins. It must be present for the production of antibodies and red blood cells. It helps regulate body fluids and aids in healthy muscle formation and functioning. It is associated with hormonal balance and, because of its importance in digestion and healthy muscles, deficiency is often associated with nausea and leg cramps in pregnancy. Depression may also be caused by a B6 deficiency.

B6 is destroyed by heat and ultraviolet light. Rich food sources include brown rice, wheat bran and germ, blackstrap molasses, nutritional yeast, bananas, salmon, and organ meats.

*B12* is needed for healthy nerve tissue, fetal brain development, the production of genetic material, proper cell division, and the metabolism of many nutrients.

Because plants do not require B12 for their growth, plant foods—unless they have been fermented (encouraging the growth of bacteria that contain and help our bodies to synthesize B12) or fortified—rarely contain this vitamin. Therefore, those on strictly vegan diets, containing absolutely no animal products, should consider using vitamin B12. Foods that do contain B12 include dairy products (with the exception of butter) and meats. Vegetarian sources include tempeh, miso, and B12-fortified nutritional yeast. However, tempeh and miso contain variable and, according to some, unreliable amounts of B12. Because our bodies need only small amounts of B12, the addition of a small daily amount of dairy or other animal products to the diet will supply enough, as will a prenatal vitamin. Maintaining healthy intestinal flora with yogurt will also help with intrinsic B12 production.

The fact that our bodies store B12 for years is in some ways an advantage, but could also prevent deficiency signs from showing up for five or six years. Signs of B12 deficiency include a glossy, sore tongue, indigestion, abdominal pains, and diarrhea or constipation. Left untreated, serious mental and nervous problems may develop, and eventually death may occur. Megaloblastic and pernicious anemia are terms used to describe deficiencies associated with vitamin B12.

*Folic acid* is a water-soluble member of the B-complex group. It is essential for the formation of red blood cells and antibodies that prevent infection. A lack of folic acid can result in severe anemia in the mother and neural tube defects in the baby (such as anencephaly, a congenital absence of the forebrain, and spina bifida, an opening along the spine). Folic acid is used in the breakdown and utilization of protein and is essential for healthy brain development. Digestive, mental, and emotional health are all related to folic acid intake. Folic acid is needed in much greater amounts during pregnancy, acting as a safeguard against anemia, miscarriage, premature birth, and birth defects. It is available in green leafy vegetables, wheat germ, nutritional yeast, eggs, whole grains, lentils, nuts, milk, and liver. As it is lost in the cooking process, care must be taken to eat raw leafy green vegetables daily and to regularly include several of these other sources in your diet.

### VITAMIN C (ASCORBIC ACID)

Vitamin C is essential for the production of collagen, a protein needed for forming connective tissue in bones, ligaments, and skin, as well as in the healing of wounds and burns. It is needed to produce a healthy placenta, capillaries, and cell walls, and helps to prevent varicosities and hemorrhage. Vitamin C greatly aids in the assimilation of other nutrients, such as folic acid, iron, vitamins A and E, and certain amino acids. It is very helpful in preventing and healing infections and is quickly used up during stressful times. During pregnancy, the daily dosage should not exceed 2,000 mg, as it can lead to miscarriage in early pregnancy, and can cause a vitamin C dependency in the baby, which can lead to scurvy in the newborn.

Found in most fresh fruits and vegetables, vitamin C is destroyed by heat, air, and light, and is also lost in cooking water. At least two servings of vitamin C–rich foods should be eaten each day. Excellent sources include green leafy vegetables such as raw or lightly cooked kale and collard greens, strawberries, peppers, citrus fruits, cantaloupe, alfalfa sprouts, and tomatoes.

Herbal sources include rose hips, watercress, dandelion greens, red clover, burdock, nettle, and alfalfa.

### VITAMIN D

Vitamin D is a fat-soluble vitamin, mainly available through exposure to sunlight and ingestion of fatty fish and fish liver oils, with smaller amounts to be found in butter, milk from grazed cows, and egg yolks. Fortified commercial milk is rich in a synthetic form of vitamin D.

Vitamin D aids in the absorption of calcium from the intestines and the breakdown and assimilation of phosphorous, both necessary for bone formation. It helps maintain a healthy nervous system, normal heart functioning, and normal clotting responses by helping the body absorb calcium. Deficiencies of this nutrient can lead to bone deformities and excesses of it can lead to dizziness, nausea, and weakness, similar to what is experienced from overexposure to the sun.

Herbal sources include alfalfa and nettle.

### VITAMIN E

This is another fat-soluble vitamin. The most common form is alpha-tocopherol, which literally means "the substance required to bring forth normal births." Vitamin E prevents the destruction of cells and vital nutrients, and it enables body tissue to function with less oxygen, thereby increasing endurance and stamina. It is essential to certain types of metabolism, aids in cell division, and promotes health and healing of body tissue. Vitamin E helps prevent abnormal blood clotting and is said to increase the pain threshold.

It is abundant in whole grains, nuts, oils, eggs, wheat germ, legumes, and green leafy vegetables. Caution should be taken with any vitamin E supplementation during pregnancy as excesses may cause abnormal adherence of the placenta. Vitamin E can also be dangerous for those with heart or blood pressure problems, so any supplementation should be done carefully and intelligently.

# Minerals

## CALCIUM

The most abundant mineral in the body, calcium is needed in the formation of a baby's bones and teeth, and in maintaining the health of the mother's bones, teeth, and connective tissue. It is essential in controlling the coagulation of blood. Muscles cannot contract and release without it. Calcium helps maintain healthy nerves, normal metabolism, mineral balance throughout the body, and regular heartbeat. It is said to increase the pain threshold, and its effectiveness in promoting nerve and muscular relaxation prevents and reduces insomnia. Signs of calcium deficiency include irritability, insomnia, and leg cramps. Sources of calcium are milk, hard cheeses, yogurt, leafy green vegetables, almonds, sea vegetables, salmon, and blackstrap molasses. It is important to maintain a balance of calcium and phosphorus in the diet as excess of either will cause losses of both. Also, calcium and magnesium work together, and when you supplement calcium, take a supplement that contains both of these minerals. Be sure to eat four servings of calcium-rich foods each day.

Herbal sources include alfalfa, red clover, red raspberry leaves, nettle, chamomile, dandelion, kelp, and dulse.

## IRON

Iron is present in every living cell. Its major function is to combine with other nutrients to create hemoglobin, which brings oxygen to all the tissues of the body. Iron helps to build the blood, increases resistance to stress and disease, and allows for proper muscle contraction. It aids in protein metabolism, helps to improve respiration, and prevents hemorrhage.

Sources of iron include leafy dark green vegetables, dried fruits (raisins, apricots, black mission figs, prunes, currants, and cherries), blackstrap molasses, sea vegetables, dried beans and legumes, whole grains, eggs, red meat, and liver. You will need to eat several iron-rich foods daily.

Herbal sources include nettle, dandelion, yellow dock, kelp, alfalfa, watercress, and fennel.

> *"We tend to think that a baby in utero is entirely cut off from the world that lies just beyond a thin layer of skin. We seldom consider the child within as a conscious being, capable of responding to sounds and the inner environment the mother creates through her sense of well-being or lack of it."*
>
> —*Joy Gardner*

### IODINE

Iodine is needed for the healthy function of the thyroid gland, which is responsible for the rate of metabolism, growth and development, and mental balance. Deficiency may be signaled by frequent infections, weakness, nervous system problems, and low activity levels.

Iodine is found in seafood—fish and sea vegetables (kelp or kombu, dulse, alaria or wakame, hijiki, and nori)—and in iodized salt and sea salt. A few vegetables contain small amounts of iodine.

Herbal sources include watercress, kelp, dulse, and Irish moss.

### PHOSPHORUS

Usually found in abundance in most diets, phosphorus is important for bone development, healthy teeth, and the healthy growth of fetal cells.

Herbal sources include alfalfa, red raspberry leaves, dandelion, watercress, caraway seeds, and comfrey.

### ZINC

Zinc is essential for normal immune system functioning, healthy hormone production, organ development, healthy reproduction, and release of vitamin A from the liver. It also protects the bones and joints, as well as the prostate gland and sexual fluids in males.

Sources include oysters, other shellfish, herring, nuts, seeds, beef, eggs, chicken, turkey, fruits, and vegetables.

Herbal sources include watercress.

### SODIUM

Sodium is an essential mineral for maintaining health during pregnancy. A deficiency of sodium is associated with swelling and toxemia in pregnancy. It is necessary for maintaining both fluid and electrolyte balance, as well as preventing muscular irritability. It is available in common salt, sea salt, and many foods. Pregnant women should reduce their consumption of junk foods, which are heavily salted, but should salt their other foods to taste using a natural form of salt such as sea salt.

### OTHER MINERALS

Other minerals, such as potassium, which is needed for strong muscle contraction, and many trace minerals should all be available to you in your diet if you are eating the quantity and variety of foods already mentioned.

## *Essential Fatty Acids*

Essential fatty acids (EFAs) are critical and overlooked nutrients needed for optimal brain development in the fetus. The breast milk of mothers in the United States is among the lowest in essential fatty acids in the world, indicating that pregnant women in this country are likely very deficient in EFAs, as are their babies. Inadequate intake of EFAs has been associated with decreased mental development, increased rates of allergies and asthma, and other atopic diseases. Essential fatty acids are found in high amounts in walnuts and walnut oil; flaxseeds and flaxseed oil; deepwater fish such as salmon, tuna, and cod; and avocados. During pregnancy, if one chooses to supplement, it is advisable to use both an evening primrose oil supplement and a high-quality fish oil supplement in order to get a balance of both omega-3 and omega-6 fatty acids. It is not necessary to supplement with fish oil if fish is eaten as a regular part of the weekly diet. However, the American Academy of Pediatrics and the American Academy of Obstetrics and Gynecology do recommend that pregnant women not consume deepsea fish more than once or twice weekly to avoid excessive consumption of mercury contamination from fish, which may be transferred to the developing fetus.

# Vegetarian and Other Natural Foods Diets

There are four common variations on the basic vegetarian diet: the vegetarian who occasionally eats fish or chicken, but relies primarily on nonmeat sources for nutrients; the lacto-ovo vegetarian who eats no meats but does eat dairy products and eggs; the lacto vegetarian who eats dairy but no meats or eggs; and the vegan who includes absolutely no animal products in the diet whatsoever and frequently excludes honey as well.

A person on a macrobiotic diet eats whole grains, beans, vegetables, occasional fruits in season, sea vegetables, seeds, and nuts, with the occasional inclusion of fish. Such a person relies on the concept of yin and yang to create balanced menus to meet individual health needs and create harmony in the body, mind, and spirit.

A person on a raw-food diet believes that humans, like animals, should eat foods in a raw state. Emphasis is placed on fruits, vegetables, fresh juices, sprouts, nuts, and seeds (preferably sprouted). The idea is that cooked foods cause impurities in the body.

It is possible to meet your nutritional needs on any of these diets during pregnancy, if you give close attention to meeting these needs. Vegetarian diets that include a variety of foods are likely to include much less fat as well as fewer, if any, chemical additives and fewer overprocessed foods. Be open to your needs and don't get stuck on a preconceived idea. Respect your intuition whether you are a vegetarian wanting a piece of chicken, a vegan wanting a cheese sandwich, or a macrobiotic wanting a grapefruit in the middle of winter in Boston. The danger lies in becoming an extremist (admittedly, I consider a raw-foods diet extreme) and in excluding foods that might be just what your body needs. Of course there are many vegetarian ways to meet your needs if you choose to be strictly vegetarian—you must be willing to educate yourself about your nutritional needs.

Many natural foods diets are based on the idea that the body is dirty and needs cleansing through fasting. This is untrue and potentially very dangerous for pregnant women. Our bodies are capable of digesting meat, dairy products (unless a specific intolerance exists), and other foods often considered taboo. The key is moderation and balance. Also, foods serve different purposes. For example, fruits and raw foods cool us down and promote elimination while heavy carbohydrates and proteins warm us and help us to build our bodies. We must recognize what is appropriate for different seasons of the year and of our lives. Pregnancy is a time of building and nourishing, with elimination being an essential function for health, but not our primary goal.

Pregnant women need to eat with great care. They should avoid exposure to harmful additives as well as to residues from pesticides, and to antibiotics and hormones in animal products (dairy included). All pregnant women would do well to eat foods that are grown organically and are processed minimally if at all, with no additives or preservatives. Foods raised, grown, and prepared this way are not only safer to eat, but also retain more of their nutrient value than processed foods. While such good food may seem more expensive, it is actually worth the money as your body will be happy, and your medical expenses will be reduced. Chemical additives in food are associated with health problems ranging from acne to cancer. During pregnancy, additives are particularly dangerous in the first trimester as they may impact on the development of the fetus. Hormones found in dairy products may imbalance a woman's own hormones, as well as cause her baby to grow overly big. (Even without these hormones, milk encourages babies to grow large.)

Women who eat a healthy, well-balanced vegetarian diet may in fact enjoy a healthier pregnancy than women who rely heavily on the standard American diet, which is laden with sugar and fat and excludes fresh vegetables, whole grains, legumes, nuts, and seeds. The primary concern for vegetarian women is that they get ample protein; also, if dairy is not eaten, foods containing calcium should be plentiful in the diet. There are many foods that can provide these nutrients, and, in fact, in China where almost no dairy is used and a lot of dark green vegetables are consumed, the women have the lowest osteoporosis rates in the world. See "Calcium" earlier in this chapter, and refer to the bibliography for more information on calcium substitutes. I encourage women not to drink milk during pregnancy and to rely instead on nondairy calcium sources, as well as hard cheeses and active-culture yogurt.

*Growing a baby is a big job that requires you to have good materials, enough to meet your needs and your baby's.*

*—A. J. R.*

In order to obtain adequate protein from a vegetarian diet, these women must learn to combine their protein sources to create complete proteins, as discussed earlier in this section. The following shows the various ways this can be done:

1. Grains (rice, corn, wheat, millet, oats, rye, barley, and so on) can be combined with a slightly smaller amount of beans or legumes (lentils, peanuts, garbanzo beans, kidney beans, pinto beans, black beans, azuki beans, navy beans, soybeans, and so on).

2. Grains can be combined with dairy products.

3. Nuts and seeds can be combined with beans or legumes.

A few examples of complete proteins include rice and beans; macaroni and cheese; rice and tahini (sesame seed paste); pasta with peanut sauce; granola that contains oats, peanuts, and sunflower seeds; whole-wheat bread with peanut butter; and tofu on toast. You don't need to eat complete proteins every time you have a protein food, but you should get four to five servings of complete proteins each day. I have enjoyed three completely vegetarian pregnancies, and one mostly vegetarian. In my last pregnancy, I was inclined to eat fish and chicken, and so I occasionally added these foods (organic poultry only) to my diet. The main advantage for me in including dairy as a regular part of my diet was the fact that it is easy to prepare and is a filling source of energy. One can eat rice, beans, and cheese, for example, and feel more filled than by eating rice and beans alone. Yogurt, or cheese and crackers, makes a great, filling, quick snack. Also, dairy foods are complete proteins, so I didn't have to be as concerned about combining foods as I would on a vegan diet. It takes a larger quantity of vegetarian foods to satisfy the appetite than, say, a small piece of steak, but vegetarian food is also easier to digest, and not likely to result in problems such as constipation or weight gain due to the high-fiber, low-fat nature of the foods.

I recommend that pregnant women do not drink milk because babies of mothers who drink a lot of milk tend to grow very big. I feel that this is a disadvantage in birthing. Milk molecules are also hard to digest, milk is high in fat, and it also contains hormones, both naturally occurring in cows and sometimes added with cattle feed. These hormones are not beneficial to human health and may possibly be harmful.

If you are pregnant and vegetarian, I can't overemphasize how important it is to eat a wide variety of foods in order to obtain all of the nutrients you now require. I've met many well-educated vegetarians whose diets were limited to just a few foods. Some rely on packaged foods. Processing is processing—it robs foods of nutrients. Also, many vegetarian women eat a lot of fruit and drink a lot of fruit juices, filling up on empty calories. Just being a vegetarian does not ensure that you are eating a healthy diet—it may mean merely that you are not eating unhealthy foods! If you plan to raise your child as a vegetarian, now is the time to do the research and feed yourself and your baby well.

# Supplements

Busy lifestyles, daily stresses, the nutritionally depleted nature of many foods sold in supermarkets, and variable appetite levels during pregnancy may mean that many pregnant women are not getting optimal nutrients from their diets. Closely spaced pregnancies and a history of current or recent breastfeeding may also mean a pregnant woman is entering this new pregnancy nutritionally slightly under par. A prenatal nutritional mutivitamin-multimineral supplement is therefore advisable for women who do not have time to eat optimally or who are not able to eat as well as they would like to due to low appetite, which is also frequently due to inadequate nutrient intake!

Unfortunately, some pregnant women become nauseated by prenatal vitamins. I for one got extremely nauseated and even vomited after taking supplements. I therefore did not take prenatal vitamins and had to be committed to an unwavering excellent diet. Finding a prenatal supplement that does not upset the stomach may take some time and experimentation with different brands. Food-based, natural supplements are probably the healthiest source when pregnant, but may cost a bit more. Ask your care provider if she can provide prenatal vitamins to you at a wholesale cost—many practitioners are able to set up accounts with companies that sell supplements, thus allowing you to get a better price on a healthier supplement.

When a woman is pregnant and shows some stress or fatigue, or has a poor diet, a daily supplement can improve her well-being. When a woman is eating well (evidenced by her diet diary and an ongoing discussion of her eating patterns) and doesn't want to take a supplement, the addition of herbal infusions and syrups (see chapter 6, Herbs, Safety, and Pregnancy Health) as well as concentrated food sources such as blackstrap molasses, liquid chlorophyll, and spirulina (a blue-green algae) can be used to boost her nutrition. Blackstrap molasses is an excellent source of calcium, iron, and B vitamins; chlorophyll can help boost iron levels; while spirulina is a source of high-quality protein and other trace nutrients. One to two tablespoons of molasses and one tablespoon of chlorophyll daily are excellent additions to the diet. Molasses can be taken in hot water; added to a smoothie with yogurt, bananas, honey, and vanilla; eaten off the spoon; or taken in an iron tonic (see "Anemia" in chapter 14 for the recipe). Spirulina, a particularly useful supplement for vegetarians who may benefit from the extra protein, can be taken in tablets or can be added as a powder to a smoothie. If iron deficiency is a problem, refer to "Anemia" in chapter 14.

However you choose to enhance your diet, it is essential that you do so, as growing a baby is a big job that requires you to have good materials, enough to meet your needs and the baby's. Remember, though, that no supplements will substitute for good food.

# Cravings

As long as you are meeting all of your daily needs with healthy food, there is no reason that you should not enjoy an occasional ice cream, piece of cake, cookies, or a chocolate brownie. The main problems arise when you follow your urge for cravings that are downright unhealthy, such as coffee, cigarettes, sodas, or alcohol, which can interfere with nutrient absorption or may cause harm to your baby. Also, problems may arise when you use your craving as a substitute for nutritious foods. For example, if you work outside the home while you are pregnant and find yourself craving a chocolate bar at 11:00 A.M. each day, your body is really telling you that you need food energy. If you eat the candy bar, you are basically sublimating your appetite and not getting anything nutritious. You could carry a healthy snack with you to work, such as a container of yogurt and some granola, apples and peanut butter, a cheese sandwich, or a small thermos of soup, and eat this when you feel the craving. If at the end of the day you've met your daily food needs and still want a dessert, have one. But even these can be made with nutritious and wholesome ingredients.

Frequently, cravings are specific clues about our nutritional needs. Deciphering them may take a bit of detective work. For example, a pregnant mother in my practice craved the proverbial pickles and ice cream. She was busy tending to her two older children, both under three years of age, and didn't bother to eat. She then became ravenous for the pickles and ice cream. It struck me that her body perhaps needed more protein and calcium (the ice cream). As for the pickles, vinegary foods encourage our bodies to release calcium into the bloodstream. When I suggested she begin to improve her intake of protein and calcium, she reported that she had no more of those cravings. Frequently, a craving for sweets is a physical need for more protein in the diet. Cravings for chips or pretzels can be a sign that you need more salt or even fats in your diet. Try to replace junk foods with wholesome choices and see how this affects your cravings. If you're eating well and still want some ice cream, bon appétit!

# Weight Gain

Because weight is such a big mental and emotional concern for most women—thin women don't want to gain it, overweight women want to lose it, and most women compromise their eating because of it—I don't place any emphasis on weight gain in my work. The fact is, a woman can gain weight even on an inadequate diet. There-fore, I focus on what and how much a woman is eating, not how much she is gaining. I did the same for myself, weighing myself at the beginning and end of my pregnancies for curiosity's sake. When I begin to work with a woman, I will ask her if she knows her weight, and I will enter this in her chart. Then at subsequent visits I will ask her if she knows her weight, and, if she does not, I will ask her if she wants to know her weight. If she says no, we don't check her weight. What is really impor-tant is whether the baby is growing and whether she feels and looks healthy. If so, there is no need, in my opinion, to be concerned about weight.

According to typical midwifery and medical standards, an ideal weight gain for a pregnant woman is about twenty-five to thirty-five pounds. Some women will gain more, some less, especially depending upon their prepregnant weight. (Very slim women may gain as much as fifty pounds while larger women may gain less.) Women will also gain weight in unique spurts, not in neat little increments per month. Many women will gain moderately in the first months of pregnancy, only to make a big weight gain in the middle months of the pregnancy. Many women will slow down again toward the end of pregnancy, despite the fact that the baby may appear to grow rapidly during the last weeks of the pregnancy. Again, quality is more important than quantity in the area of weight gain. If knowing that you are gaining is going to make you sabotage yourself by con-sciously or unconsciously cutting back your food intake, then weighing should be abandoned. Similarly, if you go for a few weeks without gaining much weight, yet your baby is growing and your health is fine, it is wise to ascertain whether you are eating enough food, particularly if you exercise heavily. Each woman has a unique weight-gain pattern.

## Chapter 6

# Herbs, Safety, and Pregnancy Health

erbs are used to promote health, spice up our lives, and restore us when we feel ill or out of sorts. There are literally thousands of herbs used around the world by different peoples for different conditions. Traditionally, herbs have been added to foods to improve the taste, promote healthy digestion, and prevent parasites and other infectious organisms from taking hold in our bodies. Herbs can be used to improve the quantity and quality of nutrients in the diet due to their high vitamin and mineral content; they can be used to promote the health of the immune system; and they can reduce stress. Many herbs are both safe and highly effective as remedies for common health complaints and more serious conditions. Herbs and spices are consumed daily around the world by pregnant women as a natural part of the diet. Taken in small amounts and using only herbs that are known to be safe during pregnancy, they can provide relief for many minor pregnancy complaints and, in expert hands, can also be used for more complex pregnancy-related problems. However, herbs are also potent medicinal agents, and therefore great care and caution is advised for their use during pregnancy. Whenever possible, the use of herbs should be avoided during the first trimester; if it is necessary to use herbs during this time, only those herbs with no known teratogenic, mutagenic, or abortifacient properties should be used, and only in the lowest possible doses.

While many herbal remedies are gentle and safe, they are also pharmacologically active agents that should be administered with care. It is important to remember that while the human species has a long history of using herbs safely, very few studies have been done to demonstrate the safety and effectiveness of herbs during pregnancy. Consider the following key points:

- Natural is not synonymous with harmless or safe—many botanical medicines contain potent pharmacological substances.

- Many herbal constituents are capable of passing through the placenta and can therefore directly affect the fetus.

- Physiological and metabolic changes during pregnancy may influence the action of herbs in the body.

- Unless medically indicated, avoid use of herbs (and drugs) during the first trimester.

- Preventive treatment and early intervention with herbs is safer and more effective than treating advanced problems, since dosage can typically be minimized and gentler herbs applied.

- Know each herb you are using by clearly understanding side effects and contraindications for pregnant women.

If you are unsure about the safety of an herb during pregnancy, do not use it. Because the practice of herbal medicine is unregulated in the United States, anyone, whether or not they have training in herbs, can give advice on their use. This includes doctors, nurses, and midwives who may have the best of intentions but not the best information. A qualified herbalist (contact the American Herbalists Guild for information on herbal practitioners in the United States) or a health professional specially trained in the use of herbs during pregnancy (a midwife, nurse, or physician who has done specific research in this area, a licensed naturopathic physician who has graduated from a four-year naturopathic college, or a registered Chinese herbalist) can provide you with safety information. You can also contact several of the organizations that exist to provide consumers with herbal safety information, for example, the American Botanical Council or the American Herbalists Guild (see resources).

It is not hard to learn how to incorporate herbs into your daily life, but it is essential that you choose from those that are known to be safe during pregnancy. The best way to benefit from herbs is to use them regularly as a source of nourishment—not only when you are ill or uncomfortable. There are many herbs that can be used safely during pregnancy that not only provide additional vitamins and minerals to your diet, but also strengthen the womb, liver, nervous system, digestive system, and urogenital tract. Herbs derive nutrients from the soil that many of our common foods may lack. Herbs are relatively inexpensive, particularly if you buy them in bulk. Tea drinking is one way to incorporate herbs into your routine. It is a daily custom in many parts of the world and can provide a nourishing ritual during your pregnancy.

The herbs mentioned in this book can be considered safe in pregnancy as indicated by generations of safe usage, as well as by clinical studies when available. Known exceptions are noted. However, there are a few potential problems that should always be kept in mind. First of all, no two people are exactly alike and therefore you cannot know in advance the exact effect an herb will have on your body (or your baby). It is best to rely on tried-and-true herbs during pregnancy and to begin with small amounts, gradually increasing dosage as appropriate and necessary. For example, chamomile is an herb considered completely safe and free from any toxic side effects according to extensive German research, yet because of its membership in the *Compositae* family, along with herbs such as ragweed, a rare individual may have an allergic reaction to it. With all herbs, it is wise to proceed slowly and carefully.

Further, there is always a risk of contamination, adulteration, or substitution of one plant species for another in commerce. For example, in one instance, a Canadian mother thought she was taking an herb, *Eleutherococcus senticosus,* considered fairly safe for use during pregnancy. After taking the capsule product regularly during the pregnancy, she gave birth to a baby with congenital androgenism—the baby was hirsute (covered with an unnatural amount of hair). Upon scientific analysis of the product that the woman was taking, it was determined that it contained *Periploca,* another herb entirely. *Periploca* is not considered safe for use during pregnancy. It is very important to purchase herbs from reliable sources only. If you are unsure, contact an experienced herbalist in your community, or one of the national botanical medicine associations such as the American Herbalists Guild (see resources).

If you are harvesting plants yourself from the wild, make sure that you are identifying them correctly. Confusing the desired herb with a poisonous plant can be a fatal mistake—and one that is not that hard to make. Even if you purchase fresh herbs from someone who has harvested them, make sure they know their stuff—I recently heard the story of an experienced harvester who came upon a group of people harvesting herbs in the woods for inclusion in commercial products. They thought they were harvesting a medicinal herb commonly used in many products, but were inadvertently harvesting poisonous water hemlock. Fortunately, the more experienced passerby herbalist informed them of their mistake before it was too late.

When purchasing bulk herbs, be certain that the common names and the Latin names of the plants corroborate with each other so you know that you are getting what you are looking for (see appendix II). Plants have many different common names, but their Latin names are internationally accepted as a standard. Also be certain to take herbal tinctures, pills, and capsules from carefully labeled jars so that no mistakes are made. Again, this is especially important during pregnancy and with young children.

It is also essential to follow general dosage guidelines for each herb. The idea that more is better is dangerous when applied to any medication, including herbs. Although most herbs are very gentle, their effects should not be underestimated. In appendix I, Herbal Preparations, you will find general dosage guidelines. Specific guidelines accompany all herbal protocols discussed with conditions later in this book.

When you are pregnant, further considerations arise. Herbs that you take during pregnancy will usually affect your baby as well as you. Herbs contain potent chemical substances, many of which have demonstrable effects on the body. Certain herbs, for example, contain volatile oils or alkaloids that can affect the functioning of the central nervous system, and when taken during the first trimester of pregnancy can interfere with the development of the baby's nervous system. Other herbs have what are known as "emmenagogic" properties—that is, they stimulate pelvic circulation. While this may be desirable when a woman is close to the time of birth, the result earlier might be the stimulation of contractions, perhaps even premature labor. Pregnancy is a natural process, and, unless you are ill, it is unnecessary to use herbs other than as gentle toners and nourishers. If you are ill and wish to use herbs remedially, it is essential that you avoid herbs that are contraindicated during pregnancy, particularly during the first trimester. You should use herbs only according to recommended times and dosages. You should consult an experienced herbalist when you are unsure about the safety of using a particular herb during pregnancy.

## Herbs to Avoid during Pregnancy

The table that accompanies this section lists those herbs most commonly contraindicated for internal use during pregnancy. For a more exhaustive list, see the *Botanical Safety Handbook* by McGuffin et al.

There are some herbs on this list that may be used in small quantities for certain conditions, where the risks of using the herb are outweighed by the benefits, but

*"A woman is the full circle, within her is the power—to create, nurture, and transform."*

—Diane Mariechild

only with qualified supervision. An example of this would be the use of very small amounts of goldenseal for severe diarrhea during mid-pregnancy, if diarrhea was causing the mother to lose weight and become dehydrated. However, large doses of goldenseal during early pregnancy may be unsafe for the developing embryo.

## Herbs Contraindicated for Use in Pregnancy

Alder buckthorn, *Rhamnus frangula*
Aloe, *Aloe vera*
Angelica, *Angelica archangelica*
Arnica, *Arnica montana*
Autumn crocus, *Colchicum autumnale*
Barberry, *Berberis vulgaris*
Beth root, *Trillium* spp.
Black cohosh, *Cimicifuga racemosa*
Blessed thistle, *Cnicus benedictus*
Blood root, *Sanguinaria canadensis*
Blue cohosh, *Caulophyllum thalictroides*
Broom, *Sarpthamnus scoparius*
Butternut, *Juglans canadensis*
Calamus, *Acorus calamus*
Calendula, *Calendula officinalis*
Cascara sagrada, *Rhamnus purshiana*
Coltsfoot, *Tussilago farfara*
Comfrey, *Symphytum officinale*
Cotton root, *Gossypium herbaceum*
Cowslip, *Primula veris*
Damiana, *Turnera aphrodisiaca*
Dong quai, *Angelica sinensis*
Ephedra (ma huang), *Ephedra vulgaris*
Feverfew, *Tanacetum parthenium*
Ginseng, *Panax quinquefolium*
Goat's rue, *Galega officinalis*
Goldenseal, *Hydrastis canadensis*
Gotu kola, *Hydrocotyle asiatica*
Ipecac, *Ipecac ipechachuana*

Juniper berries, *Juniperis communis*
Licorice, *Glycyrrhiza glabra*
Lily of the valley, *Convallaria magalis*
Lobelia, *Lobelia inflata*
Male fern, *Dryopteris felix-mas*
Mandrake, *Podophyllum peltatum*
Mistletoe, *Viscum album*
Mugwort, *Artemesia vulgare*
Nutmeg (small amounts fine), *Myristica officinalis*
Osha, *Ligusticum porten*
Parsley (small amounts fine), *Petroselinum crispum*
Pennyroyal, *Mentha pulegium*
Periwinkle, *Vinca* spp.
Peruvian bark, *Cinchona* spp.
Pleurisy root, *Aesclepius tuberosa*
Poke root, *Phytolacca decondra*
Rhubarb, *Rheum palmatum*
Rue, *Ruta graveolens*
Sage, *Salvia officinalis*
Sarsaparilla, *Smilax officinale*
Senna, *Cassia senna*
Shepherd's purse, *Capsella bursa-pastoris*
Stillingia, *Stillingia sylvatica*
Tansy, *Tanacetum vulgare*
Thuja, *Thuja occidentalis*
Wormwood, *Artemesia absinthum*
Yarrow, *Achillea millefolium*

Also, certain herbs that are contraindicated by Western herbalists and Western scientific research for use during pregnancy are regularly used in other countries, such as dong quai prescribed as a blood tonic for pregnant women in China. It is wise to use such herbs cautiously, if at all, during pregnancy if you do not have prior herbal knowledge or the assistance of an herbalist. Pregnancy is not a good time to experiment with generally contraindicated herbs. Further, Chinese herbs, especially prepared products known as "patent products," are notoriously contaminated with herbs not listed on the package, and sometimes with pharmaceutical medications and even heavy metals. These should be avoided during pregnancy unless prescribed by a qualified herbalist or Chinese doctor familiar with clean, safe brands.

Specific categories of herbs are known to be contraindicated during pregnancy. One group of herbs that has come under scrutiny are those containing pyrrolizidine alkaloids (PAs). These are known to cause liver damage in both adults and developing fetuses. Comfrey, coltsfoot, and borage are the main culprits, containing varying amounts of these PAs. It is therefore most prudent to avoid the internal use of these herbs other than very occasionally and only after the first trimester of pregnancy. External use of comfrey in small amount for a short duration is probably safe, but PAs can cross the skin, so they should not be used for prolonged periods on broken skin.

Herbs that contain other strong alkaloids (often recognizable by their strongly bitter taste), whether they be those that strongly promote digestive functions and metabolism or those that perform other duties such as enhancing cardiac function, are to be avoided during pregnancy. Choices of gentle herbs can be applied for improving digestion. Laxative herbs that exert their effects by strongly promoting bowel peristalsis can also promote uterine contractions and so should be avoided during pregnancy. Gentler methods of promoting bowel functioning should be used, such as dietary changes, exercise, and bulk laxatives (for example, flaxseed).

Herbs with strong hormonal activity and those known to promote menstruation (known as "emmenagogues") are to be avoided completely. Strong herbs used specifically to destroy intestinal worms are contraindicated as is the internal use of all essential oils.

Certain herbs in the accompanying table are considered safe for use only during the last few weeks of pregnancy, serving as *partus preparators*. See "Herbs for Late Pregnancy and Birth Preparation" in chapter 11. Some of the late-pregnancy tonic herbs can also be used during labor, with the guidance of an experienced midwife or physician.

# Herbs to Promote and
# Maintain Pregnancy Health

Using herbs helps us to connect with the natural world. What better or more primal time is there to do this than when we are pregnant? The optimal time to begin to use herbs is at the beginning of pregnancy, being careful to choose ones that are safe during the first trimester when the baby is still forming. But it is never too late to start. Herbs may be used singly or in combinations. If you begin to use herbs early in pregnancy, one cup of tea a day will be enough, taken to the end of pregnancy. However, many of these herbs can be taken in larger quantities (as indicated). If you begin during your last trimester, you might want to increase the daily quantity of some of the nutritive herbs. This will also be indicated along with the description of the herb, preparation, and dosage.

*"To come to the dimension where you are open to receiving psychic and spiritual information and energy, you must first learn to relax and clear your body of tension."*

—*Diane Mariechild*

Late-pregnancy tonics are not included in this list. Many of the herbs that can be safely used in late pregnancy are not safe earlier when the baby is in the formative months of the first trimester, and they also can cause uterine contractions that could potentially lead to miscarriage. Herbs for late-pregnancy tonics and a discussion about these herbs can be found in chapter 11, The Month before Birth.

It is simple and enjoyable to use herbs that provide us with a harvest of color, scent, and flavor in addition to their many beneficial qualities. Appendix I, Herbal Preparations, will assist you in making infusions, oils, syrups, and other preparations, as well as in purchasing the herbs. Preparing your own tinctures, salves, and syrups is not only cost-effective, it is an empowering way to create your own supplements and medicines.

As herbs are living beings harvested for our consumption, the respect and gratitude we give to our herbal preparations will also influence their healing potential. By allowing ourselves to be receptive not only to the pharmacological constituents but also to the vital essence that remains within the plants, we are opening ourselves to forces of healing that are beyond the quantifiable or reducible, that is, to the life forces that created the plants and ourselves. By growing plants or identifying them in the wild (even just some simple weeds common to backyards), you will gain a deeper appreciation for the subtle energies that invigorate herbs, which you too will absorb when you partake of the healing plants.

The following herbs are some of my favorites for promoting and maintaining pregnancy health. I hope you will find a few favorites among these. They appear in alphabetical order, not by preference. (See appendix I for definitions of infusions and teas.)

### ALFALFA *(MEDICAGO SATIVA)*

This herb, a very mild-mannered, common plant used as an agricultural cover crop, doesn't have dramatic healing properties, great beauty, or other outstanding features. What is remarkable about alfalfa is its high content of protein, vitamins A, D, E, B6, and K, calcium, iron, magnesium, phosphorus, trace minerals, and digestive enzymes. It is the most common source of chlorophyll and is also high in carotenes. The highly nutritive nature of alfalfa makes it an excellent addition to Nourishment Tea (see page 91). The tea can be taken regularly throughout pregnancy to prevent anemia and other mineral and vitamin deficiencies, to prevent hemorrhage during childbirth, and to strengthen the many systems of the body.

### BURDOCK ROOT *(ARCTIUM LAPPA)*

Burdock's taproot grows deep down into the ground, sometimes as far as two feet, making it both mineral rich and very grounding in its energy. Burdock is a prime liver strengthener and offers gentle support for the urinary organs. It helps to balance the blood sugar because it stimulates the digestion and pancreas. It also acts as a gentle laxative, reduces skin complaints such as itching, and in its role as a blood purifier prevents outbreaks of herpes infections. It is purported to have been used for centuries as an herb to promote strength and uterine tone before and after birth. It has a sweet, slightly bitter taste.

Burdock may be taken in a variety of ways. You can take it as an infusion with other herbs, using up to ½ ounce of the dried root or 1 ounce of the fresh to 1 quart of boiling water, drinking up to 2 cups daily (it is excellent combined with dandelion root); in tincture form, about 20 drops twice a day for purely preventative use, more for remedial purposes; and

> ### Burdock Root Sauté
>
> Heat 1 tablespoon of oil in a skillet and add ½ onion, sliced. Sauté for a minute or two. Add an 8-inch piece of burdock root and 1 large carrot, both sliced into matchsticks, and sauté for a couple of minutes more. Add ¼ cup of water and 1 tablespoon of tamari (soy sauce), cover, and simmer for 20 minutes. Add a few cups of chopped kale and simmer 10 more minutes. Add more tamari to taste, and enjoy while hot. When you develop a taste for burdock, you can add a 4-inch slice of kombu (kelp) cut into small squares at the beginning of cooking, along with a few tablespoons of extra water.

as a vegetable (known as "gobo" in Japanese). In order to derive maximum nutritive benefits, use burdock regularly as an infusion and as a vegetable. Macrobiotic cookbooks will provide you with numerous recipes for the preparation of burdock root; I've included here a simple one that I love.

### CHAMOMILE *(ANTHEMIS NOBILIS; MATRICARIA CHAMOMILLA)*

This is one of my two favorite herbs (nettle being the other) when I am pregnant. Chamomile eases digestion and quells nausea, relieves heartburn, reduces insomnia, promotes gentle relaxation, relieves mental tension and headaches, reduces cramps, provides calcium, prevents constipation, prevents urinary tract infections, and improves the appetite. Chamomile, when steeped for 10 minutes in a covered vessel (1 tablespoon of the herb to 1 cup of boiling water) and then very slightly sweetened with honey, has an exquisite taste. It can be sipped each evening before bed to induce peaceful sleep, or sipped during the day as a general tonic. Baths of chamomile infusion can also be taken to promote peace and relaxation. For this purpose, I love to combine chamomile and lavender in an infusion and add this to the tub.

> CAUTION: *For women with a history of miscarriage or who have been spotting and are within the first four months of pregnancy, do not exceed one cup of tea a day, as chamomile is thought by some to promote menstruation. Also, though this is rare, persons who are allergic to ragweed may have a reaction to chamomile, which comes from the same family, so try a small amount and let it sit in your mouth. If you notice any itching or any other side effects, do not use this herb. Again, this is very rare, but the possibility should not be ignored.*

### DANDELION ROOT AND LEAVES *(TARAXACUM OFFICINALE)*

Not only is dandelion highly nutritious, but when you eat the leaves as greens or drink the root in infusion, it is a digestive tonic, liver strengthener, and kidney and bladder ally. It also helps to regulate both blood sugar and blood pressure. By promoting liver functioning, dandelion aids in making iron, stored in the liver, available in the body. In early pregnancy, dandelion tincture helps to alleviate nausea and relieve a sour feeling in the stomach, and throughout the remaining pregnancy, dandelion root relieves itching of the skin and helps to prevent such problems as gallstones, indigestion, fatigue, and possibly even toxemia. To use, add chopped fresh dandelion greens to salad or sauté them with garlic and add a dash of lemon and tamari. They are slightly bitter but delicious. The root can be taken as an infusion similar to burdock root, or combined with burdock for improved taste. Tincture of the root and leaf can also be taken for medicinal benefits, though the nutritional value will not be as great this way.

### GINGER ROOT *(ZINGIBER OFFICINALE)*

Ginger root has long been employed and is well documented to be an antinauseant, antiemetic (prevents vomiting) herb effective for the treatment of morning sickness. While it is contraindicated in large amounts (more than one to two grams a day) during pregnancy due to its strong ability to stimulate circulation in the pelvis and bring on the menses, it is also an excellent herb for sluggish circulation, nausea, chills, and diarrhea. It can be taken to reduce these symptoms and reduce respiratory congestion during colds. It is perfectly safe to sip cupfuls of a warm ginger tea once or twice day (see page 187). Ginger tea can also be made stronger and used as an invigorating foot bath for aching feet at the end of the day.

### KELP *(LAMINARIA SPP.)*

A sea vegetable, kelp is an ideal nutritive supplement for pregnancy, being rich in a variety of minerals and vitamins in abundant quantities. Kelp, often sold under the name kombu, may be cooked as a vegetable (see "Burdock Root" above). Or you can add a 4- to 8-inch piece of the whole "leaf" to soups, stews, and grain dishes. Powdered kelp can also be used, especially by those who don't particularly relish the taste. (I love the taste now, but it can take awhile to get used to it.) You can purchase kelp capsules or make your own by filling "00" capsules with powdered kelp. Two capsules, twice daily as a supplement, is the generally recommended dosage. If you are using thyroid medication, check with your care provider before beginning kelp supplementation. Other sea vegetables may also be used as a nutritive and flavorful addition to the diet.

### LAVENDER *(LAVENDULA OFFICINALIS)*

Lavender is a lovely purple flower with a strong floral fragrance. Use it as a relaxing tea and as a soothing addition to your bath. It will promote sleep, reduce anxiety, lift depression, and calm heart palpitations. It also relieves gas and indigestion, and stimulates the appetite. I generally use it by adding a pinch of lavender to my chamomile tea, or I add a few drops of lavender oil to my bath, especially if I am stressed or before I go to bed. Lavender also makes a calming addition to massage oil. To prepare lavender tea, steep 1 to 2 teaspoons of the dried blossoms in boiling water for 10 minutes, with a lid on the cup while steeping. Strain and drink plain or sweetened. The tea is delicious with chamomile and lemon balm herbs added as well.

### LEMON BALM *(MELISSA OFFICINALIS)*

Another herbal nervine, lemon balm calms the spirit, reduces tension, and promotes excellent digestion. Lemon balm has a delightful flavor that reflects its uplifting qualities. It can be added to chamomile and lavender teas, or prepared alone. Cover when steeping to retain its essences, using about 1 tablespoon of dried herb or 2 tablespoons of fresh leaves to 1 cup of boiling water. Let it sit for 15 minutes. Lemon balm can be added to other infusions and teas to improve their flavor.

### MOTHERWORT *(LEONURUS CARDIACA)*

The common name of this herb implies its use as a healing herb for mothers (*wort* means "a healing herb"), and its botanical name, *Leonurus cardiaca*—"lion hearted"—reveals its reputed ability to strengthen the heart and promote courage. This herb can be taken after the first trimester to reduce stress and to relieve heart palpitations, and, under the guidance of your care provider, may be a helpful treatment for mild hypertension. The dose is typically 10 to 30 drops at a time, up to three times in a day, and not for more than five days in a row until the last few weeks of pregnancy when the dosage may be increased.

It can be taken safely in tea form, though most will find it unpalatably bitter. Motherwort contains alkaloids that may be mildly emmenagogic. These are not extracted well in water, but may be more extractable in alcohol. Care should therefore be taken when using this herb during pregnancy, particularly when the tincture is used.

### NETTLE *(URTICA DIOICA)*

Second to none, nettle is a pregnancy herb par excellence, supplying appreciable quantities of highly usable vitamins and minerals, promoting healthy kidney function, strengthening the blood vessels, reducing varicosities, and decreasing the likelihood of hemorrhaging at the time of birth. Nettle should be a regular addition to the diet of pregnant women, as it is very effective in nourishing the blood and preventing anemia (see the recipe for Nourishment Tea on page 91). For optimal health, take infusions daily, up to one quart. To prepare, steep 1 handful of dried nettle in 1 quart of boiling water for 1 hour. Fresh nettle, the richest form of this herb for its nutrients, may also be prepared as a vegetable, similarly to dandelion greens (handle carefully as the leaves pack a sting that is painful to some), or taken freeze-dried in capsules. Nettle tincture is useful for remedial purposes but nettle in the form of infusion, juiced leaves, fresh, or freeze-dried preparations is most effective for nourishment.

### OATSTRAW (AVENA SATIVA)

This herb, which comes from the same plant as oats that we eat as a grain, is an excellent gentle nervine that is rich in calcium and magnesium. It is a component of Nourishment Tea (below), which I encourage mothers to drink regularly throughout pregnancy. Drink oatstraw tea to promote relaxed nerves and healthy muscle functioning, to increase your calcium intake, and to prevent insomnia, cramps, and other related pregnancy discomforts. For deep, reliable nervous system tonification, the tincture of fresh milky oats should be used up to 1 teaspoon three times daily.

### PARTRIDGE BERRY (MITCHELLA REPENS)

Partridge berry is considered one of the best uterine and nervous system tonics for pregnancy. It can be added to Nourishment Tea or taken as a tea alone using 1 tablespoon of this herb per quart of water, steeped 15 minutes, and taken 1 cup daily, a few times a week. Herbalists commonly use it in tincture form alone or with other herbs, in a dose of $1/2$ to 1 teaspoon, one to two times daily. It can also be used as a late-pregnancy tonic as described in chapter 11.

### RED RASPBERRY LEAVES (RUBUS IDAEUS)

Perhaps no other herb has such a highly proclaimed folk reputation for use during pregnancy as the leaves of the red raspberry plant. Rich in vitamins and minerals as well as a substance known as fragarine, which tones uterine muscles, this herb is said to nourish the muscles and prevent hemorrhage due to both its high iron content and its astringent qualities. It is one of the main ingredients in Nourishment Tea

---

### Nourishment Tea

This is my favorite beverage in pregnancy. It is a nutrient supplement (iron, calcium, and many vitamins and trace minerals), and is an overall *partus preparator* or birth preparation brew. The dried herbs can be mixed in a large batch to have on hand. The tea is delicious both hot and cold, and it can be enjoyed by your whole family. You can vary the quantities of the ingredients, or add and omit herbs from time to time. It is safe to drink this brew throughout pregnancy and during labor. It is beneficial for the postpartum as well, as it helps with milk production.

2 parts red raspberry leaf
2 parts nettle
1 part oatstraw
$1/2$ part alfalfa
$1/2$ part rose hips
$1/4$ part red clover
$1/4$ part spearmint leaf

Mix all of the dried herbs together and store in an airtight container away from heat and light. To prepare your infusion, place a heaping $1/4$ cup of the mixture in a quart-sized jar. Add boiling water to fill the jar, cover, and let steep for a minimum of 30 minutes, a maximum of 2 hours. Strain, sweeten, and drink 1 to 4 cups daily.

(see page 91), and can be taken as a tea (2 tablespoons of the dried herb per cup of boiling water; steep 20 minutes) regularly throughout pregnancy.

### ROSE HIPS *(ROSA CANINA)*

High in vitamin C, a nutrient essential to health of both the circulatory and immune systems, rose hips make a nutritious and delicious addition to Nourishment Tea (see page 91), and may be used regularly throughout pregnancy as a beverage. I particularly love rose hips and peppermint prepared as a sun tea as a summer beverage. I sometimes add lemon balm and fennel seeds to this mix as well, then sweeten it with honey for a wonderful-tasting, nutritious brew.

### ST. JOHN'S WORT *(HYPERICUM PERFORATUM)*

Though this herb is not to be used regularly as an internal remedy during pregnancy, I include this plant (also known as St. Joan's wort) because it is a fantastic external remedy when used as an oil for treating aching muscles, a sore back, sore ligaments, and sciatica. Simply put a small amount of the reddish oil into your hand and rub into the affected area. Under qualified supervision, this herb may be used internally for the prevention and treatment of viral infections, including herpes virus, for the treatment of mild depression, and for the treatment of sciatic and other nerve pain.

### YELLOW DOCK *(RUMEX CRISPUS)*

Yellow dock is an excellent liver support and supplies appreciable quantities of iron and other minerals when prepared in a syrup form. It also prevents and remedies constipation, making it a beneficial herb for many pregnant women. It can be taken as an infusion or syrup (see Iron Tonic Syrup in chapter 14, under "Anemia") for its overall beneficial properties as well as mineral content, or as a tincture, which will not provide many of the nutrients but will still support digestion, hormonal balance, health of the skin, and reduction of anemia by stimulating the liver to make iron more available throughout the body. Dosage is 1 to 2 tablespoons of syrup daily, 1 to 2 cups of infusion daily, or 15 to 30 drops of tincture two to three times a day.

## Chapter 7

# Exercise and Posture

Exercise is vitally important for health in pregnancy. It increases circulation, which promotes well-being and prevents depression; it helps oxygenate the blood, reducing fatigue; it prevents the buildup of tension in the muscles; it reduces pelvic congestion and thus cramping, low backache, ligament pain, and constipation; and it prevents congestion of blood in the lower extremities, reducing leg cramps and tension as well as varicosities. Exercise promotes tone in the muscles, making the body ready for birth, aids recovery of organ tone and placement after birth, and also prevents prolapse of the pelvic organs. There are many specific exercises and yoga postures that can be used to relieve common pregnancy discomforts.

More important, exercise will help you become comfortable in and enjoy your body. Exercise will relax you as it tones your body. Many women resist exercising because they associate it with our cultural emphasis on a thin, tightly toned body. Feeling that this cultural ideal is too hard to achieve (in fact, it is not our goal here at all), many women give up before they even try. Many women have also had discouraging experiences in school physical education classes or locker rooms that have prompted a negative association with exercise. And many women are so accustomed to being sedentary that they must muster up the will to get moving. Even fifteen minutes a few times a week can be beneficial.

One excellent way to help you overcome resistance to exercise is to refer to it as movement. In what ways do you enjoy moving your body? What feels good to you—dancing, walking, yoga, tai chi, horseback riding, swimming, tennis, aerobics? Choosing a gentle form of movement that is safe for pregnancy is the most advisable way to begin. However, if you've not ridden horses before on a regular basis, this is definitely not the time to start! Similarly, some forms of movement such as swimming (although highly beneficial for both toning and relaxing) might be difficult if you don't have access to a swimming pool or reasonably warm lake.

I can recall hiking trips I took, prior to my first pregnancy, with a heavy backpack, sweating, crying, and becoming exhausted from the weight of the load. Though I have always been physically flexible and have enjoyed bicycle riding, swimming, walking, and dancing, I had never been an athlete, muscularly developed, or particularly engaged in sports. During my pregnancies, I chose yoga as a gentle form of toning my muscles, learning how to identify those muscles and to relax them. I learned to enjoy the sensations of my body moving and the feelings of warmth, improved circulation, improved digestion, better sleep, and mental wellness that rewarded my efforts. In addition, I loved to feel my baby moving as I moved with and around my growing child. For more vigorous exercise, I took brisk walks and often turned on music with a great beat (my preference being reggae and African drumming) and let loose, dancing. The latter I did in privacy, with my kids or with my husband. Dancing freely is my favorite form of movement even now, and it is something my entire family enjoys. We put on music and dance through our housecleaning! Belly dancing, originally developed as a form of abdominal and pelvic toning for pregnant women, is also an excellent way to exercise prenatally.

In these years of having babies and making movement an enjoyable part of my life, I have really learned to appreciate and enjoy my body, and my strength and endurance have improved dramatically. How you choose to move your body while you are pregnant is less important than that you do so. Dance, play, get lively, and learn to enjoy your body, whatever size, shape, or tone you are in!

Exercise, when taken to the extreme every day, can have deleterious effects during pregnancy. First of all, childbirth requires as much the ability to release our muscles as it does muscle firmness. In fact, women with backgrounds in professional dance or athletics may have a more difficult time giving birth than those women whose muscles are looser and less toned. If conscious awareness of relaxation is not included as part of exercising, then exercise may actually be self-defeating. Intense exercise also uses up precious calories and nutrients, and if these are not replaced, then exercise can actually contribute to undernourishment. Finally, for many women, heavy exercise, particularly aerobics and similar workouts, reflects control issues and a lot of inner tension. Women may be trying to control their shape, stamina, or to prove their strength without taking the time to feel good about who they are. The ability to give birth requires an ability to yield and to let go. While this does not mean giving up the control associated with autonomy, it does mean that you must give up a sense that you can make your body do whatever you want it to do. For example, while exercise is energizing, it cannot provide you with the rejuvenation that you derive from a nap. If you need to rest, don't push your body with a workout, and don't resent your body for its physical needs. You can't exercise away your stress; you have to reduce stress in your life at its source.

Many of us experience our bodies as what we inhabit rather than what we are. Often we don't like our bodies, comparing ourselves to fashion models, whom few of us resemble. Not liking our bodies translates to not liking ourselves. Exercising in an attempt to look like somebody else is psychologically unhealthy; it disturbs your ability to appreciate yourself for your uniqueness. As your breasts, hips, and waist grow during pregnancy, you may judge yourself harshly rather than seeing yourself as a gorgeous, well-nourished pregnant mama—an image of a creation goddess. If you are not feeling positive about yourself, you are less likely to take excellent care of yourself, so do something about that attitude! It will save you a lot of pregnancy and birth problems.

Be certain to balance exertion with periods of relaxation. Swim a couple of laps, then float on your back for ten minutes, then repeat this sequence; ride your stationary bicycle or do your step aerobics, but intersperse this with a few minutes of deep relaxation. Or end your sessions with five to ten minutes of guided visualization (see chapter 8 for details) or deep relaxation in a tub. The activity followed by the rest will help you to identify areas of tension in your body that you can then deliberately and progressively release. This is perfect physical preparation for birth. As you move and relax, pay attention to the sensations of the baby moving or being still within you, and notice how this changes as you relax. All of this will better enable you to allow your baby to move easily through your pelvis and into your arms. As you both move and relax, communicate your enjoyment and love to your baby.

Remember, it is possible to hurt yourself, even with gentle forms of movement such as yoga. As your belly grows, your center of balance will change somewhat, and you may find various positions or activities more challenging. There is no need to prove anything to anyone, or to show that pregnancy doesn't slow you down. To some extent, it should! Pregnancy is a time to listen to and honor your body's messages, not ignore them.

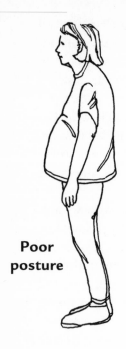

**Poor posture**

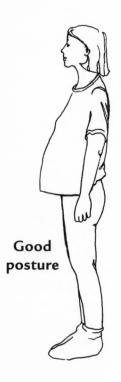

**Good posture**

# Posture

Posture is rarely discussed as an important component of prenatal health, and this is unfortunate because proper posture can prevent many pregnancy discomforts such as low back pain, shortness of breath, and indigestion. I also believe that proper posture can reduce the incidence of urinary tract infections due to stasis of urine in the ureters, as these are less likely to be compressed.

Aside from the fact that many Americans already have poor posture with a tendency to hunch their shoulders forward, pregnant women have the added tendency, as pregnancy advances, to allow the lower back be pulled forward by the weight of the growing belly. This produces the typical swayback of late pregnancy, also known as "lordosis," and accentuates the waddling gait of late pregnancy, as the legs are displaced from the hip bones being pulled forward.

While it is natural for pregnancy to affect your posture to some extent, you can learn to maintain excellent posture throughout pregnancy simply by practicing. Good posture, when standing, is as follows: Your head is held high, shoulders are held back but not stiffly, lower back does not curve forward but remains relatively straight, your tailbone is tucked under so that the tops of your hip bones are not pulled forward, and your feet should be slightly apart. When you are walking you can practice maintaining excellent posture by keeping your tailbone tucked. To keep your pelvis in a position of good posture, use your abdominal muscles to pull it up in the front and use the muscles of your buttocks to pull your tailbone down.

When you hold yourself up properly, you are lifting your diaphragm and stomach off your belly, allowing more room for breathing and for food in your stomach. You can feel the difference simply by sitting in a chair in a slouched position, and then switching to an upright, erect posture. Or if you sit down and feel either out of breath or full in your stomach, try sitting up straight. If you find yourself slouching when you sit, practice sitting taller by pushing your lower back toward the back of the chair (so that you minimize the curve in your back) and let your feet rest squarely on the floor, with your legs dropped slightly apart. If needed, you can put a small pillow behind your lower back and another behind your head and neck. This is especially good if you plan to relax in the chair. Similarly, when you are sitting up and reading in bed, sit upright, using pillows for support to prevent you from slouching.

Whenever possible, sit tailor-style on the floor. This will improve the strength of your back muscles, and you receive the added benefit of exercising your muscles as you get up and down.

When you lie down, use pillows to ensure comfort. For example, if you lie on your side, rest your bent leg on a pillow to prevent the weight of your belly from pulling on your lower back. You can also tuck a small, soft pillow under your belly to lift your belly slightly off the bed. Many women like to place a pillow between their knees when lying on their sides, rather than the pillow under their legs. Either way, it is helpful to have plenty of pillows on your bed as pregnancy advances, so that you can try a variety of positions. Comfort while you sleep will prevent you from the feelings of irritability, indigestion, and muscle aches that so often accompany a fitful sleep.

## Essential Movements for Pregnant Women

There are many excellent books on prenatal exercise and yoga, so here I will provide you with only ten prenatal exercises. These are the ten movements and poses that I have found to be beneficial to the circulation, pelvis, and digestion. They will help you identify, stretch, tone, and relax the muscles that will be called upon when you give birth. These exercises can be done individually, or as a set. The order given is a logical progression, but not from the easiest to the most difficult. You can decrease the number of repetitions if you are not accustomed to exercising, or increase them for a more vigorous workout. Use the descriptions and pictures together to best understand the movements. Begin slowly, and rest for at least five full minutes when you have completed the movements. You can follow an exercise session with a relaxation technique (see "Relaxation Techniques" in the next chapter).

I enjoy visualizing my baby surrounded with light as I do each exercise. Soothing music in the background also facilitates relaxation and concentration. I find it helpful to begin each session with a few minutes of relaxation, neck rolls, and deep breathing. Always exercise on a firm but soft surface.

## *The Standing Twist*

1. Stand upright with your feet about 12 inches apart. Extend your arms out to each side.

2. Exhaling, bend forward at the waist so that your upper body is parallel to the floor.

3. Now inhale as you resume the standing position, legs still apart and arms extended. Gently twist to your right, pivoting your right foot slightly.

4. As you exhale, bend forward over your leg, so that your upper body is again parallel to the floor.

5. Inhale and resume the standing position.

6. Repeat steps 1 and 2, again bending to the front.

7. Follow steps 3 and 4, but this time bending to your left.

8. As you inhale, return to center, and repeat step 1.

Repeat positions 1 through 8 up to 10 times.

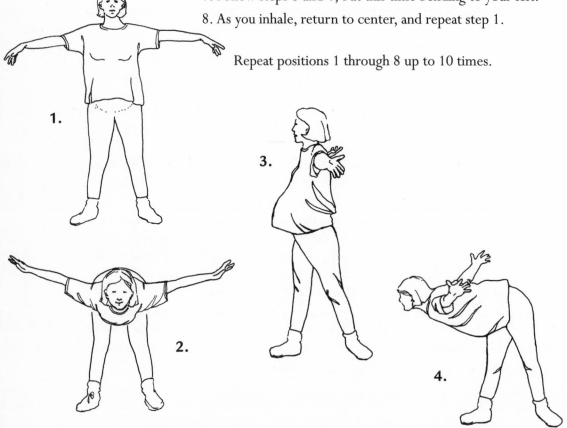

## The Yogic Squat

1. Stand upright, feet about 12 inches apart, knees slightly bent, and raise your arms over your head, with your hands joined and pointed toward the ceiling. Inhale deeply.

2. On the exhale, begin to lower your head toward the ground, one vertebra at a time, until your hands touch the floor.

3. Let your buttocks down toward the ground and, as you inhale, slowly allow your body to assume a squatting position.

4. Hold this squat for as long as you can. If you are unaccustomed to squatting, begin by holding the position for a count of 10 seconds. Eventually you will able to increase this to several minutes.

5. If you wish to repeat this exercise more than once, you can reverse the steps until you are again in a standing position with upraised arms, and begin again with step 1.

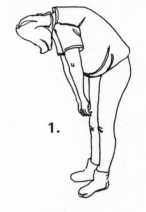

**1.**

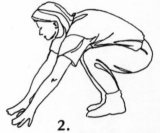

**2.**

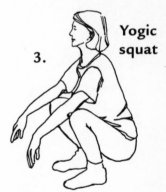

**3.** Yogic squat

## The Butterfly Pose

1. Sit upright on the floor, flat on your buttocks.

2. With your legs bent at the knees and open to the sides, bring the soles of your feet together.

3. Holding on to your feet with your hands, draw your heels as close to your crotch as possible.

4. Gently "flutter" your knees up and down, gradually bringing your knees closer to the floor.

5. Accompany this exercise with gentle inhalations and exhalations.

6. Maintain this pose for a greater length of time at each session. Draw your feet in further and bring your knees closer to the ground for increasing difficulty.

7. Optional: You can try to touch your head to your feet for an added stretch to your inner thighs. Do not try to flutter your legs while you do this.

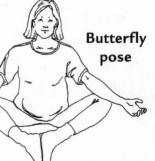

**Butterfly pose**

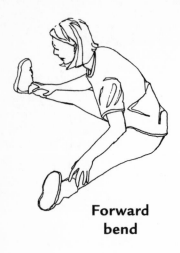

**Forward bend**

## The Forward Bend with Variation

1. Sitting upright on the floor, extend your legs to the sides, keeping them straight. Inhale deeply.

2. As you exhale, slowly lean forward, bringing your belly and chest as close to the floor in front of you as possible.

3. On your inhale, sit up straight, maintaining the leg position.

4. Repeat up to 10 times, getting closer to the floor the more you practice, and holding the forward bend longer.

5. Optional: You can also alternate bending forward over each individual leg.

## The Centaur
### (created by Jeannine Parvati Baker)

**Centaur**

1. Bend one leg under you and stretch the other straight behind you, as in the picture.

2. Your hands are in front of you as if your palms are pressing flat against an imaginary wall.

3. Hold this position for up to 2 minutes, then switch legs.

4. Optional: Maintaining the leg positions, twist your torso slowly toward the side of the extended leg, and lean back toward your foot. Switch legs and repeat on the other side.

## The Bridge

1. Lie flat on your back with your knees raised and your heels flat on the floor.

2. As you breathe in a relaxed rhythm, grasp your ankles with your hands.

3. Continue with the relaxed breathing, and slowly lift your buttocks off the floor as if an invisible string were drawing your belly button toward the ceiling.

4. Hold this position for up to 30 seconds, then lower your buttocks to the floor.

5. Repeat up to 4 times in a row.

**Bridge**

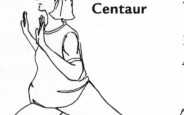

## Pelvic Rock

1. Get into a hands-and-knees position with your back parallel to the floor.

2. As you exhale, let your belly drop toward the floor.

3. Now inhale, arching your back like a cat.

4. Repeat this sequence up to 20 times, following a gentle breathing rhythm.

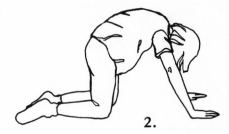

**Pelvic rock**

## Leg Extensions

1. In a hands-and-knees position, gently lift your left leg backward and upward, letting your foot reach toward the ceiling.

2. Return your knee to the floor.

3. Repeat up to 20 times, then repeat with the right leg.

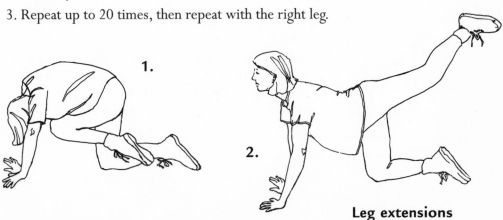

**Leg extensions**

## Leg Lifts

1. Lie on your left side.

2. Raise your right leg to the ceiling and make gentle circles in the air with your foot.

3. Lower your leg.

4. Repeat up to 20 times, then roll onto your right side and repeat with the opposite leg.

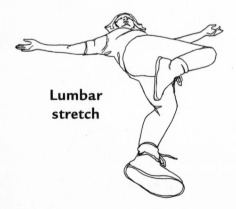

**Leg lift**

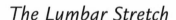

## The Lumbar Stretch

1. Lie flat on your back, legs extended and arms stretched out to the sides.

2. Slide your right foot up and bring your knee toward your chest.

3. Keeping your shoulders flat on the floor, twist your hips until your right knee touches the floor near your left hand.

4. Breathing gently, hold this position for up to 30 seconds.

5. Return to position 1, and repeat on the opposite side.

6. This can be repeated up to 3 times on each side.

**Lumbar stretch**

From this last posture you can easily go into a relaxation position, using pillows as necessary to support your legs, belly, head, and neck.

# Pelvic Health

Most women lack an understanding of their pelvic organs and muscles—where they are, what is normal and healthy, even how they look and feel. Yet this awareness can help you prepare yourself for the birth experience, as well as enable you to maintain lifelong pelvic health. Few women realize how much birth can be facilitated by the ability to consciously relax the vaginal muscles. In addition, pelvic tone will prevent a host of female problems in later life such as uterine prolapse and urinary incontinence. Sex will be improved, digestion will be healthier, and you are less likely to experience problems such as hemorrhoids. *Our Bodies, Ourselves for the New Century* by the Boston Women's Health Book Collective is perhaps the best resource for understanding your anatomy, and I encourage you to include this book in your personal library as a reference manual.

I will provide a basic idea of the structure of the pelvic bones, the yoni, and the pelvic floor muscles. Refer to the accompanying diagram for visual assistance. The pelvis is a large, bony cradle or bowl that is open at the top and bottom, with various openings within the bony structure allowing for muscles and blood vessels to pass through and attach to the bones. There are the following bones: the ileum, the two hip bones that form crests just below your waist on either side of your abdomen; the ischium, which forms the central portion of the hip bones and forms

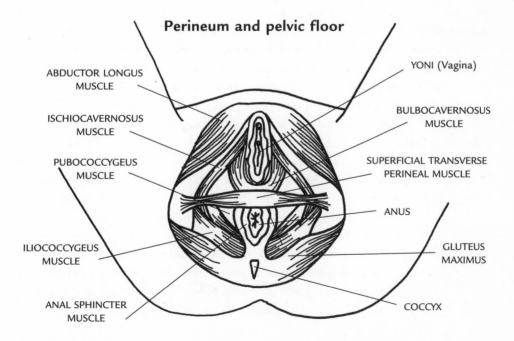

**Perineum and pelvic floor**

ABDUCTOR LONGUS MUSCLE

ISCHIOCAVERNOSUS MUSCLE

PUBOCOCCYGEUS MUSCLE

ILIOCOCCYGEUS MUSCLE

ANAL SPHINCTER MUSCLE

YONI (Vagina)

BULBOCAVERNOSUS MUSCLE

SUPERFICIAL TRANSVERSE PERINEAL MUSCLE

ANUS

GLUTEUS MAXIMUS

COCCYX

the bones commonly referred to as your "sit bones"; and the pubic bones that meet at the center of your pelvis near your pubic hair line. In the back of the pelvis are the sacrum and the coccyx, also called the tailbone. Your pelvis contains the birth canal, urethra, rectum, bladder, uterus, fallopian tubes, and ovaries. There are ligaments that connect the uterus to the front, back, and sides of the pelvis, and muscles that form a sling beneath the uterus, making up the birth canal, supporting and surrounding this and the other structures. It is these muscles that can be identified and strengthened so that you can work effectively during birth to open your pelvis and also prevent some of the health problems I've already mentioned.

In order for you to identify these muscles, collectively referred to as the "pelvic floor," you must learn to feel comfortable with your sexual organs. Look at anatomy drawings to help you understand what is what and, if you wish (I highly recommend this), look at yourself in a mirror. You can visually observe yourself tightening and releasing the muscles that surround your external genitals, the same muscles that you would tighten and release to urinate.

## The Kegel Exercise

Learning to stop and start your urine flow while you sit on the toilet is an excellent way to identify your pelvic muscles. (Always be certain to release all of the urine before you finish.) Then once you are familiar with this sensation, you can do it whenever you wish. It is known as the Kegel exercise in honor of the physician who developed it as a treatment for and prevention of urinary incontinence. For those of you in a sexual relationship, making love provides a great opportunity for practicing this tightening and releasing, with your partner confirming how tight you can squeeze your muscles during your sexual experience. (Orgasms are natural tighteners of these muscles. They also promote pelvic blood circulation. One mother I worked with referred to orgasms as "assisted Kegels.") Kegel exercises can be done up to 100 times a day (double that if you've already had problems with incontinence or prolapse).

However, tightening and releasing these muscles is not enough. Women must also learn to tighten the muscles way up in the birth canal in order to gain optimal benefit. This requires some practice, and it can be difficult and even tiring at first.

*One mother I worked with referred to orgasms as "assisted Kegels."*

*—A. J. R.*

Your midwife can help you to identify these muscles by showing you where they are in your vagina. Or you can feel for yourself. Look in books, or ask your mate to let you know when you are squeezing his fingers or penis. Try to imagine yourself tightening your muscles way up inside behind your pubic bone, not using your thigh or abdominal muscles while you squeeze.

## The Elevator Exercise

Another pelvic exercise is often called the "elevator" by midwives and childbirth educators. The basic imagery is that your yoni is an elevator shaft and you are raising an imaginary elevator from the ground floor (your vaginal opening) to the fourth floor (high inside) using just your muscles. You do this slowly floor by floor, then release slowly, floor by floor. You can also release your muscles to the basement by letting them get super relaxed, an excellent practice for totally releasing your muscles to birth your baby when she or he is crowning (the head is showing and about to be born). The elevator can be done ten times each day in addition to the above exercises.

## Happy Birthday Exercise

A final pelvic exercise, one of my favorites, I gleaned from renowned childbirth educator Sheila Kitzinger. In this exercise, you imagine that your vaginal walls are a piece of paper onto which you are writing "Happy Birthday" using your muscles to write. Beginning at the vaginal opening you "write" the *H* and continue upward tightening and moving your muscles to form all of the letters in these words. You can write any way you want to, but always cross your "t" and dot your "i." Do this ten times each day along with 100 Kegels for optimal pelvic health.

Note: In order to remember to do the above exercises, choose certain times each day to do them routinely, for example, after each time you urinate, when you wake up, go to sleep, and before each meal or snack, or every time you stop at a red light in your car or are at a checkout counter in the grocery store.

## Squatting

Squatting is another way to tone your pelvic muscles and is a great position for practicing the exercises described above. Women in traditional cultures worldwide squat daily in order to cook over fires, wash laundry in the river, and so on, naturally promoting pelvic health. The majority of women in traditional cultures are also reported to have had smooth and easy births. Try to squat for ten minutes (or more) each day, building up to it slowly if you've never squatted before. You can squat while you watch TV, play with a toddler, or read a book. Any time that you think of it, squat. Putting a book under each of your heels can help if this position hurts the back of your legs initially. By the end of your pregnancy you'll be able to squat much more easily, and much to your benefit!

# Massage: Passive Exercise

Traditionally, pregnant women were given extensive massage, often by the midwife, this being the central component of prenatal care. The pregnant woman might have been massaged weekly or more often throughout pregnancy, with a thorough massage of the belly, hips, and legs. This allowed the mother to be aware of and relaxed in her pelvis, and allowed the midwife to identify the baby's position and massage the baby into the right place if need be. I feel that this physical contact is essential for pregnant women who want to be touched soothingly, especially for women who have a low interest in sex, but still want a lot of physical contact. In addition, I am convinced that the babies love to be massaged even while in the womb, much as children love it all throughout childhood. (And what adult would turn down a massage?)

## *Benefits of Prenatal Massage*

This healing modality is nearly absent from the care of pregnant women in our culture, and this is a great loss. Prenatal massage has numerous benefits. Being a form of passive exercise, it promotes circulation which in turn oxygenates the mother's (and baby's) entire body, reducing sluggishness, nausea, fatigue, and depression. It also promotes the release of nutrients stored or stagnant in various parts of the body, and helps to relieve congestion of blood, which can result in varicosities and aches. (Warning: varicosities should never be directly massaged as this may release a blood clot, which can result in a dangerous embolism.) Massage gently tones the muscles and helps the mother relax deeply. It can be an excellent sleep promoter for women having sleeping difficulties. It encourages good posture, which in turn prevents both backache and overstretching of the anterior uterine ligaments. But most important, massage helps a woman get in touch with her body. It is an inwardly focused experience that allows her to feel comfortable physically and provides a time and place for identifying and relaxing muscular tension. This is a very important preparation for birth.

Ideally, the father of the baby will massage his partner regularly throughout her pregnancy, even if it is simply a nightly belly rub or foot massage (the latter being my favorite way to fall asleep late in pregnancy). One needn't be a professional masseuse in order to rub someone firmly and strongly or softly and tenderly, depending upon individual preferences. One only has to be receptive, willing, and sensitive to areas of tension. Massage provides a wonderful opportunity for partners to show their wives how much they appreciate them and is also a ripe time for the dad to feel and talk to the baby. If there is no partner in the picture, another friend can give you a massage periodically—as a gift or as a trade. (Nonpregnant friends would probably appreciate a back rub or foot massage, and this is nice way for pregnant women to give loving energy too.) Or you can treat yourself to an occasional professional massage.

Midwives can learn to incorporate massage, taking time at least in a couple of prenatal visits to rub a mom out. This can help to develop the feeling of trust and relaxation between you. It also provides an opportunity to teach the pregnant woman's partner how to give her a massage, and identify areas where she may be holding tension, helping her to release these. It may provide the mother with much-needed touch, especially if she is single or is the mother of young children and is putting out energy all day but has little time to replenish herself.

## General Tips on Giving a Massage

Giving an effective massage is really quite simple. The first thing to do is to create a relaxing atmosphere. You will need a dimly lit room that is warm, with a quiet and comfortable spot in which a pregnant woman can relax—plenty of pillows on hand will enable even women in late stages of pregnancy to find a workable position. Soothing music such as the sound of rain or another natural element can help induce a relaxed state.

If the woman will be removing her clothing, then you will need to provide a sheet with which she can cover herself. You will need to expose only small areas at a time, such as an arm, a leg, or her back. This will reduce her feeling of vulnerability and provide her with some warmth.

While it beyond the limits of this book to offer thorough instructions for massage, I will provide you with a general idea of how to proceed with a full-body massage. Always remember that for a general relaxing massage (in contrast to a specifically remedial massage) your sensitivity, gentleness, and willingness to listen to the mother's needs are all it takes.

Before you begin, remind the mother to use the bathroom, otherwise you can be sure she'll have to get up at some point to pee, or she'll be holding onto her muscles, preventing complete relaxation. Then help her to find a comfortable position—lying on her side with one leg over a pillow works well. Now, using a small amount of massage oil, begin by rubbing her feet gently. If the mother wants a firmer and deeper massage you can then press more deeply, but in each area begin gently to allow the muscles to respond and relax to your touch. Work your way up the legs, then proceed to massaging the neck and shoulders. Next, position the mother on her side, if she isn't already, so that you can rub her back. Gently work down her back and over her buttocks. Afterward, you can gently massage the mother's belly, rubbing your hands over it to help her relax her abdominal muscles. If at any time the woman falls asleep, let her rest.

If you wish to massage just one area, such as her feet, simply massage that area more minutely. When massaging the belly, always remember the baby, speak to the baby, and massage her or him too!

## Chapter 8

# The Need for Rest

My partner's grandmother, when she was in her late eighties, would always comment whenever she saw one of my babies napping, "Oh, he (or she) is going to grow another inch." She believed that sleeping helps babies grow. There may be scientific evidence that supports this idea, as our metabolism and hormonal levels do differ between waking and sleeping states. Nevertheless, when we rest, we are taking the energy that we would normally use outwardly to be productive in the world and turning it inward so that this same energy may be used for rejuvenation, repair, rebuilding, and regrouping. This is true on many levels, from rebuilding cells or healing from illness or injury, to taking time out or making space for our thoughts and feelings.

At no time is this need for rest greater in your life than when you are pregnant. Your body is doing an incredible amount of work growing a baby. Your physical output is great, your hormonal levels are extremely high, and you also tend to be losing sleep. If you have young children, you are already even more likely to be exhausted. You must be careful to rest when the older kids nap, or when Dad or a friend or relative takes the kids for a while. (This is the responsibility of fathers and other members of your community. Anyone who has the right to brag about the kids should also help take responsibility for them.) I cannot overstate the importance of allowing yourself to rest each day of your pregnancy. If you don't allow yourself to rest, you will be more likely to experience fatigue, nausea, indigestion, constipation, lethargy, irritability, emotional swings, and depression. Exhaustion also makes birth and postpartum infinitely more challenging.

# Relaxation Techniques

Taking time to rest does not necessarily mean taking time to relax. Relaxation specifically means letting go of mental stress and physical tensions, at least during the time you are relaxing. You can't make economic difficulties or a leaking roof disappear by relaxing, but you can call a twenty-minute moratorium on worrying, long enough to tune in to who you really are. Since most of us store our anxieties in our muscular, nervous, and skeletal systems, learning to release your worries will help to unlock areas of physical tension as well.

In addition, learning to relax is an essential skill for moving through the birth experience and into parenting with grace and joy. Learning to relax will allow your birth canal to be the path of least resistance. The following exercises are a small sampling of ways to learn to relax. (For deeper stresses and anxieties refer to "Insomnia and Anxiety" in chapter 14, and whenever necessary seek out supportive listeners or professional counselors.)

- Find a comfortable, quiet place where you'll be uninterrupted. (Remember to turn off the ringer on your telephone.)

- Put on quiet, peaceful music to help create a relaxed mood.

- If you have insomnia or find it difficult to relax, try these techniques: first take a warm bath and drink a cup of your favorite relaxing herb tea (a chamomile and lavender combination is excellent).

- If you are a restless type, do yoga or even take a brisk walk. This can help relieve your body of excess energy. Exercise is also a great way to relieve muscular tension, and relaxation is a perfect follow-up to any exercise.

- Empty your bladder before you begin so you're not interrupted by the need to urinate for at least thirty minutes.

- Be certain to prop yourself adequately with pillows so that you don't become uncomfortable lying on your back. These exercises can also be done in a chair or lying on your side.

## *Deep Breathing*

Close your eyes and imagine your baby floating or snuggled happily in your pelvis, surrounded by a golden pink glow. Now take a deep breath in through your nose and imagine that breath traveling down through your body to your womb. Let the breath encircle the baby, washing gently over her or him, then let it rise slowly back up through your chest, through your throat, and back out of your nose or your mouth. Repeat this eight or ten times, feeling yourself with each breath being washed over with your baby's love. You can continue to repeat this until you feel deeply rested or until you fall asleep. You can also follow this up with another relaxation practice.

## *Progressive Relaxation*

Close your eyes and take a few deep breaths, strongly blowing the air out of your mouth after each breath. Continue to take deep, gentle breaths, allowing a slow and gentle exhale after each inhale, as if your breaths are coming and going as waves gently lapping against the seashore.

Now, beginning at your toes, let a warm, tingly, and comfortable feeling spread over each toe. Wiggle your toes slightly, one at a time or all together. Now let that warm feeling spread s-l-o-w-l-y over your feet. Feel all tension and fatigue leaving with your next exhalation. . . .

Work your way over your entire body, continuing from your feet up to your head. Relax each area of your body slowly, deliberately releasing your muscles as you go along. Imagine your breath as fingers that are massaging away tension in specific spots. (You can also begin at your head and work your way down to your feet.) Pay extra attention to releasing the muscles in your pelvis, abdomen, and buttocks, areas where women tend to hold tension. Many times you'll find that you've fallen asleep before you get all the way from your feet to your head or vice versa. This is fine and good.

## *Creative Visualization*

This process also emphasizes the qualities of using your imagination. Creative visualization, however, focuses on using imagery to induce inner processes for facing and resolving dilemmas, or for imagining yourself how you would like yourself to be. There are many audio tapes now available that have visualizations with lovely music in the background. You can also have someone read a guided visualization to you or tape-record your own. Some excellent visualizations can be found in the books

### Releasing Anxiety: A Creative Visualization

Imagine yourself in a place that is your idea of absolute beauty, security, comfort, and safety. It can be any setting you like—the beach, the mountains, or a cozy chair in a favorite room. This is a place you can return to in your mind whenever you wish to do so.

Here in this space you can safely allow your worries to surface, knowing that they cannot harm you. Now take each image, worry, fear, or anxiety, and, one at a time, watch it grow smaller and smaller. Help it to dissolve before your eyes, let it be washed away by rain or waves, or let the wind whisk it far away. The images are dissolving until they no longer exist. These fears can no longer harm you; they are released from your heart. Feel yourself lighter, relieved of unnecessary burdens.

And now imagine your most cherished ideal for yourself and your family. Whatever it is that you consider nourishing and important, conjure up this vision. Let this vision grow larger and larger. Let yourself be filled with the joy of this image. (Pause for a few minutes until you feel filled with this sensation.)

These positive feelings will grow and develop as you nourish them each day. They are a part of you now and always.

When you are ready, you can return to your regular awareness filled with the joy of nourishing yourself and your baby. Slowly open your eyes, and take a few minutes to breathe deeply before you get up.

*Transformation through Birth* by Claudia Panuthos, *Silent Knife* by Nancy Cohen and Lois Estner, *Pregnancy as Healing* by Gayle Peterson and Lewis Mehl, and *MotherWit* by Diane Mariechild.

The accompanying box provides an example of a visualization you can do for letting go of anxieties. I was inspired to create this after reading *MotherWit*. To begin, follow the general relaxation instructions and a brief version of the progressive relaxation to bring you into a more deeply receptive state.

## Spending Time Out-of-Doors

Pregnant women are a living metaphor for the Earth, which carries and sustains us from her very body. In a sense, a pregnant woman becomes a microcosmic representation of the Earth.

Natural pregnancy health is facilitated by spending time in fresh air. Walk barefoot; feel the sun on your face and the wind in your hair. Sit on the Earth and feel the pull of gravity drawing you close to her, work in a garden, stroll along the beach, or take a walk in the cool, quiet woods. There is no greater recipe for pregnancy health—for confidence in your body and clarity of mind—than recognizing your relationship with the forces of nature.

Too often women become accustomed to a sedentary daily routine, lived mostly in the confines of houses, offices, cars, stores, and so on, going out primarily when it is necessary to go from one place to the next. This type of lifestyle can cause you to become mentally and emotionally contracted, dwelling on fears, anxieties, stresses, and the mundane details of housework and other responsibilities. While I acknowledge that not all of you who are reading this book will have access to pristine natural settings in which to expand your awareness of the world around you, most women can take a walk in a park, along a river, or near a pond. I myself grew up in an inner city and know that some connection with nature is always possible—even if it's just admiring a tree or the clouds in the sky, or enjoying the purifying sensation of rain on our faces. Being close to nature is a reminder that you, too, are a beautiful part of the miracle of life.

## Chapter 9

# Physical Changes during Pregnancy

While every woman is unique in her pregnancy, there are certain physiological changes that occur regardless of body type, size of the baby, or other factors. The degree to which these changes become uncomfortable, however, can be influenced by nutritional habits, exercise, heredity, available support, and personal outlook. Understanding the changes you are experiencing can help you relate to your body with acceptance and approval, knowing that it is adjusting just as it should. Of course you should feel free to discuss all questions you have about your body with your midwife or other health-care practitioner.

## Your Breasts

The increasing hormones in your bloodstream can cause breast sensitivity and even extreme tingling or tenderness soon after you conceive and even before you miss your first period. These sensations usually quickly abate, though you may experience heightened sensitivity in your nipples throughout pregnancy and breastfeeding.

As pregnancy advances, women will notice small raised bumps around the areola (the dark area surrounding the nipple). Called Montgomery's tubercles, these are small oil-secreting glands that keep the nipple lubricated. The nipple and areola will also become darker. As pregnancy progresses, some women notice a yellowish or cream-colored discharge coming from their nipples, a wet spot on their bed sheets near their breasts, or a bit of crusted matter in their nipples. This is colostrum, the first "milk" that is in the breasts, which will last for the first few days after birth until your real milk comes in. During pregnancy you will want to look at your nipples to see if they are erect, flat, or inverted. If they become erect in cool air or when you feel sexually aroused, then you are ready for breastfeeding; if they are flat or actually dimple inward even when squeezed or stimulated, then speak with your midwife or a La Leche League leader to learn how to prepare your nipples for nursing. There are simple things that you can do that will enable your baby to latch onto your nipples with greater ease, but these should be done before the birth for an optimal transition to breastfeeding your baby. Flat and inverted nipples need not prevent you from nursing your baby.

Your breast size may increase substantially during pregnancy, which can lead to discomfort, especially if you already had large breasts. If this is the case, a supportive bra in the appropriate size can be helpful, even if you haven't worn one before. You may notice that the veins on your breasts and on your chest are more visible, appearing like the blue lines on a map that mark the location of rivers. As your breasts increase in size and weight, you may notice silvery lines: these are stretch marks.

It is also normal for the breasts to feel slightly lumpy due to enlargement of the alveoli (the milk glands). However, it is sensible to feel any lumps carefully to be certain that they are part of normal breast changes. Learning to massage your breasts can be part of a regular practice of loving your breasts and will help you to recognize cyclical changes as you become more familiar with your body. In this way you are likely to notice any problems, should they arise, without the anxiety that a formal breast exam conjures up. Of course, any suspicious lumps should be further palpated by your midwife or other health-care practitioner, and, if necessary, further information should be sought to determine the nature of the lump, as pregnancy does not prevent breast cancer (though according to research studies, extended breastfeeding substantially decreases the risk of developing this disease). Remember, however, that most breast lumps are not cancer.

During pregnancy it is important that you be honest with yourself about how you regard your breasts. Many women harbor anxieties, measuring their breasts against cultural standards. If you are unhappy about your breasts, this can hinder breastfeeding. For example, if you have always felt that your breasts are small and inadequate, you may also worry whether you can produce enough milk (small breasts can produce as much milk as large breasts), or if you are embarrassed about your breasts you may hesitate to nurse your baby in public and may feel uncomfortable and inhibited in general. Talking to your midwife or a La Leche League leader can be helpful.

# Your Yoni

Vaginal changes also occur early in pregnancy, with the birth canal becoming a purplish color and the amount of vaginal discharge increasing. The yoni and vulva become quite engorged during pregnancy due to increased blood flow to the area. This can greatly increase sexual sensitivity and pleasure. The increased amount of discharge can cause considerable wetness, to the point of it being completely normal to change your underwear during the day.

Increased wetness can also promote the growth of vaginal organisms such as yeast. This can lead to itching, burning, or irritation, increased need to urinate, and discomfort during lovemaking. Depending upon the type of organism, it can also cause the discharge to become thicker, with a creamy, yellowish or greenish color and an odor ranging from a mild "bread-yeast" smell to a strongly unpleasant fishy odor. (See "Vaginal Infections" in chapter 14 for treatment suggestions.)

In addition to the birth canal and vulva becoming engorged, so does the cervix. It also becomes softer and more likely to bleed if it is touched or scraped. Therefore, it is not uncommon for pregnant women to notice a few spots of blood or pink-tinged vaginal mucus after sex.

# Digestive Changes

Most pregnant women are familiar with the digestive changes that pregnancy brings—an increased sensitivity to smell, a change in food preferences, slower digestion, nausea, indigestion, lack of appetite, and bowel changes. Most of these changes are due to increases of progesterone and estrogen and to the increasing pressure of your growing baby and uterus on your digestive organs. There might be increased sponginess of the gums—hormonal changes cause them to bleed more easily. Pregnant women should take care to brush and floss regularly but gently, and to maintain an excellent diet rich in iron, vitamin C, and bioflavonoids.

To some extent, some of the digestive changes of pregnancy are unavoidable and normal. However, with excellent nutrition and attention to rest and exercise, many prenatal digestive discomforts can be reduced or prevented.

# Urinary Tract

Due to increased blood volume, pressure from your growing womb, hormonal changes, and incorrect posture, pregnant women experience a marked increase in the need to urinate. This can be as frequently as every couple of hours during the first trimester and even more frequently during the last months. Most women will also need to urinate at least once during the night, but sometimes as often as two or three times in late pregnancy. You may also need to go when you stand after having been sitting for a while, and as soon as you get in the car to go on a long journey! Most pregnant women will notice that they don't urinate quite as frequently during the second trimester. This is because the weight of the uterus has lifted somewhat off the bladder. If you are experiencing extreme urinary frequency, discomfort when you urinate, backache, frequent uterine contractions, or flulike symptoms, see "Urinary Tract Infections" in chapter 14. It is beneficial to use herbs such as dandelion, nettle, and chamomile regularly, as they promote kidney health, prevent urinary tract infections, and have general nutritive value.

Due to the pressure of the womb on your bladder, you may notice that you occasionally dribble a bit of urine when you sneeze or if you run or jump. This may also be due to weakness of the pelvic floor muscles. It is to your long-term advantage to begin now to strengthen your pelvic muscles to prevent later problems of incontinence or prolapse of your pelvic organs (see "Urinary Incontinence" in chapter 14).

# Uterus and Belly

The most obvious change your body goes through during pregnancy is uterine growth. This transformation is generally very exciting, though at times anxieties may arise. You may wonder how much more you can really stretch, or whether you will ever be able to see your toes without bending over. A pregnant woman's belly receives a great deal of public attention as well, some of it welcome, some unsolicited and unwelcome. Strangers and friends alike rarely fail to comment on how big or small a pregnant woman is, on whether she carries her baby like it's a boy or a girl, and so on. With all of this attention, it is easy to overlook the incredible miracle that your body is manifesting.

The uterus grows from the size of a small a pear to a large watermelon. Your womb increases in weight from a couple of ounces to about two pounds. It is an incredible structure capable of growing to such a size and then returning to its pre-pregnant size in a matter of weeks. In addition, it serves the marvelous purpose of sending your baby forth from your body and into the world. The layers of the uterus also have built-in mechanisms for contraction that prevent excessive bleeding after the birth.

Your womb will grow steadily throughout pregnancy, with the baby having occasional periods of more- or less-rapid growth. By about twelve weeks, the top of the uterus, called the "fundus," can be felt just above the pubic bone, and by twenty weeks the fundus is usually at about the level of your navel. At approximately thirty-six weeks, your uterus will be pushing up against your diaphragm and you'll probably be wondering how much bigger you're going to grow. Then about two weeks before the baby is likely to be born, the baby will drop down slightly into the pelvis. While this gives you more breathing room and room for food, you'll likely be urinating a lot again. For some women who have already given birth, this shift, known as "lightening," may not occur until labor begins.

> *"It is an honor to become a parent. A mother is the doorway through which we gain entrance into this world."*
>
> —Diane Mariechild

Of course, all of this growing means that your body is doing a lot of stretching and growing around the middle (and everywhere else). Many woman are afraid of putting on weight, fearing that they'll never lose it again. It is true that pregnancy changes our bodies. In general, we become just a little softer and certain changes such as stretch marks are permanent, though they do fade with time. If we can accept the beauty of our bodies as they are, not comparing ourselves to a cultural ideal, and commending ourselves for our incredible ability to bear children, these changes will be accepted and needless tension will dissolve. In fact, if we could redefine the standards of beauty for women's bodies, our whole culture would be healthier and more sane. It is up to women to claim our pregnant bodies as beautiful and powerful. Only by each one of us changing our attitudes can society change its attitudes. We are not meant to be teenagers forever—we are meant to become women, with all of the aging and stretching that goes along with this transformation.

During pregnancy you may notice periodic and irregular tightenings or contractions of your uterus. This is not generally an uncomfortable sensation; you may merely notice that your belly feels very hard for a matter of seconds. These contractions may get more frequent or last longer as you get closer to the time of labor. They are more likely to be noticeable in your second or succeeding pregnancies. You are also likely to notice such contractions after orgasms. These contractions are in fact beneficial as they serve to tone your uterus and help to regulate pelvic blood flow. Only if they become regular, of stronger intensity, or progressively closer together more than three weeks before you are due will there be any need to contact your midwife or health-care practitioner to try to stop the contractions.

# Skin and Hair

For most women, pregnancy brings enhanced hair and nail growth, with hair becoming lush and thick for the duration of the pregnancy. I've also heard stories of women's hair changing color during pregnancy, generally becoming darker, though I've never heard any scientific reason for this phenomenon, nor have I seen it. Many women will notice accelerated underarm and pubic hair growth as well. This usually stops after the birth, and in fact much of the new growth may fall out during the first year after birth.

Your skin can also go through a variety of changes during pregnancy, ranging from darkening of the nipples, development of the line of pregnancy that extends over your abdomen, and the mask of pregnancy, a brownish discoloration over the eyes and on the forehead that resembles a mask (and is perhaps a sign of folic acid deficiency), to an increase or a decrease of preexisting skin troubles such as acne or eczema. Itching may also be noticeable, particularly as pregnancy becomes advanced. Whether the problems clear up or are exacerbated depends upon your diet. The healthy functioning of your liver will help to process the hormones that can trigger skin troubles. Healthy bowel and kidney functioning will also help to reduce skin problems as the task of elimination will not rest so heavily on the skin if your other systems are performing their eliminatory functions optimally.

During pregnancy and through the first months after birth, women generally sweat much more than usual and with a stronger odor. This increase in sweat is both due to hormones stimulating the sweat glands and due to the extra heat of pregnancy from increased metabolism and subsequent sweating, a cooling mechanism. Again, a healthy diet with good elimination should reduce strong body odors, and a natural deodorant (one that contains no aluminum, is based on natural ingredients, and is not an antiperspirant) may also help. In her book *Holistic Midwifery,* Anne Frye suggests taking 1 to 2 tablespoons daily of liquid chlorophyll to help reduce body odor and provide extra nutrients at the same time.

# Bones and Muscles

Contrary to popular assumptions, pregnant women do not suffer bone loss or tooth demineralization if they eat a well-balanced diet. In fact, pregnancy enhances calcium uptake, and though some bone loss may occur during lactation, this is replaced when your child stops nursing. Of course, a nourishing diet rich in minerals is essential.

Due to the influence of hormones, in late pregnancy you will notice that your joints, especially in your pelvis, feel looser. You may notice tenderness, or outright discomfort, or a feeling of mushiness. You may even notice clicking sounds in your pelvis as you walk or roll over in bed. It is this same loosening effect that allows the pelvic bones to separate slightly to accommodate the baby's head. You should pay attention to your posture, as the loosening of the joints and the slight relaxation of the abdominal muscles can lead you to sway your back and consequently develop low-back pain. All of these changes are more likely to register as complaints and discomforts if your muscle tone is already lax, particularly if you've had a number of children already. Regular exercise, both before and during pregnancy, and good posture are beneficial.

# Touch, Sound, and Smell

Sensitivity to touch and sound are generally enhanced (much to the chagrin of mothers with toddlers!) as is the sense of smell. It is very common for pregnant women to be irritated by noise and sensitive to touch.

The sense of smell is greatly exaggerated, though the nasal mucosa may become engorged, leading to a slightly stuffy nose. Taste may be either enhanced or decreased, depending upon the woman, but either way it is usually noticeably altered. Spatial awareness is also frequently altered—for example, it is not uncommon for a pregnant woman to miss the last step going down a flight of stairs, when her belly prevents her from seeing the step. Her sense of balance may also be affected. Some pregnant women notice that they drop things more easily or that their short-term memory seems fuzzy at times. These are all temporary changes, may not occur at all or only rarely, and may have to do with nutritional needs—for example, anemia may affect mental clarity as less oxygen may be delivered to the brain than is optimal.

| # Chapter 10

# Emotional Changes by Trimester

Just as pregnancy changes us physically, it changes us emotionally. Such change is a normal and healthy part of becoming a mother. Because a woman is emotionally sensitive, she can reflect on her fears, anxieties, concerns, and joys. The themes that infuse women's emotional and psychological issues are very similar, often reflecting the specific stage of pregnancy the woman is in at the time.

Your emotional state can affect your health and your baby's health either beneficially or detrimentally. Stress and joy can increase or reduce tension levels, reduce or enhance immunity, change heart and respiratory rates, and so on. Therefore, your emotions deserve as much attention as your nutrition or exercise plan. Past experiences such as a miscarriage, difficult pregnancy or birth, or problems with a surviving child can all surface as anxieties, as can childhood traumas. Also, depending upon individual circumstances, women will have their own concerns, such as being a single mother, a mother who works outside the home, a mother carrying two or more babies, or a mother in a stressful partnership.

You may feel, as do many pregnant women, that you are the only one experiencing anxiety, ambivalence, fear of birth or motherhood, or sexual tensions with your partner. You may assume that your problems are overwhelming. Internalized stress is no small matter. It can lead to insomnia, poor eating habits, high blood pressure, rapid pulse, poor weight gain, and many other symptoms. Not addressing these symptoms can lead to complications in your pregnancy or in giving birth. It is vitally important that you work up the courage to talk with your midwife so that you can resolve the problem and feel good about yourself. This section is intended to let you know that most women have many anxieties during pregnancy, and that you are definitely not alone or crazy!

# First Trimester

The first trimester can be considered a time of integrating the fact that you are pregnant. For some women, this will be a joyous realization, having wanted a child. For some women, the news will be a surprise. Some women will be outright unhappy to be pregnant, having not planned or wanted a baby at the time.

Some ambivalence is usual in pregnancy and will not cause physical harm to the baby. If you are experiencing ambivalence or if you do not accept the fact that you are pregnant, you can discuss the matter with your midwife or health-care provider. She can guide you in letting your baby know that it is nothing personal, that you have some issues to work through. It may take several months to integrate the pregnancy, particularly if it was unexpected. This ambivalence is generally increased by the nausea, exhaustion, and other physical discomforts common to the first trimester. As these discomforts begin to subside, it is very common for the ambivalence to subside as well. However, it is a good idea to discuss your feelings openly with your partner, midwife, or trusted friend so that you don't overload yourself with worry or guilt.

Feelings of nausea and other physical discomforts can also cause you to feel extremely incompetent and dependent, particularly if the nausea is severe or you have other responsibilities such as children or work that you don't feel capable of doing. This can lead you to feel very discouraged about your ability to cope with pregnancy and to wish it were all over. Being dependent on your mate for extra help can also lead to tension, especially if he does not understand how terrible you feel. If both of you discuss your situation with your support person(s), it can help resolve the tension and help you get the support you need without feeling guilty for needing it.

How a partner responds to the news of your pregnancy can also influence you. You may get angry at him, feel rejected and depressed, or worry whether you may have to bear the child as a single mom. Many women find that during pregnancy they feel an intense desire to be with their partner practically all of the time to develop a very intimate connection. Unfortunately, men who are feeling anxious about the responsibility of fatherhood or who are not accustomed to such bonding may feel boxed in. Open communication and learning to feel centered are essential skills for a healthy relationship. While it is perfectly reasonable to want the baby's dad to be excited about having a child, many men experience a wide range of complex emotions and may not have the grace to show excitement so that you can feel secure in the situation. Hopefully you will both come to a place where you can joyously support each other in welcoming your child into the world. Nevertheless, you must first learn to feel secure in yourself.

The hormonal changes of pregnancy can cause strong emotional fluctuations and a heightened sensitivity that can lead to unexpected, new emotional outbursts, such as weeping, anger, taking things personally or feeling rejected (particularly with your mate), and sentimentality (such as crying over a children's story or a song on the radio that would never otherwise make you gush). Nausea, fatigue, and hunger can exacerbate some of the more unpleasant outbursts. On the brighter side, you are also likely to experience new levels of elation, sexual union, and joy, and a deep connection to living beings.

The first trimester is often accompanied by a sense of disbelief that you really are pregnant. I can recall that with each of my four pregnancies I would expect to see menstrual blood each time I wiped after urinating. Many women will wait with bated breath for any physical indications of pregnancy, and with each increase or decrease in breast tenderness or nausea will think, "Oh, I really must be pregnant" or "I guess I'm not pregnant after all." Even with a positive pregnancy test, women will wonder if it was a false reading.

If you have a history of miscarriage, you may anxiously wait until you are past the point where the miscarriage occurred in the previous pregnancy. This can be a very stressful time in which you don't allow yourself to become attached to this new little person, afraid that this baby too could be lost to you. However, the actual process of working to connect with your baby, as painful as this may seem, can help you to maintain your pregnancy. Even if the baby is not going to stay with you, a strong spiritual bond can exist for you, and you can help that being on its way. Similarly, a woman may put off bonding with her baby prenatally until she receives the results of prenatal testing (for example, amnio or alpha-fetoprotein), which confirms her baby's wellness, rather than loving the child regardless. If you are planning to keep your baby even in the presence of a potential abnormality, there is no reason to avoid developing an emotional bond with your baby prenatally, and for as long as you are gifted to enjoy his or her presence.

# Second Trimester

During mid-pregnancy, most women will feel at the peak of health and energy. At this point, your belly has become more obvious and your baby begins to move, giving you a very tangible sense of her or his presence. This movement will make the experience finally real for the father as well, enhancing your connection together. People, even strangers, may notice that you are pregnant and you may find it fun to receive the extra attention.

The second trimester, however, is not without its own emotional nuances. General concerns such as finances or other problems may still worry you, and if you are looking after other children, particularly toddlers, you may still feel more tired than you do usually. The middle trimester is often a time of reflecting on your own childhood and on your relationship with your mother. It is perfectly natural for you to need your mother's support during pregnancy, yet at the same time to evaluate what your mom did that you would or would not want to do with your own child. In this generation, many women who want to have natural pregnancies and follow natural birthing and parenting styles may find it difficult to call upon their mothers, as most women in previous generations did not have such experiences and do not know how to talk to us about nutrition, birthing consciously, or breastfeeding our babies. This can lead to you rejecting your mother, and prompt tension in a relationship that you want to be nourishing. You also may want your mom to treat you as an adult woman. But because she may give advice or treat you as a child, you may feel unacknowledged in your own transformation into motherhood. All of these feelings may be confusing, but in the long run can often bring you closer to your mom. For women who come from seriously abusive families, the complexity of issues may be greater and may have an impact on your pregnancy and parenting experience. It can be helpful to seek the support of an experienced counselor and to discuss such matters with your midwife.

Another common concern that women express during this time is a deep fear that something horrible will happen to their mate, leaving them alone with the baby. In fact, many women have such fears about birthing the baby without the dad that it will bring them to tears. This anxiety can cause these women to worry when their partner is late in arriving home and can also cause them to get angry if he didn't call to let them know he'd be late. If you are economically dependent on your partner, you

> *"Happiness, joy, awe, wonder—to think of a baby, a new life growing within—what a miracle. I had some feelings of fear especially when intense nausea and fatigue set in. Just fear like how would I be able to take care of everyone."*
>
> *—Lisa Olko, mother and midwife, journal entry*

may worry about how you would support yourself if a tragedy occurred. To reduce your anxiety, you can ask your partner to give you general notice if he won't be at an expected place at an expected time. Clear communication from you can let your partner know how important an issue this is to you.

The second trimester is also a time when women tend to become obsessive about dreams (which may be exceptionally vivid during pregnancy) and about comments people make (which are not always considerate). For example, it is not uncommon for a woman to have a dream that her baby has a deformity, nor is it uncommon for someone to tell a pregnant woman a pregnancy or birth horror story. You may find yourself wondering over and over if a worrisome dream is true or if a person's horror story is some kind of message that this is going to happen to you. While these ruminations are perfectly normal, they don't help you feel positive about your baby or pregnancy; the only purpose they serve is to help you to find your confidence and courage. Trust that you are doing your best by consciously caring for yourself and your baby.

## Third Trimester

By late pregnancy, you may be feeling more physically tired again, needing to rest in the afternoon or go to sleep earlier. If you already have kids, you may find yourself falling asleep while you put them to bed. You probably have to urinate a couple of times at night, and you may find it hard to eat much before you feel full. In general, all of these sensations may propel you to feeling ready to give birth. At the same time, you may feel overwhelmed by preparing your supplies or getting your home ready for the baby. Many women become obsessive about having a clean house, scrubbing areas that are usually overlooked such as the corners of cabinets, the base-boards, or spots on the walls. This seems to be a normal, almost instinctive need at this time. However, it is important that you are able to let go of being compulsive, trusting that you will be ready when the time is right, and that as long as your home is generally clean, the baby doesn't really care how the cabinets or baseboards look.

You may not feel obsessively worried about your mate any longer, but may now worry that you yourself may die giving birth. This seems to be a particularly worrisome thought for women who already have children. You may also worry that if you and the baby are okay, something may happen to one of your older children. Such anxieties are perfectly common and reflect how important your family is to you. They may also help you see how much you value your life and your commitment to your baby. We are too often trained to expect the worst or to feel as if we can't have it all, causing us to mistrust the future. This is, again, a time to call upon your trust in yourself that if you've done all you can (and likely you have) to be healthy, then you are healthy. It is very rare for women to die in childbirth in affluent countries such as this.

You may also feel depressed about the size of your body, uncomfortable in all of your clothes, and awkward as you engage in physical activities. Physical fatigue may cause those of you who already have children to worry how you will cope with the baby. Remember that you will have hard days and smooth days, and that the better you eat, rest, and refresh yourself emotionally, the better you will cope in the future. Sex may also feel awkward at this stage. You and your mate may need to try different positions so that you feel comfortable. If you honor the beauty of your pregnant body (and take care to exercise regularly to maintain your limberness), you will feel more comfortable in late pregnancy and have a more positive body image.

Toward the end of pregnancy many women find themselves more "spaced out" than usual. You may find yourself daydreaming about your birth or baby, or preoc-cupied with other details that you feel the need to attend to before your baby is born. While you are no less capable of dealing with concrete tasks, you may prefer to bask in a warm bath, take a long walk, or write in a journal. It is normal and actually beneficial to take the time to tune in to your more intuited needs at this time. A natural birth is best facilitated when you are able to enter into a relaxed, reflective, and intuitive state.

## Chapter 11

# The Month before Birth

During the last four to six weeks of pregnancy, you may, like many women, feel eager to prepare yourself for birth and to meet your baby. This anticipation is welcome. You may also face new discomfort now that you have become so ripe with child, such as the need to urinate frequently, difficulty in eating due to less physical space in your stomach, more fatigue if you are caring for older children or working outside the home (or both), difficulty finding a comfortable sleeping position, heartburn, indigestion, and so on. Hopefully you have read earlier sections of this book and have been able to bypass most of these complaints, or at least have found natural approaches for addressing these discomforts and so have greatly reduced them.

Late pregnancy is a transitional time in which you may feel ready to move beyond pregnancy and hold your baby in your arms. This is a healthy and natural readiness that helps to prepare you mentally to welcome birth. It is also a time when utmost patience is required, particularly as you approach your due date. Each baby comes in his or her own unique time. During these last weeks of your pregnancy, you may have many questions for your midwife or other care provider, especially about birth and caring for babies. There are no silly questions, and since you will be seeing your care provider more regularly, you can use the time to become better informed.

As the end of your pregnancy approaches, you may also begin to wonder whether you can really do it or to feel that you just aren't ready yet. This is a common anxiety, a reckoning with the forces of birth that you are about to face, and an awareness of the great responsibility of parenting. There may also be other anxieties or feelings of ambivalence. The best way to resolve these is to discuss them openly. By admitting worries and asking for help, you are more likely to facilitate your birth. By holding back, you may actually hold the birth back, as your hormones and muscles mirror your emotions. Midwives are usually prepared, willing to listen to your concerns and help you face and work through these feelings. By acknowledging and addressing your doubts, and arriving at a place of confidence before you enter labor, you will be in a stronger state of mind for birth.

How well you care for yourself during late pregnancy can strongly set the tone for your birth experience. This chapter is devoted to helping you continue caring for yourself optimally during these last weeks of pregnancy so that the tone you set is positive. It explores ways that you can prepare your body and nourish your spirit so that when the time comes for your baby to be born, you will be ready, willing, strong, and healthy.

## Nutrition and Rest during Late Pregnancy

A mother who enters labor tired and poorly nourished stands a very great chance of not being able to cope with the intensity of the process, of having a dysfunctional labor in which her uterus does not contract effectively, and of eventually requiring interventions that enable her body to birth or be delivered. Sleep and nutritional deficits are easy to prevent and even cure during pregnancy for most middle-class American women. It is therefore of tremendous importance that you pay close attention to your body's needs during this time.

### Sleep and Relaxation

When you are tired, stress seems magnified and pain is less tolerable. When you are fatigued, emotions seem to take on a life of their own and your body will function less effectively. It is standard for you to tire more easily during late pregnancy than at other times in your life; you are working constantly, even when at rest, to grow your baby. When you ignore your body's need for rest, problems begin to arise. The simple solution is to rest regularly, napping in the afternoon whenever possible and getting to bed early. (I generally recommend that women try to get to bed by 10 P.M. during the last weeks of pregnancy.) These habits will ensure that you will be well rested so that if you begin labor at two in the morning, for example, you will have had some sleep.

If you are unable to take a regular afternoon nap, a short period of deep relaxation can substitute. Chapter 8 provides several suggestions and techniques for deep relaxation. It can be done before you go to sleep at night, enhancing your sleep. It can't be overstated that you must be well rested during late pregnancy. Birthing can take a long time and you will be able to meet this challenge only if you meet your body's needs beforehand. It should be clear that fatigue can actually prolong labor.

## Nutrition

For most women, late pregnancy brings fluctuations in appetite ranging from being ravenous to not having much appetite at all. Your increased appetite will be in proportion to growth spurts that your baby has in the last weeks of pregnancy. A loss of appetite often occurs at this time because you have a sense of fullness as your growing baby presses against your stomach, leaving much less room for food than you had earlier in the pregnancy. It is important to maintain excellent nutrition throughout your pregnancy, since this will keep you in top preparation for birth, which requires an enormous expenditure of energy. If you find that you are tired of the same-old-same-old, treat yourself to a new recipe book or ask your friends or your midwife for recipe suggestions. Sometimes just having a change of foods can spark your appetite.

As your baby grows and you find it difficult to eat a quantity of food at one sitting, you may want to eat small but frequent meals throughout the day and into the evening, avoiding foods that might contribute to heartburn (tomatoes and peppers are common culprits). It is very important to eat sufficient complex carbohydrates, proteins, and iron foods at the end of pregnancy. The complex carbohydrates will help maintain stable blood sugar levels, keeping your energy levels steady as well. The increased protein and iron are essential, the protein for the rapid development of the baby's brain, and the iron for storing in the baby's body for the first six months of life. If you have a consistently poor appetite, anemia may be an underlying cause, and should be treated using the recommendations found in chapter 14, under "Anemia."

# Herbs for Late Pregnancy and Birth Preparation

*Partus preparators* (*partus* meaning "labor"; *preparators* meaning "preparatory") are herbs historically used during the last weeks of pregnancy to tone and prepare the uterus for labor with the hope of "ensuring a speedy delivery." Classic *partus prepara-tors* include blue cohosh *(Caulophyllum thalictrodes),* black cohosh *(Actaea racemosa* syn *Cimicifuga racemosa),* partridge berry *(Mitchella repens),* and spikenard *(Aralia race-mosa).* The use of such herbs to prepare women for labor begs the question of why one would use an herbal preparation to ready the body for something it naturally knows how to do. Furthermore, the safety of these herbs prior to the onset of labor is questionable. At least one report published in the 1998 issue of the *Journal of Pedi-atrics* implicates the late pregnancy use of blue cohosh in the myocardial infarction of a neonate at birth. This herb contains a number of potent chemicals called alka-loids and cardiac glycosides including methylcystine and anagyrine, the latter of which is known to have an effect on cardiac muscle activity. It is therefore prudent to entirely avoid the use of *partus preparators* containing blue cohosh during preg-nancy and, unless there is a reason to suspect otherwise, to trust the body to enter labor naturally and in its own time.

In the case of postdates pregnancy (when the mother is two or more weeks overdue), where labor stimulation is medically indicated, caution must again be exercised in the use of herbs to initiate or augment labor, but this can be done effec-tively with qualified supervision. With careful monitoring of the uterus for intensity of contractions, along with diligent monitoring of the fetal heart rate, certain herbs such as blue cohosh and black cohosh may be judiciously employed with perhaps greater safety and less intervention than other augmenting agents such as oxytocin and misoprostol. Self-medication by patients is not recommended, and the expert guidance of an obstetrician or midwife trained in the use of botanical medicines is advised.

Below I provide information on herbs that are considered *partus preparators,* as they are popular for use and are commonly recommended by both direct-entry midwives and certified nurse-midwives. Again, I do not recommend their use for general purposes, but at least readers may obtain a basic knowledge of the herbs fre-quently included in such formulas. *Partus preps* are typically only used during the last three weeks of pregnancy because of their ability to stimulate labor; therefore use them only after thirty-six weeks of pregnancy, and only as recommended by an experienced herbalist.

Also included in the discussion below are several herbs that can be used to relieve late-pregnancy discomforts and safely tone and relax uterine muscles. The right balance of relaxation and tone is necessary for effective labor. The use of many such herbs was taught to us by Native American women, who have long used herbs in late pregnancy for the purpose of easing birth, and was widely used and popularized by a group of physicians practicing in the 1800s into the early 1900s, called the Eclectic Physicians. Two recipes for late-pregnancy tonics are included here as well. You can also create your own formulas. Refer to chapter 14 for herbs that address specific complaints, such as leg cramps or insomnia, which may also occur during late pregnancy.

*Black cohosh* is not botanically related to blue cohosh, though the two are commonly used together. *Cohosh* is simply the Algonquin word for "gnarly root." Black cohosh has a vastly different physical action than blue cohosh, though in the classic botanical literature, the actions of the two are often confused and overlaid, leading to contractions frequently being attributed to black cohosh.

Black cohosh actually helps to relax the cervix and uterine muscles, relieve irregular uterine contractions and promote more regular ones, and reduce blood pressure by dilating peripheral blood vessels. Black cohosh is classically used when there is aching in the back of the legs and in the pelvis. The herb is commonly included in late-pregnancy tonics and should be used with some caution as it can cause side effects such as headaches, dizziness, and nausea. These adverse effects will cease when use is discontinued. The best method for dosing with black cohosh is small and frequent doses of $1/4$ to $1/2$ teaspoon of the tincture every fifteen to twenty minutes for premature uterine contractions to $1/2$ to 1 teaspoon every two to four hours for other conditions and for improving uterine activity during labor.

*Blue cohosh* has developed a strong reputation for its effectiveness as a late-pregnancy uterine tonic, preparing the uterine muscles for birth and stimulating contractions when a woman has gone past her due date. However, as mentioned above, blue cohosh has been implicated in at least one and possibly several incidences of cardiac problems in newborns, including myocardial infarction (heart attack), when taken by pregnant mothers in the last three weeks of pregnancy, even when used in generally recommended doses. It has not been associated in the medical literature with problems when used short-term during labor, but the potential for such problems cannot be entirely discounted. Again, the use of blue cohosh as a general late-pregnancy tonic is not advisable, it should never be taken prior to three weeks before the due date, and its use is best left to qualified health professionals.

*Chamomile* can be steeped into a delicious tea that is taken daily to reduce both muscular and nervous tension, bringing a definite sense of calm, reducing aching, anxiety, insomnia, and possibly elevated blood pressure. This herb can also be used in tincture form, alone or combined with other herbs such as passionflower for relaxation, wild yam for uterine or intestinal spasms, and dandelion root, slippery elm, and spearmint for stomach upset and heartburn. I frequently went to sleep in late pregnancy after a warm cup of chamomile tea, which induces enough relaxation to promote a gentle sleep. However, this herb can be used freely during the day without slowing your reflexes or making you sleepy. I also enjoy the beneficial effects of chamomile tea during labor. As it is considered by some to be an emmenagogue, it is best to avoid if you have had late-pregnancy bleeding.

*Cramp bark* has properties that you might expect based on its name. While it tones the uterine muscles in preparation for birth, it generally serves to promote muscular relaxation, relieving uterine cramping and spasms, leg cramps, and low-back pain, as well as pressure in the groin. It can be used during pregnancy and makes an excellent addition to a late-pregnancy tonic. It is used as a tincture, $^1/_4$ to 1 teaspoon repeated as needed, based on the condition being treated. Black haw, which may be slightly stronger, can be used interchangeably with cramp bark. These herbs may help to reduce arterial blood pressure, relieve anxiety, and prevent irregular uterine contractions. As it is a hypotensive, women may feel slightly dizzy if they stand up too quickly when taking this herb for prolonged periods.

*False unicorn* has classically been used as an overall excellent uterine and hormonal tonic and can be a beneficial addition to a late-pregnancy routine. Typically used in tincture or tea form, this herb is largely endangered in the wild and is notoriously hard to cultivate. Therefore, herbalists discourage its use from a conservation perspective.

> *As for remedies, yes, the herbs are powerful healers in and of themselves, but healing is deeper and more than the plant. Healing is will and intention—the strong desire for life.*
>
> —*A. J. R.*

*Partridge berry* is highly esteemed for preparing a woman's body for birth. It tones the uterine muscles while promoting gentle relaxation. It helps to reduce backaches, leg cramps, anxiety, and tension, and also tones the urinary tract and the bowels, making it an all-around ally for women in late pregnancy. It can be taken in infusion or tincture form (for the latter, dose is 20 to 35 drops two to three times daily), and you will find it in the formulas listed below. While it can be used throughout pregnancy, it is most beneficial in the last four to six weeks. It is a particularly valuable herb to consider when a woman has a history of recurrent urinary tract infections, and it combines well with wild yam to both tone and reduce spasms of the urinary bladder.

*Motherwort,* already mentioned several times throughout this book for its wonderful ability to promote relaxation and reduce emotional anxiety as well as to strengthen the heart and prevent hypertension, can be used during late pregnancy for all of these same purposes. Before thirty-six weeks, it should be used sparingly, or in infusion rather than in tincture form, as it contains substances that can stimulate the uterus. It can be used in slightly larger amounts in late pregnancy. As it is very bitter, a tincture is the most palatable form for using this herb. Take up to 20 drops at a time for anxiety or high blood pressure, not to exceed four doses daily, five days a week. Hypertension should not be self-treated during pregnancy; treatment of hypertension requires the supervision of a qualified health-care provider.

*Nettle* throughout pregnancy maintains kidney health, prevents late-pregnancy urinary tract infections, prevents excessive fluid retention, and helps to regulate the blood sugar. Using nettle infusion regularly throughout late pregnancy may also prevent anemia and heavy bleeding at birth, and may promote a healthy adaptability to stress. Up to a quart a day of the infusion can be taken.

## Late-Pregnancy Tonic Recipes

Late-pregnancy tonic recipes should include herbs that both tone and relax your uterine muscles as well as your nerves, helping you to stay relaxed and well rested while preparing your body to give birth. Here are two formulas:

Combine 1 part each of red raspberry leaf, partridge berry, blue vervain, and cramp bark, and add $1/4$ part of wild yam and motherwort. Steep 4 to 6 tablespoons of these herbs in one quart of boiling water for 30 minutes. Strain and drink 1 to 2 cups daily. The taste will be quite bitter.

Take 10 drops each of the following tinctures two to three times daily during the last three weeks of pregnancy, increasing the dosage to 20 drops each, two to three times daily during the last week before you are due: partridge berry, blue vervain, motherwort, wild yam, and cramp bark.

In addition to one of these formulas, take 500 mg of evening primrose oil or black currant oil daily for the last four weeks of your pregnancy. Do not increase the dosage unless you are overdue and your cervix is "unripe" (not yet soft) according to a vaginal exam. In this case, you may double the amount, but do not take more than this. These oils contain substances that support prostaglandin production, a hormone in our bodies responsible for cervical ripening. Semen also contains prostaglandins, and regular intercourse in late pregnancy can help to prepare the cervix for birth.

***Wild yam*** is an excellent herb for treating an irritable uterus, which can be particularly bothersome in late pregnancy, causing insomnia and anxiety. It is very effective combined with cramp bark in equal parts. Typical dose is $^1/_4$ to $^1/_2$ teaspoon of each tincture given as often as every one to four hours, depending upon the level of discomfort.

# Preparing Your Body for Birth

Your body, unhindered, knows exactly how to give birth and nourish a baby. There are several ways that you can promote and enhance these natural abilities, including vaginal muscle awareness, the use of herbs, and regular body movement, which should be emphasized in the last four to six weeks of your pregnancy.

Vaginal muscle awareness was touched upon in chapter 7; refer to this chapter for a full discussion of the muscles involved in birth, as well as the importance of Kegel exercises. During late pregnancy, you can increase this awareness by practicing vaginal muscle massage. This technique is commonly referred to as perineal massage; you or your partner massage and stretch the external vaginal muscles to enhance suppleness and to prepare you for the sensation of your baby stretching you during the crowning of its head when it is about to be born. Unfortunately, emphasis has become placed on using this technique to prevent tears. Tears are best prevented when the woman has the ability to relax the yoni, not by having it stretched. I have offered this technique to help you to become comfortable with your vagina, identify areas where you may be holding pelvic tension, and learn to relax your muscles.

Perineal massage is frequently recommended by midwives and childbirth educators as a way to prepare your vaginal canal for birth. Similar to taking herbs to ensure a "speedy labor," there may be some distrust of a woman's ability to birth implicit in the idea of having to do perineal massage for birth to go more smoothly. Indeed, both the vaginal canal and perineum are perfectly designed to relax and open for the baby to be born. Further, there is little proof that perineal massage prior to labor reduces the risk of anything but very insignificant tears. Reduction of more significant tears has not been demonstrated. The advantage of perineal massage is that it provides an opportunity for women to get comfortable being relaxed and open about their vaginal area, which is very good emotional preparation for birth. If you would like to practice perineal massage, your midwife can provide instruction at a prenatal visit, particularly at a visit to your home if a home birth is planned, or if this is where you feel most relaxed. You can do vaginal massage on yourself by inserting your index and middle fingers into your birth canal either while you are in a bath or while standing with one leg on a chair. If you are quite supple, you might be able to do it lying in bed, propped on pillows. Your mate can also help you by doing the massage. The idea is to identify areas that feel tight both in the vaginal canal and along the perineum, and gently massage them while you deliberately try to relax these muscles. This will help you relax these muscles during birth, allowing your baby to be born with minimal resistance.

Vaginal massage can be done a few times a week or even daily, using either plain vegetable oil, a mild massage oil, or an oil that is specifically made for perineal massage, sometimes available through mail-order birthing supply companies. An excellent blend can be made at home following the instructions in appendix I for making an oil. Chamomile, St. John's wort, lavender, and calendula are some herbs that may be included in such an oil. Vitamin E oil also makes an excellent addition since it benefits the skin.

Lovemaking is also an excellent way to prepare your yoni for birth if this is something you enjoy during late pregnancy. You may have to be creative in finding positions in which you are comfortable, but the movements of your pelvis are excellent for toning your uterus and your vaginal muscles. Lovemaking can be creative in other ways, without intercourse, if intercourse is too uncomfortable for you.

As discussed in chapter 7, regular movement during pregnancy in the form of dance, yoga, swimming, walking, or other gentle but strengthening activities helps you become closely attuned to your body. This is essential preparation for an active and positive birth in which you are able to work cooperatively with the birth energy. Late pregnancy may require you to slow down some or to modify your activities, but it is highly beneficial for women to remain physically active even until the last minutes of pregnancy. Physical activity will keep your heart and lungs prepared for the work of labor, and will help to keep your blood pressure steady, your circulation excellent, and your stamina and endurance up. However, physical activity is effective only if it continues to be in harmony with your physical needs and your baby's needs. Such exercise should help you get loose and relax and tone your muscles.

## Preparing for Breastfeeding

Breastfeeding provides your baby with both perfect nourishment and the continuity of closeness with which your baby is so familiar. Many women wonder whether they will be able to nurse their babies—whether they will have enough milk, whether they have the right nipples for nursing, and so on. These concerns arise more from internalized cultural messages than reality. Most well-nourished women will have a plentiful supply of milk for their babies and most women's nipples are just fine for breastfeeding. Occasionally a woman will have flat or inverted nipples, where the nipples do not become erect when stimulated by touch or cold, or they actually dimple inward. Women with flat nipples will usually be able to nurse without any prenatal preparation of their nipples other than massaging the area around the nipple (on the areola, the dark circle around the nipple) to break up any tissue adhesions that might prevent the nipple from protruding. Frequently women will have flat nipples before their first baby is breastfed, but will have erect nipples after having nursed their first child.

If you have truly inverted nipples, you will want to consult with a La Leche League leader or a lactation consultant for information on how to prepare your breasts for nursing. Nipple shields, small plastic cups with a hole in the inner layer, which are worn over the nipples for a period of time each day, exert gentle traction on the nipples, encouraging them to come out before the baby is born. You may also need a bit of extra support with nursing after your baby is born, but even if you have fully inverted nipples, you can nurse successfully—it may just take a bit more determination.

There is no need to "toughen" your nipples by rubbing them vigorously with a towel or any such technique, but you may wish to go without a bra periodically, if you are comfortable doing so, and let your shirt rub against your breasts. Also, if you are able to expose your nipples to a bit of sunshine now and then, even through a window (but preferably directly), this may be beneficial. Again, none of these steps are necessary for successful breastfeeding. Excessive nipple stimulation can actually cause contractions!

If milk production is a problem, refer to my book *Naturally Healthy Babies and Children* for a comprehensive discussion and suggestions that are highly effective.

## What You Need after the Baby Is Born

While this book is not about postpartum care, there are certain preparations for the days immediately after birth that you will need to have made during your pregnancy. Late pregnancy is the time to make sure that you have the supplies you will need for your baby, as well as the support you will need for caring for yourself, the baby, and the other members of your household while you are recuperating from the birth.

## Baby Supplies

I've never been a big supporter of baby paraphernalia. There is very little equipment that you need for your baby during the first months of life. A car seat is essential, as there is substantial evidence that babies in car seats are the safest passengers in moving vehicles, but aside from that, all you really need are cloth diapers and diaper covers, appropriate clothing (you will need very few newborn-size things since most breastfed babies will outgrow these in the first week or so), a baby hat (babies lose a lot of heat when their heads are exposed), a diaper bag, a baby blanket, a few receiving blankets, and a handful of soft washcloths. A sling baby carrier is a useful addition to this list. Later on, a high chair or Sassy seat is helpful, and simple toys. A backpack for carrying a baby, in my opinion, is indispensable. Playpens, cribs, a host of plastic toys, bath tub inserts, pacifiers, bottles, and so on are really unnecessary if you are going to be with your baby and breastfeed. Baby stuff is big business, not necessities.

## Help after the Birth

During pregnancy, I have my clients consider who of their friends or relatives might be able to come to their home a few hours after the birth to help prepare a nourishing meal for the couple or the family, to run linens that might have been used at the birth through the washer and dryer, and to look after the other children. This allows both the mother and father the freedom to rest and bask in the presence of their newborn without interruption, and ensures that everyone will be well cared for. While, for most women, birth is not a traumatic event (in fact, you may feel very energetic immediately after the birth), it is important that you allow people to cater to you. This is a time for you to allow yourself to be nourished by those who care for you.

If you would prefer not to have company in the immediate hours after birth, you can still prearrange for a friend to leave a meal outside your front door, so that all your mate or midwife has to do is warm it and serve it to you. You can also have meals in the freezer that merely need to be defrosted and heated. You can prepare and freeze these in advance, or ask friends and relatives to gift you with meals that can be frozen. One of my clients was given a casserole shower by her friends. Guests brought a dish for the mother to freeze for both her late pregnancy when she might not have the energy for cooking, and also for after the birth. This was very liberating for the both the mother and her mate, as dinners did not have to be a concern for several weeks after the birth.

If you have older children, particularly if they are under seven years old, you will also want to have someone at home with you at least for the first week after the birth who can tend to their needs. This will help the children feel cared for, as well as prevent you from becoming exhausted.

If you are in a situation where you live far from relatives, or have just moved to a new town and don't know many people and can't easily arrange for support, you might want to hire a doula, a woman whose profession is to provide postpartum care for mothers. A doula will come to your home for the number of hours that you agree upon and will do the housekeeping, grocery shopping, meal preparation, and laundry. Some will even pick children up from school and bring them home. Most doulas also have basic knowledge about newborn care, breastfeeding, and the needs of new mothers, and can therefore provide valuable emotional support and answer some questions that may arise. To find a doula in your area, ask local midwives, obstetricians, or La Leche League leaders. The address for Doulas of North America is listed in Resources.

# Celebrating Pregnancy

Pregnancy provides a wonderful opportunity to celebrate not only the coming of your baby, but the transformation of your own life as well. In our country, the traditional form of celebration is to give the mother a shower shortly before the baby is due, passing on to her positive stories of birth and motherhood, as well as giving her everything she needs (and sometimes doesn't need) for the baby. While this ritual has the potential to be a time to disseminate valuable information as well as to encourage and empower a woman about to cross through the doorway that is birth, it is often less relevant, though still a memorable occasion. In addition to this celebration, or in lieu of it, I'd like to share with you the tradition called the Blessingway. I also want to share an enjoyable activity—making a belly mask—that results in a terrific conversation piece as well as a long-lasting objet d'art that tangibly honors your pregnancy experience.

## The Blessingway

The term Blessingway derives from the Diné (Navaho) culture and language, but such rituals are germane to peoples all over the world. This ritual, taught to me by my mentor, Jeannine Parvati Baker, has become popular among midwives across North America as we have sought to reclaim and create meaningful rituals and beautiful celebrations for our life cycles.

The Blessingway is a ritual that can be done to honor, celebrate, direct, and emphasize any significant life changes that are occurring, such as a new job, a move, a marriage, a graduation, the onset of the first menses, menopause, a birthday, and so on. While it is a celebration, it is not a party; it is a ritual, a time of focus and concentration on the subject(s) for whom the ritual is being created, and a time to give birth in an atmosphere that reflects the purpose of the ceremony.

*"As you do unto your unborn children, so they will do unto the world."*

*—Thomas Verny, M.D., from a workshop on prenatal psychology*

The Blessingway has three basic parts: the opening of the ritual, the body of the ritual, and the completion of the ritual. While there are certain elements that are commonly included, they are not fixed. You can create your own ceremony using original ideas or those you glean from other sources. There are several useful books in the bibliography and many others to be found in bookstores. Singing is an important and uplifting aspect of the Blessingway. Look for CDs and tapes at women's bookstores. There are many beautiful recordings of chants, spiritual songs, and even songs for ceremonies and rituals. Many of these songs are quite simple and have repetitions that make it easy to follow along in a large group, even if people haven't heard them before.

The Blessingway does not need to follow any specific faith tradition. You can infuse the ritual with your own religion, but if you are not part of any organized religion you can extract elements from a variety of cultures and religions or create a nature-centered ritual.

A Blessingway can be given by a close friend, a relative, or your midwife, or it can be done by yourself or with your mate and children. It is usually done in the weeks just prior to your due time. Blessingway guests should include only those people with whom you are very close and with whom you feel positive and comfortable. Blessingways can be women only, women only except for your mate, or mixed. A small group is better with Blessingways, as it is easier to remain focused.

Supplies for a Blessingway vary, but the main ingredients are objects that symbolize pregnancy, life, babies, relationships, the powers of nature and Earth, and so on, which can be used to create an altar or centerpiece for the gathering. Guests can bring gifts to decorate the altar. Additionally, there should be lit candles, flowers, comfortable seating (lots of floor pillows and soft chairs), and a special area arranged for the guest of honor, the mother. To the Blessingway, each guest should bring a small gift for the mother, preferably homemade, or of simple and natural materials if purchased. This gift can be a poem that is appropriate, a new hairbrush or hair clip so that she has something new and personal for herself after the baby is born, a gift for the baby, or even the promise of several meals or help with older children just before or after the new baby is born. Each guest should also bring a dish to contribute to a potluck meal or snack after the ritual. Ideally, one person will get a list from the mom as to whom she wants at her Blessingway, and this person will then call the guests and tell them what to bring. The Blessingway should not cause extra work for the pregnant woman unless, of course, you are planning the Blessingway yourself.

Before you begin the Blessingway, create an atmosphere in the area that invites peace, contemplation, and comfort. You are creating a sacred space. Let people know exactly when you will begin, as latecomers can disrupt the energy of the ritual once it gets going. I find that Blessingways done indoors are facilitated by semidarkness and candlelight. Blessingways held outside are quite beautiful as well.

### OPENING THE RITUAL

Opening the Blessingway involves several aspects or actions on the part of the person facilitating the ritual: welcoming everyone and explaining what the ritual is about and why you are doing it. You needn't be historically accurate; simply explain your intention to create a meaningful way of honoring and supporting—Blessing the Way—of your friend who is about to give birth. (If you are doing this ritual by yourself or with your mate, you may wish to mention your intentions for this ritual rather than the explanation.) This explanation can also help anyone unfamiliar with the idea of ritual, who may associate it with horror movies or something scary. Let folks know that the Blessingway is a participatory event, that you are just helping to keep it focused on the purpose of blessing the mother.

Next comes a purification. I prefer the technique known as smudging. I use smoke to ritually remove any energy, thoughts, or feelings that may be negatively influencing any of the guests or the mother, and to welcome in positive and loving energy. To smudge, you light the herbs cedar and sage and allow the smoke to circulate around each person by holding the lit herbs near their body (use a bowl or a large shell to contain the sparks and ashes). You can blow on the herbs to direct the smoke around the person's body. A nice way to smudge is to have each person smudge the person to their left, going clockwise around a circle. To order smudge sticks that are made for this purpose, see resources. If you know other purification techniques, you can substitute your own methods.

Finally, the invocation is spoken, that is, a prayer to invite and welcome all of those spiritual forces (use your own terms: angels of birth, spirit guides, your own higher powers, forces of nature, Great Mother, Heavenly Father, God, whatever your belief system holds for you) that will assist this mother on her path. The tone should be reverent, the room receptive to these spiritual allies, and the prayer slow and eloquent.

This invocation can be given by the person organizing the ritual or someone else in the group. During the smudging or purification, songs can be sung.

## THE BODY OF THE RITUAL

This part of the ritual is focused on nurturing the mother, encouraging her sense of support and empowerment, and creating a collective positive intention for her safe and joyous experience of birth. It is a time for each guest to share his or her love individually and as a group for the mother and baby. These are the steps that I usually follow when giving a Blessingway. They are open to your own creative input.

> *waters rising*
> *moon filling me*
> *this vessels holds firm*
> *but is ready to*
> *overflow at any time.*
> *so ready for my baby*
> *to be born*
>
> *—A. J. R.*

Note: After each step in the ritual, it is pleasant to punctuate the celebration with singing. My friend Lisa Olko created handwritten lyrics sheets almost ten years ago that I continue to use at Blessingways. You can write your own by jotting down the words to several songs that you might want to sing. Then photocopy enough pages to hand out to the guests so that each person can follow along. Hand drums, rattles, and other simple percussion instruments can help set the tempo for the music. These are easy to play and add richness to the singing. You can ask guests to bring instruments if they have any. In fact, when I plan a Blessingway, I call each guest about a week before the gathering and let them know that they can contribute to the ritual by bringing items for the altar, flowers, and a verse, poem, song, or thought to share.

1. Going around the circle clockwise, each guest introduces herself and tells why she came and what she would like to contribute to this ritual. Each person should have the opportunity to place something special on the altar should she so desire.

2. The person facilitating the group can lead the guests on a guided visualization, perhaps of imagining giving birth as they would wish it to be. Begin the visualization with a deep relaxation exercise so that everyone has the opportunity to relax and benefit from the ritual. (*MotherWit* by Diane Mariechild is an excellent book filled with relaxation and visualization exercises that can be adapted for rituals.)

3. Give everyone the chance to return to a sitting position in the circle and introduce the idea of grooming the mother. This involves massaging the mother's

feet in a foot bath, brushing her hair, and generally doting on her. Utmost sensitivity to the mother's needs and sense of personal space is essential. For the foot bath, use a rectangular bucket wide enough for her feet and with enough water to reach her ankles. Add herbal oils to scent the water and float a handful of herbal potpourri in the bucket, or prepare a strong herbal infusion and let her soak her feet in this. Lavender, rose petals, calendula, mint, lemon balm, and other aromatic herbs are wonderful. While her feet are soaking and massaged by two of the guests, a third person, perhaps the mother's closest friend, sister, or mother, will brush the pregnant woman's hair (sprinkle a few drops of lavender or rose oil on the brush for added effect) and then style it using hair clips, ribbons, and so on. This is symbolic of preparing her "head space" to be ready for birth and mothering. A flower garland, easily homemade with a bouquet of flowers and wire, makes a perfect crown after her hair is completely groomed. I also have a special Blessingway gown that was a gift to me, that each mother dons at the beginning of the grooming part of the ritual. After each Blessingway, it is washed and put away until the next Blessingway.

After the hair is done and the feet massaged, the two women at her feet rub cornmeal over the woman's feet rather than drying them with a towel. This gives the feet a nice glow and symbolizes wishes of luck, protection, and prosperity for the mother as she walks along her path.

4. When the grooming is complete and all of the grooming supplies set aside, the next step is the Give-away, when each guest has the opportunity to address the mother. I like to go around the circle clockwise once more and have each guest say something special and positive that she remembers from her own experience of giving birth. If she has never given birth, she can relate some other special experience. Each person will then present her gift, either reading a poem she may have brought or explaining the gift. This is often a teary experience, so give plenty of time for each person to speak. However, if anyone starts getting negative or goes on and on, you may have to graciously move the energy along.

Another lovely thing to do, taught to me by midwife Diane Bartlett (Whapio), is to create a basket of good wishes, decorated with colorful ribbons. Have some strips of ribbon available for decorating the basket. Give each person a slip of paper and a pen and have each write a prayer, wish, or blessing for the mother and baby on her paper, then pass around a small basket. All wishes should be for the highest good of the mother and baby. Tell each guest to read her wish aloud in turn and, as she does, put the paper in the basket and attach ribbons to the basket. When this is completed, you will have a beautifully decorated wish basket that the mom can look at for inspiration whenever she desires. It will also be a beautiful keepsake for the baby. The actual gift giving can be done when the basket has been completed.

**COMPLETING THE RITUAL**

To complete the ritual, the facilitator can ask if anyone has anything further to share. It is nice if all of the guests hold hands and sing. Although I don't know who wrote it, a very special song that was taught to me is this:

Dear ones, Dear ones,
Can I tell you how I feel?
You have given me such treasures,
I love you so.
*This is sung to the tune of "Soul Cakes," a familiar old folk song.*

Once done, thank all of the participants, most especially all of the helping angels and other beneficent beings who have blessed the mother's way. Welcome everyone to join in a feast and celebration. You have completed the Blessingway ritual.

## Making a Belly Mask

This simple, inexpensive project is the creation of an actual plaster cast of your belly, best done in late pregnancy for full effect. It is made with the same techniques and materials you use for making plaster face masks. Here's how to do it:

Purchase about three rolls of plaster gauze at a local craft store. This is plaster impregnated gauze used for making face masks. You will also need a small jar of Vaseline, an old plastic bucket, and a few rags.

Because it is a messy project, it is best done either out-of-doors where the rain or a garden hose can wash away the drips of plaster, or indoors on a drop cloth or inexpensive shower curtain liner. It is preferable to have someone help you with the process.

To begin, assemble all of your supplies and fill the bucket with warm water. Take your clothes off (you can leave a bra or short tank top on) and stand on the plastic or drop cloth. Measuring horizontally across the areas to be covered, cut strips of the gauze in pieces long enough to cover your belly (and torso if your want to include your breasts), and additional gauze to add two to three layers of thickness.

Now smear a thin layer of Vaseline onto the areas that you will be plastering. This will prevent the materials from sticking to you or hurting when you pull them off.

You don't need to smear Vaseline onto your pubic hair—the plaster doesn't stick well to hair. Then, following the directions on the package of gauze, dip the strips into the warm water and begin applying them to your belly. The general idea is to make overlapping horizontal layers leaving no places uncovered and continuing until you achieve the shape of the belly that you want. When you are finished applying the strips, allow the cast to dry for about five minutes, then remove it from your belly, smooth out the edges by folding them back a bit, and put in a dry, protected spot to harden completely. It will take about twenty-four hours to be dry enough to paint.

Paint with acrylic paints, and have someone spray or paint it with a lacquer or glaze for extra protection. If you must spray it yourself, do so only in a well-ventilated area, preferably outdoors.

# Chapter 12

# Pregnancy as a Rite of Passage

*I*n many cultures, including our own as evidenced by first communions, bar mitzvahs and bat mitzvahs, graduations, weddings, baby showers, and other celebrations, it is important to mark life transitions in tangible ways as rites of passage. The ceremony is a marker indicating that a person has learned what is necessary or has grown to a stage of development that gives him or her the privilege of entering a new stage. In traditional cultures, rites of passage are used to mark the transition from youth to adult responsibility in a tribe, village, or community. During this time, the initiate must demonstrate her or his ability to withstand or endure certain challenges and will also receive knowledge imparted by elders about the new stage to come.

In our society, little recognition is given to the major transformative nature of pregnancy, which, along with its culmination in the birth of a child, is a lengthy rite of passage into becoming a mother. One can call pregnancy a liminal stage, that is, "a phase of becoming." Women becoming mothers are neither given the special recognition as initiates, nor imparted the skills that teach and support them to be strong women and capable mothers through the teachings of elders. But we can change all this by acknowledging the important transformative qualities that pregnancy has in a woman's life.

By viewing pregnancy as a rite of passage, you can take it upon yourself to make the most of the process, looking at the entire pregnancy experience not simply as a means to an end (the birth and the baby) but as a valuable process in and of itself. You can make a firm and courageous attempt to become a powerful woman, learning to trust your body and your innate wisdom. By doing so, you will come to realize that filling and surrounding yourself with the aura of strength and wellness will infuse the baby with these qualities as well.

## An Opportunity for Personal Growth

Pregnancy can be viewed as an opportunity to resolve conflicts from the past that may hinder your sense of empowerment. Pregnancy is a time of heightened emotional sensitivity, a perfect time to learn to work with your emotions. It is a time to develop the strength to deal with your issues with grace, confidence, and determination. These are the same attributes that will see you through birth.

It is perfectly natural and healthy to expect that, as we walk through the doorway of pregnancy and birth, we will feel fear—we are, after all, facing the unknown. This is inevitably challenging as we grasp the enormous responsibility of motherhood, as well as recognizing the intensity of the birth experience. And there seem to be benefits in what I refer to as "the work of worrying." I've noticed that women who do some healthy worrying during pregnancy and admit to having fears or anxieties are actually engaged in resolving conflicts. Women who deny—either consciously or unconsciously—that they have fears about birth, the baby, motherhood, their marriage, and so on tend to have a more difficult experience of birth. If you can actively look at a particular concern, prepare or educate yourself about it, and then let it go once you've done what you can to address, resolve, or at least contemplate it, then you are actively working out your fears. It is by addressing such fears or concerns that you can find the inner strength for creative problem solving. For example, if you already have toddlers and find yourself pregnant, you may feel anxiety about how you will handle all these responsibilities. Creative problem solving might include arranging support for a while after the birth, making menus or freezing foods during your pregnancy to have for after the birth, and affirming each day your ability to nurture yourself so that you maintain the energy to care for your family.

You might also choose to relieve bouts of anxiety by writing in a journal, nurturing yourself with tea and a bath by candlelight, crying on your mate's shoulder, or drawing a picture of yourself with images of abundant love being showered down upon you by an imagined loving mother. Such visualizing can help to increase your sense of greater energy and support.

# Self-Empowerment

Empowerment refers to the ability to know what one needs and to feel confident to meet those needs. However, for many women, trained since childhood to be accommodating and passive, this is no simple feat. For a pregnant woman to give herself and her child the best care possible, she must relinquish passivity and empower herself to make choices in her health care.

In the present health-care system that denies individuality for the sake of efficiency, predictability, and cost-effectiveness, women must become empowered if we are to receive the care we want for ourselves and our families. To accept treatment that is not truly in our best interest is to allow ourselves to become victims. When one chooses something, this is empowerment; when one allows oneself to be manipulated, coerced, or frightened into accepting something, this is victimization. I always remind my clients that they are the ones in charge of their health-care decisions, not the midwife, doctor, or anyone else. Short of an emergency situation, it is your voice and your needs that should determine the care you receive.

So how do you become empowered to make health-care choices? Often it takes a difficult experience before a woman is empowered. But you don't have to have an initial experience in which you have felt victimized to bring about such revelation. Determination to trust your body and gradually learning to do so is an excellent place to start. Trusting your inner voice, your intellectual abilities, and your mental competence, and then speaking up for yourself or following your feelings, are also ways to empowerment. Telling a doctor, for example, that you didn't like a negative comment he or she made about pregnancy, birth, or your body, or asking a neighbor not to tell you negative birthing stories is empowerment. Rather than meekly accepting a negative comment for the sake of being polite or for fear of offending someone, you must protect and care for yourself.

Listening to your body, an important aspect of empowerment, means taking the time to be body-centered each day. Because pregnancy brings so many new sensations, this is a ripe time for becoming aware of your body. As you respond more readily to your body's cues, they will become more apparent. In the same way, you will increasingly trust your intuition and common sense. You have to trust that you know what is best for you. You can elicit information, advice, opinions, and support, but then you will have to decide how you feel about things.

Experience too, is empowering. Many women have never had the opportunity to spend time with babies and young children, have never seen a woman breastfeed, and have never changed a diaper. Therefore many women enter motherhood feeling that they lack the skills necessary to care for their young. While much of mothering is highly intuitive, not all of it is. It does help to spend time around babies. The opportunity to assist another mom with the care of her baby, letting her know that you want to be familiar with the feel of a newborn and to feel comfortable with changing diapers and caring for a child, can raise your level of confidence and your sense of empowerment. Reading books to educate yourself about the basic facts about pregnancy, birth, and parenting can be empowering. Learning infant massage, infant CPR, or other skills, and hearing about other women's positive birth experiences also can be empowering.

> *"In my life the physical acts of birthing have been an incredible means for sourcing my power."*
>
> —Diane Mariechild

Empowerment is taking an active stand that acknowledges your intrinsic worth as a human being and honors your right to choose whether to say yes or no. It is choosing to replace self-doubt and undermining behaviors with self-loving actions, protective of both you and your family. It is only by each of us actively making self-empowering choices that we will create the attitude in our culture that pregnant women know best what they and their babies need for optimal well-being.

## Affirmations for Nurturing Yourself

Affirmations are a powerful tool for personal transformation. Repeating these messages to yourself is a way throughout your day to consciously and deliberately create an inner sense of well-being: the best times are when you wake, during the course of your day, and before you sleep. By repeating affirmations, you slowly but surely remake your thought processes into those that foster wellness. Affirmations are not used to suppress or deny concerns, but rather to dispel nagging anxieties that do not benefit you. They are useful for dispelling the negative messages we have all internalized—for example, that our bodies are not trustworthy, that our intuitive awareness is inferior to science and technology, that we are unworthy of joy and success, and so on. The following list of affirmations is a sampling of what you might use:

- I am a strong and capable woman.
- My body knows exactly how to nourish my baby.
- I have enough love to share.
- I give myself the right to accept love and nourishment from others.
- My baby is healthy and beautiful.
- I love my pregnant body.

- I will let my labor and birth be its own unique experience.
- I embrace the concept of healthy pain.
- I trust my ability to give birth with strength and power.

If you find yourself countering an affirmation—for example, if you tell yourself, "I am a strong and healthy woman" but a little voice pops into your mind saying, "no you're not, you're weak"—try to figure out whose voice you have internalized and how that happened. Even if you can't figure it out, you may gain an interesting insight. Don't let such negative messages undermine your efforts. As you persist in the affirmations, you will replace the old, self-defeating messages. Remember, language not only expresses your thoughts, it shapes both your thoughts and our culture. Merely by shifting your attention to the positive, without denying your concerns, you can nurture health and enthusiasm.

Because pregnancy is a time of great sensitivity and a portal into a new phase in life, it offers you the opportunity to recognize and release your fullest potential as a woman. This in turn will nurture your confidence as a mother, and as an advocate for other pregnant women and other mothers. By holding the intention to be healthy and joyous, and by admitting to and resolving doubts, old beliefs, and negative internal messages, you can grow joyously through this rite of pregnancy, becoming stronger and more powerful in the process.

For further suggestions on honoring pregnancy, see "Celebrating Pregnancy" in the preceding chapter. For more on the healing and transformative powers of pregnancy, as well as releasing emotional and psychological blockages, I recommend the following books: *Transformation through Birth* by Claudia Panuthos, *Pregnant Feelings* by Rahima Baldwin and Terra Palmarini, *Birthing Normally* by Gayle Peterson, *Silent Knife* by Nancy Cohen and Lois Estner, *Open Season* by Nancy Cohen, and *Pregnancy as Healing* by Gayle Peterson and Lewis Mehl, all listed in the bibliography.

## *Spirituality*

Each of us has our own spirituality. For some, this might be the religious experience they have in a synagogue, church, mosque, or sweat lodge. For some, spirituality might be experienced during a walk through a sunlit wood, through hearing waves crash against the shore, or by listening to the sound of rain. The experience of spirit often connects us to something that includes but is somehow larger than our individual selves. Pregnancy offers you an opportunity to experience a heightened sense of your spirituality because during the precious months of pregnancy you are an individual, yet you are also more than this. It is a period of time during which your connection with something beyond yourself is more apparent than in a nonpregnant state—it is at once physical and transcendental.

The awareness that you are participating in the process of creating life may also enhance your spiritual awareness, as you may find yourself connected to the realm that your baby is in, a realm that is at once physical and at the same time mysterious and unseen. Even ultrasound testing, which makes a baby visible during pregnancy, does not explain the mystery and miracle of the pregnancy process.

You may also experience a heightened awareness of spirituality if you find yourself dreaming about angelic realms, "hearing" your baby talking to you, or experiencing an unexplainable "knowing" of who your baby is and what your baby needs, or have other insights about your pregnancy, birth, or child. I find that during my own pregnancies I also have increased experiences of precognition, for example, thinking of an old friend minutes before she phones or receiving a letter from her in the mail. This section discusses ways in which you can develop the spiritual aspects of your life during your pregnancy, and how you might use your spirituality to bring you closer to your intuitive awareness, as well as closer to your strength as a woman.

## Nourishing Your "Womanplace"

There is eminent value in taking time regularly throughout your pregnancy to create a sacred space where and when you take time to honor yourself, other women, family, babies, pregnancy, and birth, and affirm and nourish your great strength as a woman.

Within each of us resides what writer and midwife Nancy Cohen has referred to in *Open Season* as our "womanplace." This term refers to the part of us that innately knows how to be pregnant, nourish our babies, birth, and live our lives in a creative, empowered, and intuitive way. It is impossible to deny even by scientific standards that we are capable of what can be termed intuition or extrasensory perception. Pregnant women, as do all women, have access to this womanplace for information. But first, each of us must identify and then nourish this place. Depending on the ways that you express yourself creatively, you may identify your womanplace as residing in a distinct area of your body—for example, an artist may identify with her hands, a gardener with her feet planted firmly on the ground, another woman with her heart or womb. To make your womanplace come alive for you, you must nourish and call forth this part of yourself.

You can make this place real within you by actively awakening it through ritual and creative expression. Ritual is simply a time set aside regularly for active attention to your womanplace and for creative expression. How do you like to be nourished with beauty and what kindles your soul? I enjoy putting on music that makes me dance, and after working up a sweat, I like to feel that creative place strong and alive within. I also like to sing and drum in a dark room with lit candles, or in my garden. I enjoy drawing. Do whatever nourishes your sense of strength and brings you closer to your true self, where you feel a sense of spirit beyond your mundane self and where you feel strongly attuned to your body. It could be a walk in the woods, planting flowers in a garden, making love, or having a water fight with your kids. Visualize your womanplace, even draw what it should look like. Set up a special place in your home, perhaps on the top of a bureau or night table, to remind you of your womanplace. Place objects there that reflect the strength of women and the power and beauty of nature, pregnant women, and mothers. This will serve as a visual reminder of your strength and connectedness with other women and the forces of nature. Nourish that place of creativity and aliveness often and it will be alive for you when you birth and when your kids are little and you need to find your inner resources of energy and patience. By doing so, you also give your children the great gift of energy, as they see your vitality and are supported by you in developing their own place within.

*A particular mother had developed a sacred time of connection with her baby and very late in her pregnancy (over a week past her due date) had the distinct feeling that her baby was going to be born in the caul, that is, with its water bag still intact around the baby. I told her that some cultures consider this an auspicious sign, and that it is certainly possible, though very rare. That night she began labor, and a few hours later she gave birth to her daughter—in the caul as she'd predicted!*

## Support of the Women's Spirituality Movement

The women's spirituality movement can also help you to move closer to your womanplace. Through the writings of such women as Merlin Stone, Marija Gimbutas, Riane Eisler, Vicki Noble, Anne Kent Rush, Starhawk, Jeannine Parvati Baker, Elizabeth Davis, and many others, and through our own spiritual practices and social commitments, we reawaken to the divinity and strength of women. Ancient traditions reveal that long before written history, female deities were recognized and revered as much as "God the Father" is now. To reclaim the self-respect we deserve for our varied roles and talents as both nurturers and women of social power is incredibly revitalizing. Similarly, awareness of women's great contributions to political and environmental change also gives us a sense of collective strength, pride, and power. We come to realize that spirituality, politics, and women's status are all intimately connected to the environment we create for pregnancy, birth, and motherhood, and that, in reclaiming our strength and wisdom, we can make this world a healthier place in which to live, birth, and raise children.

## Chapter 13

# Your Changing Family

Whether this is your first baby or your sixth, each pregnancy and baby brings changes to the family structure as you and your mate adjust to your changing needs and the needs of other family members. Older children may be delighted or they may groan, the youngest has to adjust to the idea of a sibling, and your family budget has to stretch just a little bit more. Approached with a healthy awareness of the stresses involved, the changes of pregnancy need not be overwhelming. Pregnancy can be a joyous time of celebration, anticipation, and integration of this new being into your life.

## Your Relationship with Your Mate

Regardless of how long a couple has been together, pregnancy and a baby change your roles, expectations, and needs. Women who have careers and who now choose to be home as well as women who have never had a job may begin to feel dependent upon their mates and lose their sense of competence and value, both so important in the transition to motherhood. These feelings may cause a woman to act more child-like or cling to her partner or, conversely, to withdraw. For men, pregnancy will hopefully bring a sense of increased responsibility, but along with this may come the shadow of feeling burdened, overwhelmed, or scared. This may cause him to withdraw from his partner, seeing her as the object or cause of these feelings.

In school we are not taught "Communication Skills 101" or "Relationship Skills for Sophomores" (literally, "wise fools"), and we therefore all too often go bumbling through our relationships. Of course, not all marriages work out and it isn't always healthy for women and men to put up with intolerable or abusive situations for the sake of commitment. But many marriages began as loving relationships, and it is often merely a lack of relationship skills along with mundane pressures that cause marriages to fall apart.

## Common Sources of Tension

Because pregnancy causes parents to feel new concerns and pressures, as well as causing them to reevaluate their needs and expectations for support, this can be a time of stress. In addition, parents may begin to discuss and disagree about how to raise the child—for example, parenting styles, religion, how and where to birth, whom to choose as a care provider, and so on.

A common source of tension for pregnant couples is how the pregnant woman's physical and emotional needs should be met. For example, when a woman feels consumed by nausea in the first trimester, she may feel too ill to keep up with the responsibilities she typically attends to and may want her mate to help out more. He may respond with irritation, even accusing her of exaggerating her illness in order to shirk her responsibilities. She may then become angry at him in addition to blaming herself for feeling so horrible. Such tension can cause the relationship to suffer throughout the pregnancy.

As a pregnant woman's body grows and changes, she may feel insecure about her appearance and may look to her husband for reassurance. While it is important for a woman to like her own body regardless of another's opinion, her mate's attraction to or rejection of her will influence her sense of self. If a woman perceives that her mate is rejecting her pregnant body, or if he actually is, this can be a very painful situation. It seems to me very sad that any man wouldn't find his pregnant mate beautiful; however, this issue often arises for couples. The man may be confused by finding himself attracted to a mother—a new way of seeing his sexual partner. Usually, a frank discussion facilitated by a counselor or a midwife will clear the air and resolve misconceptions.

Sexual needs are also a common source of stress. A pregnant woman may not feel like having sex during the first couple of months, if she is extremely nauseated or fatigued, or very late in the pregnancy. If suddenly she isn't interested in intimacy, he may take this as rejection. Other pregnant women may feel like having sex more often than ever. If he is not a person who wants to make love frequently, she may take this as rejection. If either partner is afraid to hurt the baby or feels embarrassed making love "with the baby there," this can create sexual tension. A useful guidebook to lovemaking during pregnancy is *Making Love during Pregnancy* by Elizabeth Bing and Libby Colman. For ideas on creative relationships as well as intimacy, see *The Couple's Comfort Book* by Jennifer Louden.

## Healing Tensions

If you are both committed to being together, you can learn skills that will enable you to integrate your differences and transcend the difficulties in order to create a vital, dynamic, committed loving relationship. The book by Jennifer Louden mentioned above has many creative ideas for improving communication, rejuvenating a relationship, and enhancing intimacy both sexually and in general.

The foundation of any marriage has to be two strong individuals who agree to be together because they love each other and enjoy each other's company. Each of you must work on your own ability to be loving, compassionate, strong, caring, and sensitive. Then you can give love because you want to, without your entire sense of self resting upon your partner's response. However, a healthy marriage must be mutually satisfying; if the responses you receive do not nurture you, this will not be a mutually happy situation.

A couple must be able to communicate their needs and expectations openly and truthfully. Both partners must feel free to express themselves and must be able to listen to the other with the heart. It is not fair to have expectations that are not expressed, then resent the other for not meeting these expectations. You cannot expect someone to read your mind, a common mistake that pregnant women make when they want their mates to anticipate their needs. It is fair, however, to expect your partner to see your needs as important, since you are carrying this child for both of you. How one expresses needs can also have an impact on whether they are heard. "Love, would you please rub my back" sounds vastly different than "Why don't you ever offer me a back rub? You know I'm tired!" While an empathetic partner might respond lovingly to either message, the first is certainly more likely to elicit the desired response. Again, expressing messages clearly and from your loving heart is essential, especially if you want to be heard by a loving heart. "The Man's Point of View," a section later in this chapter, provides further insights on the importance of the father's (or mate's) role in the relationship during pregnancy, and should be read by both of you.

# When You Already Have Children

Pregnancy the first time around is quite a different experience than when you have other children to care for. Most first-time moms do not have the same amount of household work and demands that a mother who already has children may face. If you already have children, particularly if they are young, you are apt to be more tired than when you were having your first baby. Yet so many women seem to forget this simple truth and berate themselves for falling asleep at eight o'clock when their four-year-old goes to bed, letting housework slide a bit more than usual, or eating peanut butter and jelly for lunch instead of a high-protein meal with a fresh green salad.

I am writing this section to simply remind you of the importance of taking good care of yourself. It is important to learn to ask for help and to be easy on yourself. Do let your toddler watch an afternoon movie so that you can take a nap. Let your husband help you prepare meals, and enlist older kids in getting household chores done. While P.B. and J. sandwiches are okay once in a while, by all means don't skimp on your meals. Fatigue can be reduced by eating well and getting plenty of rest, but if you try to be a supermom you'll probably be exhausted no matter what you do, and your pregnancy and birth may be more difficult for you. Learn to set limits without feeling guilty, and trust that you are a good mom and deserve time to nourish yourself and the baby.

## Involving Siblings in the Pregnancy

I can barely describe the magic and wonder on a child's face when she or he sees a newborn sibling for the first time. As a midwife, this is one of my favorite moments. Yet not all siblings react with keen interest when they meet a new brother or sister. Much resistance can be prevented and even melted away by integrating and welcoming children into the life of the baby before it is born.

*The baby moves around so much each day. It feels wonderful to have this reminder that we are welcoming this new little one into our family.*

*—A. J. R.*

As a baby's life begins at conception, the best time to tell older children that you are pregnant is soon after you find out. Should you miscarry, you can explain this to your children gently in a nonthreatening and age-appropriate way. By making your children insiders in the process and sharing the pregnancy as a family experience, you will give them months to integrate the idea of a new family member. This will also help to keep your children from being confused by your mood changes or your changing body. You will not only be allowing your children to feel secure in the knowledge that they are important, respected members of the family, worthy of knowing such important news, but you will be providing essential education in the pregnancy process. Children who have a realistic perspective on pregnancy and parenting may be more thoughtful in preparing for their own families, and may choose to do so in a more responsible fashion than those who have never been involved in a pregnancy or the care of a young child.

When children are involved in the pregnancy from the beginning, they tend to marvel with you at the changes in your belly, the kicks and rolls of the baby in your womb, and the sound of your baby's heartbeat. Children will usually, if not either pushed with the idea or protected from it, develop a healthy anticipation and eagerness to meet this little being inside you.

A lengthy discussion about having siblings present at the birth is beyond the scope of this book, but if you plan to have your child attend the birth, there is no finer preparation than being included in the prenatal care, becoming familiar with your birth attendants, and being exposed to your naked pregnant body. If you view pregnancy as a normal fact of life, so too will your children, and if you extend this view to the birth, your child will do the same.

It is empowering to young children to feel that they are capable people and important members of your household. You can ask your toddler to help you prepare a meal for you both and let him or her know that this feeds the baby as well. You can ask your older child to watch a toddler for an hour while you rest or stretch, or you can invite your children to stretch along with you. You can teach them with books and videos about how the baby lives in your belly. You can ask your midwife or physician to help the children feel the baby's head, feet, or bottom when she palpates your belly at prenatal visits. Of course, if your child is shy about this, she or he should not be forced to participate. If you have been open with your older children all along, they are likely to want to be involved, and most toddlers love to be in on the action.

When children attend prenatal visits with their parents, I always invite them to feel and listen to the baby. I've even done a mock prenatal on little ones who insist that they are also pregnant. I've had little ones hug me when I've left their homes after a sibling has been born, and thank me without being prompted for helping their mommy with the birth. This always moves me to tears. And as I watch the closeness of these children with their younger siblings, I am reminded of the value of welcoming siblings into the process of pregnancy.

# The Man's Point of View
## *by Tracy Romm*

*A woman's experience of pregnancy can be enhanced by the participation of a loving support person, whether it be her mate or another close friend. This section was written by my partner and the father of our four children, Tracy Romm. He offers ideas on how to support your pregnant partner, how to meet your own needs, and how to honor your changing role as you become a father.*

While it takes both a man and a woman to conceive a child, that is the point when any biological necessity for male participation in this sacred act ends. The fact is that women can grow and birth a child independently of the father. Sadly, an increasing number of women in our modern societies are compelled to do exactly that.

Just because men do not bear or birth babies themselves, however, does not mean that we don't have a vital role to play in childbearing. When we help to conceive a child, when we become a father, we assume a host of lifelong responsibilities to both mother and child. Although many men define this role primarily in material terms—being the breadwinner—it is clear that other men are searching for more.

Pregnancy and birth present men with a powerful opportunity to cultivate our nurturing qualities and to bond in deep and lasting ways with our mates and children. The benefits of fathers' active participation in childbearing for optimal maternal, child, and overall family health has been amply documented in the research literature. Nowadays, childbirth educators routinely expect fathers to attend classes, and some childbirth systems assign to fathers a key role at birth. In sum, all signs point to a shift in the way men perceive their place in the childbearing cycle.

Yet how ill-prepared so many of us are. I remember all too well the dominant images of fathers in my formative years. One of the Desi Arnaz and Lucille Ball shows depicted an almost hysterical Desi trying desperately to cater to the every need of an almost equally hysterical Lucy—to the point of an all-hours search for the proverbial pickles and ice cream. Yet where did it get him? At the birth, he became the stereotypical figure of the pacing father in a cramped waiting room, pockets full of cigars, grasping for any word from any white-clothed figure with authority.

There are reasons to wonder whether our current Hollywood models are any better prepared to show us the way. The movie *Nine Months* featured a successful psychologist who took almost the full term of his mate's pregnancy to willingly make a commitment to mother and child. In the end, it required the video image of an ultrasound to win him over, convincing him that the fetus was a child worth loving and working for. In the end, however, he was reduced to a bumbling idiot as he rushed his wife to the hospital, culminating in an adrenaline-induced brawl with another expectant father in the delivery room at the very moment his wife gave birth. At least we men have made it to the birthing chamber!

This section acknowledges the unique and important role for fathers in pregnancy. When all is said and done, we are usually the single most significant other in the life of our mates. As they grow this baby, they look to us for many types of support—emotional and spiritual no less than material. Pregnancy is a dance, admittedly a new one for many of us, and it often takes a while to learn the steps. Take heart. To paraphrase an African proverb, if you can walk you can dance; if you can talk you can sing.

## Becoming a Father

You become a father when you conceive a child. There should be no debate about this assertion. Whatever the conflicting medical and spiritual positions about when life begins, it is certain that at the moment of conception a man enters into a deeper and more intimate relationship with a woman. She now carries within herself a part of his biological essence merged with hers—and the whole is greater than the sum of its parts. The relationship now has a tangible nature that cannot be simply wished away or erased. (How many men who have experienced the loss of a child through abortion, for example, can really forget that event, even if they supported or encouraged the abortion in the first place?) This realization can be exhilarating or terrifying. For most of us, it is both.

When Aviva and I confirmed the conception of our first child, I was truly exhilarated. I felt as if I were walking on air—literally. All of the pressing concerns of my life seemed to melt away in the rosy glow of those first days. Perhaps I was more fortunate than many because I knew that I wanted this child. For a man who feels ambivalence about assuming the responsibility of fatherhood or even about his commitment to the mother, it must be much more difficult. One point to keep in mind is that doubts are common and most men experience them.

Am I ready to be a father? Will this child interfere with my life? Can I afford this (another) child? Do I really want to be in a lifelong relationship with this woman? Will the child be healthy? It is okay to let yourself ask these questions and others. In fact, it is probably healthier in the long run to begin to face your shadows at the outset rather than to deny them. Many men report that becoming a father unleashed emotions and thoughts that were not usually part of their waking consciousness. You might find yourself, for example, reflecting more deeply on your own childhood, and specifically on your father's place in your early years. Remember that pregnancy is a process that lasts nine months and that you have time to grow. At the same time, don't get lost in your doubts; don't forget to enjoy the moment, for the glow can grow faint at times.

Pregnancy produces some of the most profound changes to a woman's body and psyche that I can imagine. These changes are often so gradual that at any one moment they are imperceptible. The result is that it is often easy to forget what is really going on. We get so caught up in the stresses of day-to-day living that we forget we are in the midst of this extraordinary experience that is like nothing we have ever faced before. There are no simple road maps; no one person, not even this book, can fully prepare you for what lies ahead. If you expect the familiar, particularly if you are a first-time father, forget it.

## Supporting Your Pregnant Partner

Pregnancy requires surrender. Unfortunately this word has negative connotations for most men in our culture. Surrender implies giving up to a stronger person or position; it implies defeat. This is decidedly not what I am trying to convey here.

To say that pregnancy requires surrender is to acknowledge and even honor the fact that the childbearing woman must—by biological necessity—accept that many aspects of her life are no longer under her control. It is a 24/7 task: twenty-four hours a day and seven days a week she is growing this baby inside of her belly. Everything about her life may be in a state of flux, of change. The predictable is fleeting, whether we are speaking of sleeping patterns, eating habits, emotions, or clothing styles and sizes. Anyone who has experienced pregnancy with his partner remembers the restaurant where she ordered a delectable meal, only to turn it away after the first bite. Or the new urgency in finding access to a public bathroom and in packing snacks for excursions out of the home, particularly in late pregnancy. In my many years of marriage to a practicing midwife, I have noticed that the women who do not surrender to these pregnancy changes, these new needs and desires, frequently have the most difficult transitions into birth and motherhood.

What does this mean for the new father? A number of years ago, I came across a slim volume entitled *Your Baby Is Your First Guru*. Translated literally, *guru* means "spiritual guide." The kernel of wisdom I gathered from this book is that learning to cheerfully accept the needs of your mate and baby and to make them a priority in your life develops your inner strength and your ability to face the ups and downs of life generally. We all know that life is not a straight line; we do not start and end, traveling along a predictable path as in a board game. There will be crossroads of decision and detours, as well as peaks and valleys. We will never have total control over all of the challenges life presents to us. We do have some measure of control over the attitude with which we face them. What better place to start than with our own mate and child?

At the same time, to surrender does not mean that fathers have to mimic the pregnancy experience itself. Although many men report sympathetic changes in their own biology during pregnancy—such as morning sickness, insomnia, and weight gain—the ideal model of partnership during pregnancy focuses on supporting the childbearing mother. Rather than mimicking her symptoms, we would be wiser to envision ourselves as the willow tree. Willows are renowned for their flexibility when the winds are gusting, yet they are rarely uprooted. Our task is to bend to our mate's needs, yet not to lose our sense of rootedness. Our mates will be looking to us throughout pregnancy, as well as during birth, for steadiness and reassurance. How can we provide these to her if we are so caught up in our own changes?

The downside is the danger that you may begin to feel unsupported. If mother and baby become the center of your universe, who will fill your needs? In the process, aren't you becoming henpecked, tied to your wife's apron strings, less of a man? Please know that the surfacing of resentments is a very common experience for expectant fathers. It would be surprising otherwise in a culture where male programming calls for men to be in control and to wear the pants in the family. Even those of you who are not bound by these stereotypes may feel resentful at times of the incredible amount of effort that pregnancy demands of your mate and thus of you. Being pregnant together, in the fullest sense of the word *together,* does not mean that you and your mate have to do everything alike and at exactly the same time. As you nurture your partner, do not forget to nurture yourself. While pregnancy is not a time to go out to sow your oats in a last-chance fling at freedom, it is okay to continue to cultivate your interests and to meet your needs.

The key is to align yourself with your mate and baby in total love and understanding. Assume your full responsibilities as their protector. I know this notion may strike many as sex-role stereotyping, but my experience is otherwise. Becoming a father activates our protective instincts; most women want us to be protective at this time if for no other reason than they are incredibly preoccupied by the internal demands of pregnancy, including being fiercely protective of the child growing within them. But

> *"The path of the mother should be given its deserved value as a sacred and powerful spiritual path."*
>
> —Tsultrim Allione

being protective does not mean that we have to dwell in the land of fight or flight. Perhaps "advocate" imparts a truer sense of our role than "protector."

As an advocate, you are acting in the service of your pregnant mate to ensure that her best interests are always the priority. This requires your willingness to listen and to respond to her expressed needs. Even though male programming may tell you that you know better, you must maintain an open mind, affirm your mate's best intentions, and be fully prepared to yield to her requests. And, if necessary, you must offer your mate a gentle reminder when pregnancy calls on her to grow or change in ways she may resist or does not see. The fruits of this attentiveness and caring are a healthier mother and pregnancy, as well as improved communication and a deeper trust that will continue to nurture your relationship through the demands of raising a family together.

## Becoming a Part of the Pregnancy

Serving as an advocate allows fathers to assume an active and full involvement in the pregnancy process. This course of action requires the total involvement of both heart and mind. To act as an advocate, however, we must be knowledgeable about what we advocate. In other words, we must educate ourselves about pregnancy. Be truthful with yourself, how many of you have read this book carefully? I know that I knew very little about pregnancy and childbirth before the birth of our first child, despite having attended two home births previously and being married to a midwife. My life was busy; pregnancy was her field. Yet there is no way that I could advocate on behalf of Aviva and our babies if I didn't educate myself about the needs of pregnant women and the prenatal experiences of babies. When your partner puts those books in front of you, don't say "later." Turn off the television; quiet the music; put down your book. With all of the excellent material available today, which our forefathers didn't have access to, we have no excuse. If we remain uninformed, we are choosing to remain ignorant; what we are conveying is nothing less than disinterest.

As you attune your mind to pregnancy, you can act from the heart with mindfulness. During pregnancy, loving your mate is the best way of loving your baby. In this dance, actions clearly speak louder than words, and it is often the simple, everyday actions that speak the loudest. Support your mate in caring for herself and the baby, for example, by bringing her a glass of fresh juice or water before she asks for it. Keep an eye on the refrigerator and ensure that it is well stocked with a variety of healthful foods. Exercise is something you can do together, whether it's a brisk walk or a session of yoga. Remember that pregnancy requires extra sleep. If your mate is at home full-time, she might need to be reminded that it is okay to let the housework wait—she's not being lazy. Be resourceful: there are countless ways that you can show her that you recognize and appreciate all of her hard work growing your baby.

For those of you who already have children, the challenges can be far greater. I never realized how much easier the first pregnancy was until we experienced subsequent ones. With our first child, Aviva could eat and rest when her body signaled; in later pregnancies, she had to juggle the competing demands of children and the in-utero baby. Fathers often have to be even more energetic in supporting these pregnant moms. There were times when I felt that coming home from work was like going to a second job. Fathers really need to be proactive with later pregnancies. Taking care of the children while your mate rests, preparing evening meals, pitching in with the housework—each of these acts serves not only to give her a break but to remind her that you care.

Be involved with your mate's prenatal care. This means more than just attending the regularly scheduled prenatal visits. Educate yourself about the various complications of pregnancy, and be ready to question a health-care provider about any tests that are recommended. Pregnancy can activate many fears for a woman, especially about the well-being of her baby, and a father has a responsibility to deflect unwarranted pressures on his mate to submit to any procedures. The best health-care providers welcome questions from fathers who are sincerely trying to become part of the pregnancy.

It is critically important that you continue to nurture your relationship with your mate. While this sounds easy, often you may get so busy with added responsibilities around the house that you forget to connect directly with her. You may even begin to feel imposed upon if, despite your contributions, she still wants to spend more time with you. Intimacy shared during pregnancy creates a reservoir of trust that can be drawn upon when you need it most—for example, during birth or after.

Massage is probably one of the easiest and most effective ways to connect two people, and its value in a healthy pregnancy cannot be overstated. You do not have to be a massage therapist to give a massage. More than anything else, what is required is sensitivity to your partner. Ask her what feels good, work lightly, and let her signal if she wants you to work harder on an area; give her the choice of using a massage oil or not. If you keep the lines of communication open and allow your heart to guide your hands, you will not go wrong. There is nothing that a pregnant mom enjoys more than to feel you loving your baby as you rub her belly. Gently stroke your child, even speak with him or her. What the child feels or hears perinatally is a question of current scientific research. My sense in the matter is clear: with each child I felt a certain familiarity and bonding from the first moments after the birth. If nothing else, rubbing Aviva's belly on a regular basis gave me the confidence that our child felt truly loved and wanted by both of us, and that I knew how to hold and touch him or her in nurturing ways.

By no means is this section exhaustive of the ways fathers can become a part of pregnancy. Needs and life circumstances vary. Through each of our four children, I feel that I have grown to be a more supportive and loving partner in pregnancy. But I have made mistakes, stemming primarily from an inability to listen and to yield to Aviva. I share this observation with you as both an encouragement and a reminder. It is possible to grow into the kind of man you envision and value, despite the lack of role models in our culture. In the process, you may inspire others and thereby contribute to the evolution of new models of manhood. Just remember that your opportunities to experience pregnancy are limited: most of us have only a handful of chances to be this close to the miracle of life. Cherish the occasion.

Part II

# Common Concerns during Pregnancy

## Chapter 14

# A Guide to Common Pregnancy Issues

Pregnancy is a normal process that our bodies are quite capable of accomplishing. It is also a process that transforms our bodies and our lives, and sometimes the changes that are part of this transformation can be difficult for a pregnant woman to integrate into her familiar existence. For instance, some of the physiological changes of pregnancy can lead to discomfort. Your growing uterus may cause your stomach to be displaced upward. This change, along with decreased gastric motility, can lead to heartburn. Or a woman who works on her feet all day may get severe backaches. By means of some suggestions and natural remedies, many such discomforts common to pregnancy can be prevented, alleviated, or at least minimized. It is also true that by paying early attention to some common complaints, such as vomiting or a bladder infection, a woman can prevent these conditions from worsening into more severe problems, such as clinical dehydration or kidney infection.

As a midwife and herbalist, I emphasize natural healing techniques. These are what I have experience using, and I've made every effort to present remedies that have been widely used with efficacy and safety. No deleterious effects are known to occur when the techniques described in this chapter are used as directed. When there may be a risk associated with a health concern, I have noted it and indicated the standard medical protocol currently in use. The descriptions of natural healing techniques in this chapter are also accompanied by any potential side effects. Always remember that any therapy—natural or otherwise—should be used carefully. Of course, every woman is unique, so please always give utmost attention to how you feel when trying anything new, and do consult your health-care practitioner if you suspect a problem or need help in determining which treatment you should try. Refer to chapter 6 for further information on the safety of herbs during pregnancy.

May these suggestions assist you in enjoying a healthy and comfortable pregnancy.

# Anemia

Anemia is a reduction in the number of red blood cells in the bloodstream. Because red blood cells carry oxygen throughout the body, this reduction decreases the efficiency of the body's oxygenation processes and causes a number of symptoms, including dizziness, shortness of breath, general weakness, paleness (of the skin, fingernail beds, and mucous membranes), loss of appetite, heart palpitations, and gastrointestinal disturbances including constipation and abdominal pain. Frequent colds or infections may also be a sign that you are anemic. Anemia is not a disease; it is a symptom of an insufficient number of red blood cells. The cause of anemia is in most cases a nutritional deficiency. Sometimes anemia is caused by sickle-cell disease or a chronic infection. Anemia may also occur as a result of blood loss or hemorrhage, such as chronic bleeding gums, which also may be nutritionally related.

Three types of nutritional anemias are most likely to occur during pregnancy: iron-deficiency anemia; folic acid deficiency, known as "megaloblastic anemia"; and pernicious anemia, which is a deficiency of vitamin $B_{12}$. In most cases, a healthy diet with appropriate supplementation will prevent and rectify nutritional deficiencies. Left untreated, anemia can lead to a variety of discomforts and medical problems for both mother and baby. The childbearing cycle is an excellent time for laying the foundation for a lifetime of nutritional health. Refer to chapter 5 for further nutritional information. If your condition doesn't respond to dietary improvements, seek medical evaluation.

## *Folic Acid Anemia*

Folic acid is one of the B vitamins. It is found primarily in leafy green vegetables as well as in wheat germ, molasses, nutritional yeast, whole grains, root vegetables, beans, milk, and liver. Animal liver contains high concentrations of environmental and systemic toxins, so I normally do not suggest it for pregnant women. Only in the case of severe deficiency do I sometimes suggest it, but then only if the liver comes from an organically raised animal.

Spirulina, according to midwife and author Anne Frye, is exceptionally high in folic acid as well as other nutrients, including easily assimilable protein.

To obtain the maximum amount of folic acid from vegetables, eat them raw, steamed, or lightly sautéed. When they are boiled, folic acid is leached out in the cooking water and most of it is discarded. All pregnant women should be certain to eat at least two large portions of leafy green vegetables daily as well as an ample amount of other foods that contain folic acid.

Symptoms of folic acid deficiency include the mask of pregnancy and other skin pigment changes, appetite loss, vomiting, persistent vaginal infections, and, because other B-complex vitamins may also be deficient, a host of nervous system complaints. Babies are more likely to be born with neural tube defects (such as spina bifida) when mothers are deficient in folic acid.

Herbs that contain folic acid include amaranth, watercress, parsley, chicory, nettle, dandelion leaves, and lamb's quarter greens. Most of these can be eaten as vegetables or steeped to make tea, though parsley should only be used in limited quantities as a vegetable, not as a tea, during pregnancy.

## Vitamin B12 Deficiency

This deficiency is not common because vitamin $B_{12}$ is manufactured by bacteria in our intestines. We need only minute amounts daily, and that is usually available in most diets. It is stored in the liver and becomes available as needed by our bodies. Several factors can lead to inadequate intake or absorption of this nutrient:

- A vegetarian diet that contains no dairy products may cause problems. It may take up to five years to use up stores of $B_{12}$ in the liver, and that long for a deficiency to appear.
- Stored $B_{12}$ may not cross the placenta (or breast milk) and therefore the baby may be deficient.
- Stomach acids that aid in the breakdown, absorption, and stimulation of $B_{12}$ production may be insufficient.
- The content of vitamin $B_{12}$ may be depleted in foods produced by poor agricultural practices and nutrient depletion in soils, particularly of the mineral cobalt, an essential component of vitamin $B_{12}$. Nutrient loss in soils affects the levels of $B_{12}$ in both animal and vegetable foods.

Symptoms of vitamin B12 deficiency include weakness and gastrointestinal disturbances such as loss of appetite and diarrhea; a sore tongue; slight yellowing of the skin; nervous system disturbances including soreness, weakness, or coordination problems in the fingers, arms, legs, and feet; diminished reflex response and sensory perception; difficulty in walking and speaking (stammering); and nerve deterioration. If you have these symptoms, you should seek medical diagnosis. Treatment of an existing B12 deficiency includes an injection of vitamin B12 twice in one year. It is considered safe, has no side effects, and is very effective. Left untreated, B12 deficiency can result in permanent mental impairment and paralysis.

You can usually get enough vitamin B12 by eating a wide variety of high-quality foods (particularly organically grown foods where there tends to be attention to soil quality), including ample amounts of vegetables, fruits, nuts, seeds, whole grains, and the regular consumption of some dairy products, preferably yogurt and hard cheeses, on a daily basis. Small amounts of meat on an occasional basis can ensure that you are also getting a concentrated source of the nutrient. Fermented foods such as miso and tempeh may contain small amounts of B12 and may also improve the intestinal production of this vitamin, which grows much like yeast and penicillin. Nutritional yeast can serve as a B12 supplement. Pregnant women need more B12 than nonpregnant women (see chapter 5). Adequate amounts may serve to prevent infection as well as aid in nervous irritability, memory impairment, depression, and insomnia.

## Iron-Deficiency Anemia

Iron deficiency is common in women because we lose blood every month through our menses, and we often don't take enough time and care to replenish ourselves. Women may begin their pregnancies deficient in iron. Iron is essential during pregnancy for the adequate transport of oxygen through the mother and to the baby. The baby will store enough iron in its liver during the last couple of months of gestation to last for up to six months after birth. This is nature's way of assuring that the baby has enough iron reserves because breast milk is low in iron. If the mother is anemic, the baby may have insufficient iron stores and may also become anemic. Iron-deficient mothers may also have more difficulty with bleeding during birth than those who are well nourished, and are more prone to fatigue and repeated illness as well as more susceptible to infection.

A simple blood test, done by just having your finger pricked by your midwife or physician and an on-the-spot analysis, can reveal your hemoglobin or hematocrit (depending upon the test performed), indicating whether you are anemic. If you are iron deficient, you may experience symptoms including pallor of the skin, fingernail beds, and the lining of the eyelids; weakness; fatigue and irritability; nausea and appetite loss (particularly when prolonged past the first trimester); constipation; shortness of breath; heart palpitations; pica (cravings for nonfood items such as cornstarch, clay, dirt, and ice); and an uncomfortable, irritable feeling in your legs at night. Hemoglobin is the oxygen-carrying portion of the red blood cell. As the amount of blood plasma increases in mid-pregnancy, the concentration of hemoglobin decreases, causing the hemoglobin count to drop slightly, though the actual amount of hemoglobin in the blood has not changed. This is a desirable effect referred to as "hemodilution." If the hemoglobin is below 11mg in mid-pregnancy, herbal and nutritional approaches can be used to improve the levels. A low hemoglobin count (below 12 mg) in early or late pregnancy is considered indicative of anemia.

> **Bonnie had fatigue, skin pallor, and shortness of breath. A blood test confirmed mild anemia. She began to increase her dietary iron, and added herbal iron supplementation to her diet. Within a month her symptoms were relieved and her blood tests normal. Her overall quality of life also improved dramatically as she began to have more energy and feel better.**
>
>

During the second trimester, at about twenty weeks, a pregnant woman's blood volume should expand to about 50 percent more than it was before. Most midwives feel that a hemoglobin count of 12 is ideal at the end of pregnancy. In fact, a high hemoglobin (over 13.5 mg) might actually be a sign of a contracted blood volume, in which case you may need to increase your protein, fluid, and salt intake. If this is the case, discuss the situation with your midwife or other care provider, and refer to books by midwife Anne Frye (see bibliography) for a complete discussion of this subject.

You don't need to reduce your diet to numbers and milligrams to avoid iron-deficiency anemia. Eating a well-balanced diet based on whole foods provides an excellent nutritional foundation. To ensure that you are obtaining adequate supplies of iron, eat iron-rich foods on a daily basis and choose from the selection of herbs that provide the extra boost you need. You can also use the following suggestions for the prevention and treatment of iron-deficiency anemia prior to conception and throughout pregnancy. You can also use them during the time after birth, especially if you've had any significant bleeding. If you are already anemic, you can expect to see noticeable improvement after two to three weeks of diligent work to build your blood.

## Dietary Recommendations

- Iron supplements are hard for the body to assimilate and should not take the place of nutrient-rich foods. Therefore, it is important to include daily portions of iron-rich foods in your diet. These include dark green leafy vegetables, sunflower and pumpkin seeds, organic unsulphured dried fruits (raisins, prunes, black mission figs, apricots, and cherries), blackstrap molasses, beets, red beans, dark turkey meat, and eggs. Beef, which contains a very highly absorbable form of iron called "heme" iron, taken as a stew prepared with vegetables, organic beef, and a tomato base, eaten three times per week, can help to rapidly improve iron levels. Also, many of the plants listed under "Herbal Recommendations" below can be used as vegetables.

- Seaweeds, most notably kelp (kombu) and dulse, are very rich sources of iron. They can be eaten as vegetables (refer to macrobiotic cookbooks, available at natural food stores, for recipes); in powdered or flaked form, they can be sprinkled on foods; or, if you can't tolerate the taste, they can be taken in capsules. Take 1 to 2 tablespoons of flakes or powder, or approximately 8 "00" capsules daily.

- Take your iron-rich foods and iron supplements with vitamin C (250 to 500 mg of C each time you take your iron-supplements, but do not exceed 2,000 mg per day). Vitamin C assists in the absorption of iron. Of course, all nutrients work in concert, so be certain that your overall diet is well-balanced.

- Dairy products may inhibit iron absorption, so have iron-rich meals and dairy-rich meals at different times. Don't take your iron supplements with dairy products.

- Caffeine and phosphates in soda interfere with iron absorption (and inhibit appetite, preventing adequate nutritional intake), so decrease your consumption or omit soda from your diet.

- Cooking in cast-iron pots increases the iron content of foods, so use them whenever possible.

- Regular exercise increases the body's demand for oxygen. This causes a response in the body that allows iron to be absorbed more easily, as iron occurs in the red blood cells as part of the oxygen-carrying capacity.

- If you do choose to take an iron supplement, use a chelated iron. ("Chelated" means that the mineral is chemically bound to another substance that the body can more easily absorb than the mineral itself, thus acting as a vehicle for the absorption of the mineral.) Ferrous gluconate, ferrous fumerate, and ferrous lactate are considered the most easily absorbable forms of iron.

- Iron supplements may be most easily digested when taken with a meal, particularly with dinner if you are prone to nausea earlier in the day.

> NOTE: *Commercial and prescription iron supplements may do more harm than good, particularly if they are causing constipation or other digestive upsets. In fact, I have often recommended that pregnant women discontinue iron pills because assimilating them is too taxing on the body. Herbal and dietary approaches to increasing your blood levels of iron are usually more effective.*

## Herbal Recommendations

- An excellent iron tonic for pregnant women is the humble herb nettle. Not only is this plant rich in iron and other minerals, it also strengthens the blood vessels, the kidneys, and the adrenal glands. You can take it daily throughout pregnancy to increase your blood count. My own preference is for a very dark green and strong-tasting brew, made by steeping a large handful of the dried herb in 1 quart of boiling water for a couple of hours. If you prefer a milder brew, steep 3 to 4 tablespoons of the herb per quart of boiling water for 30 minutes. Drink between 1 and 4 cups daily depending on your needs.

- Yellow dock and dandelion root tinctures can be taken twice a day on those occasions when you are unable to carry your syrup with you—for example, if you are traveling. Take 30 drops of each twice daily. However, this is not a long-term substitute for the syrup because the alcohol extract

---

### Iron Tonic Syrup

This version of yellow dock and dandelion syrup increases iron supplies and encourages iron to be liberated from the liver. It also eases the constipation associated with both anemia and commercial iron supplements. Place $1/2$ ounce each of yellow dock and dandelion roots into a quart jar and fill with boiling water. Cover the jar and steep for 4 to 8 hours. Strain the liquid into a small stainless steel or glass pot, and simmer uncovered until the liquid is reduced to 1 cup. Add $1/4$ cup of blackstrap molasses (also high in iron), stir well, and turn off the heat. Pour into a jar, cool to room temperature, label the jar, and store it in the refrigerator. It will keep for many months. Dosage is 1 to 2 tablespoons daily. Take each dose with 250 mg of vitamin C for enhanced iron absorption.

does not contain substantial amounts of iron. The alcohol extract, though, does assist your body in better assimilating the iron that is available and liberates iron stored in your liver, making it more available in your general circulation.

- Liquid chlorophyll, usually derived from alfalfa, is another herbal source of iron. Take 1 tablespoon daily (not more unless so directed on the product label) as a supplement.

- Floradix Iron and Herbs is a supplement made from iron and extracts of dried fruits and herbs. It is delicious, easy to take, and can be purchased at most natural food stores. Many women have good results when using it along with the dietary recommendations and perhaps another of the herbal recommendations included here. Take according to the directions on the bottle.

- Chinese herbal formulas, such as dong quai and peony formula, can be beneficial for women with a history of anemia. Seek the assistance of a person trained in Chinese diagnosis and herbal prescription. See resources for the National Certification Commission for Acupuncture and Oriental Medicine.

## Anxiety

(*See* "Insomnia and Anxiety")

## Backaches and Sciatica

Pregnant women get backaches for many reasons: the weight of the baby and uterine contents placing stress on the lower back muscles, constipation, poor posture, standing for long periods of time, urinary tract infections, and the stress of overwork. Sciatica, a severe back pain that radiates into the legs, can occur from the growing baby and womb placing pressure on the sciatic nerve (located in the space between the hip bone and sacrum). In many cases, backaches and sciatica can be alleviated with the sensible use of exercise, nutrition, and herbs.

Pregnancy adds to the workload of your kidneys, which must filter both your wastes and your baby's wastes as well as maintain your expanding blood volume. The enlargement of your uterus can add physical pressure on the urinary tract, leading to infection, which in turn can cause backache. Speak with your care provider if you are experiencing backache—you may have a urinary tract infection. (If so, refer to "Urinary Tract Infections.")

# General Recommendations

- Good posture can prevent sciatic nerve discomfort and backache. Many pregnant women have a tendency to sway their bellies forward to handle the weight of the baby. This posture, known as "lordosis," allows the lower back to sway forward, straining and eventually weakening the muscles in the lower back, leading to discomfort as well as strain on the abdominal muscles. Likewise, many women will slouch their shoulders forward, which leads to neck, shoulder, and upper-back discomfort.

- To improve your posture, and therefore greatly improve how you feel (your digestion will improve and you will find it easier to breathe and eat), stand up very straight and tall—but not stiffly. Tuck your tailbone under so that your pelvis does not tilt forward and your back doesn't sway. Wear flat, comfortable shoes, and sit up straight in chairs and when you drive. Over time, good posture will become second nature to you because you will have strengthened your muscles. (See chapter 7, Exercise and Posture.)

- Take a walk every day and do exercises like leg lifts and lunges. Exercise is a great way to reduce both emotional and muscular tension and can significantly improve back problems. Swimming is a wonderful way to become weightless for a short time and get low-impact exercise. Yoga is useful for many problems. Many yoga centers now offer classes for pregnant women, and books and videos on pregnancy and yoga are readily available.

- Passionate lovemaking is great for relieving pelvic congestion, and if you rock your hips, you will also reduce lower back discomforts.

- Eliminating constipation is a must, because constipation can lead directly to lower backaches and pelvic discomfort. See "Constipation" in this section.

- Be certain that you are getting enough minerals from your diet. Insufficient calcium and magnesium, for example, can lead to muscle aches and a lowered threshold of discomfort. See chapter 5 for information on nutrition.

- Elevate your legs periodically, preferably for twenty minutes a day, to improve circulation in your legs. You can put your feet up on a chair or lie down and put them up on two pillows.

## Dietary Recommendations

- If you are experiencing lower backache, try these suggestions. Keep cold foods and raw foods to a minimum in your diet, since they place increased strain on your kidneys. If you've been eating a lot of salads, you might try more steamed greens and other vegetables. Fruits such as grapes, pears, and apples are the least watery of the commonly available fruits and place the least strain on the kidneys. Minimize your use of fruit juices, and eliminate caffeinated items—like coffee, black tea, chocolate, cocoa, and soda—from your diet. While they may give you a burst of energy, they do so in part because the chemicals they contain act like adrenaline. Overstimulation by adrenaline will aggravate kidney and adrenal problems, and over time cause a weakening of these organs.

## Herbal Recommendations

- If you are tired, overworked, or stressed, you could be experiencing adrenal gland deficiency. The best herb for nourishing the adrenals during pregnancy is strong a infusion of nettle leaf tea. Additionally, adaptogenic herbs such as schisandra berries, eleuthero, and very small doses of American ginseng can be used, generally in tincture form. They are highly nutritive and are safe for pregnant women to take in small amounts on a regular basis. They can help regulate blood sugar, and nettle supports with nutritive benefits as well. For nettle infusion, steep $1/2$ ounce of the dried herb (1 ounce if fresh) in 1 quart water for up to 2 hours; strain and drink. To make this tea more pleasant tasting, add 1 teaspoon of fennel or anise seeds and a few pieces of dried orange peel or a tablespoon of spearmint leaves. Drink up to 2 cups daily. To use the other herbs mentioned, add $1/2$ teaspoon of any one of them, or $1/2$ teaspoon total of a combination of two or three of these herbs, twice daily, to your nettle infusion or to warm water.

- Many herbs can reduce aches and pains. My two favorite herbs to be taken internally for deep backache and sciatica are skullcap and St. John's wort. Together these herbs form a dynamic duo that can be taken as a tincture, 30 drops of each two to three times daily over the course of a few weeks, and, if necessary, a similar dose during acute discomfort. These tinctures can be added to a cup of hot chamomile or lemon balm tea for added relaxation and pain-reduction qualities.

- Black haw or cramp bark tincture can be taken, 25 drops of either, up to every half hour for two hours for acute spasm, or up to four times a day preventatively, to relieve backache.

- Apply a combination of arnica and St. John's wort oils externally to relieve tension, promote healing of muscles, and reduce nerve tenderness, preferably having someone massage them into the affected areas. Put a warm water bottle over the treated area, and take time to consciously visualize yourself becoming loose and free of tension. You can do this daily. St. John's wort is said to contain substances that are able to penetrate to the endings of nerve fibers and promote their healing.

- Here are two recipes for external use that you can easily make at home with wonderful results.

---

### Deep Ache Ointment

Melt $1/2$ cup of coconut oil together with 2 tablespoons sweet almond oil. Let cool slightly and add 1 teaspoon each of lobelia tincture, St. John's wort tincture, and cramp bark tincture. Pour into a clean, wide-mouth jar, let cool, cap, label, and apply as needed. This is one of the most effective oils I've found for deep aches, sprains, sciatica, frozen and stiff joints, and even arthritis. Use liberally as needed.

---

### Muscle Ache Oil

To 1 cup of olive oil, add $1/2$ teaspoon of each of the following: cinnamon oil, spearmint oil, rosemary oil, and lavender oil. Shake vigorously and apply as needed. These oils stimulate circulation in the area to which they are applied, relieving circulatory congestion, promoting warmth, and inducing gentle muscle relaxation.

---

**NOTE:** *The herbs in these oils burn mucous membranes, so keep them away from sensitive areas such as your eyes. Essential oils are highly toxic if ingested, so store bottles out of the reach of children.*

- Take a hot bath to which you have added Epsom salts or any of a number of essential oils or herbal infusions. Some possibilities are wintergreen, lavender, or rosemary oil; chamomile, lavender, or lemon balm; or a combination of these.

# Bleeding and Cramping in Early Pregnancy

Little is more disheartening than vaginal bleeding during pregnancy. Yet many women experience some bleeding during the first trimester, ranging from mild to heavy spotting, and they do not miscarry. Bleeding can occur after sexual activity or merely from a vaginal examination. Other causes include implantation of the fertilized egg in the uterine wall, bleeding caused by fluctuating hormonal levels occurring when you would normally have your period (some women will experience this for the first month or so of pregnancy and, very rarely, throughout the entire pregnancy), polyps on the cervix (if necessary, a physician can remove them), and a condition known as a "friable cervix" in which the tissue of the cervix is easily split. (This can usually be improved with a high-quality diet.) The amount of bleeding you are experiencing can help you to determine the type of care you should seek. If you are spotting or bleeding mildly, especially if the blood is brown, you can call your health-care provider and elicit her opinion. Frequently you will be told to wait and watch for further possible signs of miscarriage (discussed below).

> **WARNING:** *If you are hemorrhaging (bleeding heavily and steadily—for example, soaking a large menstrual pad in a half hour or less), if you have been bleeding for a prolonged period of time, or if the blood is bright red (meaning that it is fresh blood), seek the help of your midwife or physician, or go right to the hospital emergency room.*

If you feel your uterus cramping, it does not mean you will miscarry. There are other causes of the cramping, including stretching of the round ligaments (supporting the uterus), gas, constipation, and insufficient intake of calcium and magnesium. Cramping occurs in many pregnancies and, even when accompanied by spotting, does not necessarily mean that miscarriage is occurring.

Another lesser-known cause of bleeding and cramping during pregnancy is a urinary tract infection (UTI). I have seen several pregnant women bleed profusely and have regular uterine contractions caused by a UTI. Your lower abdomen or low back may ache, your urine may burn, and you may experience flulike symptoms or malaise (depression and lack of motivation). You can have your midwife or physician check your urine (or check it yourself with urinalysis sticks) for the presence of leukocytes (white blood cells) or nitrites (a by-product of bacterial breakdown). The appearance of these together is a positive sign for a UTI and is a noninvasive method for testing. See "Urinary Tract Infections," later in this chapter, for treatment suggestions.

Perhaps the most dangerous cause of cramping in early pregnancy, sometimes accompanied by vaginal bleeding, is an ectopic pregnancy, which will be discussed later in this chapter.

## General Recommendations

- Try to calmly assess the situation and seek help if necessary.
- Take a warm bath and relax in bed afterward.
- Contact your health-care support person and ask for her recommendations.
- Avoid intercourse, heavy lifting, and strenuous activity for several days after bleeding has ceased.
- Light massage may help relieve muscular cramping and spasms.
- If you are troubled by gas and constipation, you should address these complaints.
- If you determine that cramping is due to round ligament pain, gentle stretching can be effective. Touching your toes, lying on your back with your legs pulled up to your chest, or alternating toe touches while sitting with your legs stretched in front of you can all be effective.

## Dietary Recommendations

- Be certain that you are getting enough minerals in your diet, especially calcium and magnesium, which are essential for the healthy functioning of muscular tissue and for preventing spasms. A dietary supplement may be in order if you are experiencing chronic problems, but your first recourse should always be to improve your diet and use beneficial herbs. Helpful foods include green leafy vegetables, almonds, sesame seeds, deep-sea fish (salmon is excellent), sea vegetables (kelp, dulse, hijiki), beans, whole grains, and small amounts of yogurt and hard cheeses. Refer to the section on nutrition for further information.
- Excessive intake of dairy, particularly milk, may actually interfere with optimal calcium absorption and therefore should be avoided. Likewise, chocolate and other caffeinated products (soda, coffee) inhibit absorption of calcium.
- For a cervix that tends to bleed or be lacerated easily or for a weakness of the placental bed, add 1,000 mg of vitamin C with bioflavonoids to your daily diet. Vitamin C plays an integral role in the health and strength of the blood vessels.

Lisa had a history of miscarriages and very much wanted to have this baby. Nonetheless, she began spotting and contracting ten weeks into her pregnancy. She began regular consumption of an infusion to prevent miscarriage and, by twenty-four hours later, the symptoms had abated. One week later, she again began to spot and have mild contractions. She resumed the infusion and confirmed that the baby was still alive by having the baby's heartbeat listened to by a midwife who had a doppler, which can detect heartbeat this early in pregnancy. She continued the infusion for another week, had no further problems, and gave birth to a healthy baby a few days after her due date.

To improve dietary intake of vitamin C, eat dark green leafy vegetables, raw cabbage, cantaloupe, strawberries, grapefruits, and oranges. Many of the foods you already enjoy may be rich in vitamin C; refer to chapter 5 for an extensive list.

- Vitamin E (alpha-tocopherol) may improve the placental attachment to the uterus, reducing spotting. It should be taken in doses of up to 400 IU each day for up to three weeks. Prolonged or excessive use may result in the placenta becoming abnormally attached to the uterine wall. Therefore, do not exceed this dosage, and do not prolong your intake past this time. If you have heart disease, do not exceed 50 IU per day without discussing it with your physician.

- Excessive cramping and bleeding can be caused by overconsumption of foods and beverages that are cold in nature because they cause constriction of blood vessels and poor blood circulation. Examples of cold foods are those coming directly from the refrigerator or freezer as well as those produced in climates that are hotter than the one in which you live. For example, bananas and citrus would be considered extremely cooling for one who lives in New York, even more so in autumn or winter. It is also important to eat foods and drink beverages at room temperature or slightly warmed. Avoid cold beverages and foods such as smoothies and ice cream if cramping has been a problem.

## Herbal Recommendations

- Black haw, cramp bark, and wild yam are all excellent antispasmodics that may be used safely during the first trimester to reduce cramping. Take $^1/_4$ to 1 teaspoon of one of the tinctures, or preferably a combination of black haw or cramp bark with the wild yam, up to every thirty minutes in the lower dosage, or every two hours in the higher dosage, depending on the frequency and severity of the cramping.

- I've included here an example of a formula for cramping that contains some of the herbs just mentioned. You can also use it as a basis to create your own formula of favorite herbs.

> ### Formula for Cramping
>
> *1 ounce cramp bark tincture*
> *1 ounce wild yam tincture*
> *$^1/_2$ ounce black cohosh tincture*
> *$^1/_2$ ounce chamomile tincture*
>
> Mix all of the tinctures together and put into a clean tincture bottle (or refill and relabel the bottles the tinctures came from). Take $^1/_4$ to 1 teaspoon of the combination as needed, not to exceed 6 teaspoons in 1 day. Consult with your care provider if contractions persist and seek immediate medical care if symptoms increase.

## Bleeding, Late-Pregnancy

With the exception of spotting in early pregnancy and blood-tinged discharge preceding or during labor, if you begin to bleed, call your midwife or physician immediately. If bleeding is profuse, head to the nearest emergency room!

Sometimes a woman may see some streaks of blood in her vaginal mucus (on toilet tissue or underwear) after intercourse. This is no cause for alarm. It occurs if the cervix was slightly jarred. Bleeding later in pregnancy may be related to a placental problem, such as a placenta previa, a condition in which the placenta partially or completely covers the cervix, or a placental abruption, in which the placenta separates, to varying degrees, from the uterine wall. These two situations require immediate medical attention. A blood loss that causes you to soak a medium-size sanitary pad within thirty minutes is termed a hemorrhage. All bleeding that occurs during pregnancy should be traced to the cause. Calm your mind, assess the situation, and be certain you and the baby are not endangered.

> **CAUTION:** *Heavy or steady bleeding during the first four months of pregnancy usually signals a threatened miscarriage. Call your health-care provider. See "Miscarriage" later in this chapter.*

Always remember that even in an emergency room you can find caring and supportive people and that you can maintain your sense of power and authority over your body. Always bring a support person to act as an advocate for yourself when you seek medical care.

# Breasts, Sore

As early as the first few weeks of pregnancy, you may notice that your breasts are tender, sore, or tingly, and that your nipples are unusually sensitive. This is due to the usual breast enlargement that occurs as a result of hormonal changes accompanying pregnancy. It may remind you of those years in junior high school when your growing breasts were highly tender and sensitive. The hormones of pregnancy also help ready the breasts for breastfeeding. While the acute sensitivity usually subsides after a short time, your breasts, because of their increased size, may feel heavy and tender throughout pregnancy.

## General Recommendations

- When you are reclining, go braless to avoid friction.

- When you are out and about, particularly as you get farther along in your pregnancy, wear a bra that offers you support and helps prevent your breasts from feeling heavy.

- Hot soaks in the tub, with the water at a level over your breasts, can help to relieve discomfort and heaviness.

- See "Preparing for Breastfeeding" in chapter 11 for more information on breast care during pregnancy.

## Herbal Recommendations

- For tenderness in early pregnancy, massage the following soothing and lovely scented oil into your breasts once or twice daily:

    To 3 ounces sweet almond oil, add $^1/_2$ ounce each of St. John's wort and arnica oils. Also add $^1/_2$ teaspoon each of lavender essential oil, rosemary essential oil, and rose geranium essential oil.

**Visualization is a wonderful tool for gently affecting physical change. Mary had been trying various techniques to change her baby to a head-down position, but to no avail. Her baby was consistently in a position where the shoulder was presenting. We decided to try a visualization—beginning with deep muscular relaxation. I then guided her through imagining her baby's head in her pelvis. We also told the baby that this head-down position would allow it to be born safely. By the end of the visualization, the baby's head had moved downward, and it stayed that way until her baby was born, vaginally at home.**

# Breech Births

Your body knows how to birth, even if the baby is in a bottom-first position. Actually, breech births are not uncommon. Many babies are in breech position until well into the pregnancy, even as late as the eighth month. For example, I recently worked with a woman whose baby didn't turn head down until thirty-eight weeks of pregnancy, just two weeks before birth, which she then did spontaneously.

If everything seems normal, but your baby insists on remaining bottom first, then be as determined as your baby is in your desire for a vaginal birth. Many obstetricians support vaginal births of breech babies, so seek a supportive care provider. Some midwives will assist in breech births at home if the mother has had babies before and if the baby seems healthy and is not too big for the mother's pelvis. Sometimes an ultrasound will be recommended to make sure the umbilical cord is not wrapped around the baby in a way that will interfere with birth. Occasionally a breech is caused by congenital anomalies that prevent the baby from fitting head down in the pelvis or by a deformity or variation of the pelvis or uterus that also prevents a head-down position. A discussion of breech birth is beyond the scope of this book but can be found in other childbirth literature. An excellent video on breech births is available from Ina May Gaskin at The Farm (see resources).

## *Suggestions for Turning a Breech Baby*

At thirty-two to thirty-four weeks, you can begin taking gentle measures to encourage your baby to turn:

- Spend time each day imagining your baby head down. Put pictures around your home of head-down babies in their mothers' bellies. Tell the baby that it's safe to turn and that it would help you relax if he or she would do so. Look closely at your own fears of birth and motherhood as well as any stresses in your life that might cause tight pelvic or abdominal muscles.

- Pelvic tilts are simple to do and quite an effective method to encourage a baby to turn. Rest a board (any sturdy board of sufficient width to support you) at a 45-degree angle, putting one end on the floor and the other on the edge of a chair or sofa. Lie on the board with your head near the floor and your feet near the top of the board. Ten minutes in this position twice a day is the recommended length of time. If you practice yoga and can handle them, headstands are also effective. If you are a swimmer, you can do headstands in the water. Of course, you should not attempt headstands unless you are already adept at them.

- Moxibustion, a traditional Chinese treatment, is highly regarded and has recently been written up in the *Journal of the American Medical Association* for its ability to cause a breech baby to turn. It involves holding a lighted "cigar" made of the herb mugwort over a specific acupuncture point on the pinkie toe. This is done for ten to twenty minutes on each toe at a session. The heat stimulates energy in the point. The Chinese doctor from whom I learned this technique witnessed its effectiveness when his sister's baby was breech. I've since employed it and have found it useful as part of an overall approach but have done no studies on its effectiveness as a solitary treatment. It is simple to do and can be done at home.

  You will need to purchase a couple of moxa sticks. Unless you purchase the "little-smoke" moxa sticks, perform the entire treatment in a well-ventilated room. Unwrap and remove the outer paper, leaving the inner white paper in place. Next, light the end of the stick with a match or candle and blow on the lit end until it glows like a coal. Hold the lit end one-half to two inches away from the outside edge of the little toe, near the toenail. It does not matter whether you begin on the left or right foot. Maintain the heat on the point for ten to twenty minutes; then do the same spot on the other foot. If at any time you feel a burning sensation, simply pull the moxa a bit farther away from the spot. Repeat this procedure twice each day until the baby turns.

- The external turning of the baby to a head-down position is frequently an effective method, but it is not without risks and should therefore only be done by a skilled midwife or physician who can carefully monitor the baby's heartbeat while he or she is being turned. An ultrasound will be done before and during the procedure to be sure the baby does not become tangled in the umbilical cord in the turning process. If he or she is already wrapped in the cord, the procedure will not be attempted to avoid harming the baby. The procedure is not without significant risk and is therefore done in the hospital should an emergency cesarean be required.

Remember, if the baby does not turn despite all your efforts and if neither you nor the baby seem to have a physical problem causing the breech or inhibiting birth, in all likelihood you will be able to birth your baby vaginally. Finding a supportive obstetrician or midwife will likely be the most difficult part of your job!

# Colds, Flu, and Mild Illnesses

Colds and flu generally pose no threat to the mom or baby as long as the mother remains well nourished with foods and fluids. During a severe illness—for example, with high fever (over 103°F), prolonged fever (longer than two or three days), or symptoms such as frequent and violent vomiting, diarrhea, and persistent coughing—it is wise to consult an experienced midwife or a physician. Herbs that you have used for treating colds when you were not pregnant may not be safe now, so refer to "Herbs to Avoid during Pregnancy" in chapter 6 before you begin any treatment. Never take any herbs if you are not certain they are safe during pregnancy.

Many women find that they have an increased resistance to illness and infection during pregnancy. Getting adequate rest, eating highly nutritious and natural foods, getting moderate exercise, and maintaining a generally adventuresome, positive outlook on life may go a long way toward keeping our resistance to illness strong. Yet this may be easier said than done if you are already busy with children, a career, or the many stresses that plague human beings in our fast-paced society. Anxieties about money, relationships, and time constraints can open the door to illness. Treatment of colds and other simple illnesses (such as an intestinal virus, for example) must therefore always include reflection on what is going on in your life that may have left you susceptible and what this illness can show you about your lifestyle that might serve you in the long run. This is not an invitation to blame yourself or anyone else; rather, it is an opportunity to be introspective and aware of your needs. Perhaps you can find practical ways to reduce stress in your life and create the space to care for yourself, your health, and your growing baby.

## General and Dietary Recommendations

- As soon as you feel the first signs of illness—fatigue, chills, loose bowels, or constipation—try to excuse yourself from your daily responsibilities and get some rest. This is the perfect time to turn off your telephone, ask for help with your kids, take a sick day (what I refer to as a "health day"—a day off to prevent yourself from getting really sick), and nurture yourself. Do what is comforting: take a warm bath with a few drops of relaxing oils such as lavender or rose and a few drops of antiseptic oils such as rosemary, thyme, or eucalyptus. The latter help clear respiratory congestion. Then put yourself to bed with a cup of hot herbal tea and perhaps a book you've been wanting to read (if it is relaxing), soothing music, or just a soft pillow and a cozy blanket and let yourself sleep.

Fatigue is a prime reason for illness to occur, so let yourself rest as long as you feel you need to without feeling guilty.

- Often when we are ill, we lose our appetite. Indeed, this is the body's way of resting the digestive system and sending healing energy to other areas in your body. However, you still need to grow your baby. So if you don't feel much like eating, try broths, soups, and simple buttered toast. A well-made vegetable soup, miso soup, or chicken soup can be as medicinal as any herbal remedy and is worth preparing. Add some rice or pasta and you will have nourishing, yet light food to sustain you until your appetite returns in a day or so.

- You must drink fluids, even if you must force yourself to do so. Your baby needs amniotic fluid, and your kidneys will be taxed if you don't drink adequately. In fact, you can even begin to have contractions if you get dehydrated. A full glass of clear fluid, broth, or tea every two hours if you are not feverish, and more if you are, is adequate. Keeping yourself well hydrated is essential when you are pregnant and is moreover an important component of healing from illness.

- Be certain to dress appropriately for the weather. If you are chilled, dress warmly, but don't become overheated. Wear breathable cotton clothing and cover yourself with natural-fiber blankets if at all possible. If your fever breaks in a heavy sweat and your clothes are wet and clammy, change them swiftly so you don't get chilled.

- Take about 250 mg of vitamin C every two hours, but don't exceed 2,000 mg daily during the first trimester; after that, don't exceed 4,000 mg daily. And discontinue either dosage of vitamin C after five days.

## Herbal Recommendations

- Echinacea root tincture is a gentle but effective remedy for either a viral or bacterial infection. Combined with vitamin C, it is probably one of the best cold and flu preventions and treatments. It encourages the body's immune system to resist illness. Begin taking it at the earliest sign of sickness. Dosage is 1 drop of tincture for every 4 pounds of body weight (that is, if you weigh 120 pounds you would take about 30 drops of tincture) every four hours for general prevention and mild colds. For more acute symptoms, you can either take the tincture every two hours or you can increase the dosage to 1 drop per 2 pounds of body weight. As you recover, slowly reduce the amount and frequency of the dosage. Echinacea has been demonstrated to be safe even for long-term use during pregnancy.

- Garlic lemonade is one of my family's favorite cold and flu remedies. An excellent bactericide, garlic is effective in treating all manner of general illnesses including colds, intestinal and stomach viruses, and strep throat. It can be taken in conjunction with echinacea and vitamin C.

- Ginger tea, also an excellent cold remedy, produces a warm feeling, preventing your temperature from getting too high and reducing tension. Ginger has properties similar to those of garlic. When made into a mild tea sweetened with lemon and honey, it has a very pleasant taste.

---

### Garlic Lemonade

Steep 4 to 6 cloves of chopped raw garlic in 1 quart boiling water (cover the jar while you steep) for 30 minutes. Then add the juice of 1 or 2 lemons and honey or maple syrup to taste. Drink warm, up to 1 cup every two hours. If you don't find this tea palatable, try steeping the garlic as above, but add a couple of bouillon cubes or 1 tablespoon of miso to the tea instead of lemon and honey. This is a warming tea if you have chills but can be used at any time of the year.

---

### Ginger Tea

Steep 1 teaspoon of freshly grated raw ginger in 1 cup boiling water for 15 minutes. Steep covered to retain the volatile oils, which are antiseptic. Sweeten and add lemon if desired. You can take a hot cup of this tea every two hours. It is also soothing for a sore throat and eases respiratory congestion.

---

> **CAUTION:** *Ginger in large amounts (more than one to two grams a day) has been associated with miscarriage. Therefore, do not prepare it any stronger than directed and avoid it during the first trimester if you have a history of miscarriage.*

- Kudzu, an intruder into the southeastern landscape particularly here in Georgia where I live, yields a root high in starch, similar to arrowroot but more nutritious. This starch, available in small chunks and powder, makes an excellent tea that reduces fever, relaxes the muscles, eases stomach discomfort, and soothes inflamed mucous membranes in the throat and bronchial passages. Because of its high starch content, it is also nutritive. You can prepare kudzu root as a tea in a number of ways. I'll give you a couple of ideas, and you can choose what sounds appealing, even creating your own recipes as you go along.

At the time of Molly's first midwife visit, her skin had a yellowish green hue, her blood pressure was 120/90, and she was nauseated, had severe headaches, and hadn't had a bowel movement in two weeks. She quit her iron supplement and began to use gentler, more assimilable forms of supplementation, such as chlorophyll, spirulina, and Floradix each day, in addition to dietary improvements and prunes with bran as a drink (for iron and as a laxative, see page 190). She added fresh fruits and vegetables to her diet, as well as fresh fish and more water. Within three weeks, she was having daily bowel movements, and all of her other symptoms completely resolved. Her blood pressure stabilized at 118/70.

---

### Garlic-Onion-Ginger-Kudzu Tea

This is really more of a soup, taught to me by an acupuncturist friend, and is one of my personal favorites when I feel a cold coming on or if I feel chilled. Sauté $^1/_2$ onion, 2 cloves of chopped fresh garlic, and $^1/_2$ inch of chopped fresh ginger root in 1 tablespoon of olive or sesame oil for 2 to 3 minutes. Add 3 cups of water, cover, bring to a boil, and simmer for about 20 minutes. Then add 1 tablespoon of miso paste and stir. In a small cup, dilute 2 teaspoons of kudzu starch in $^1/_4$ cup cold water (if you try to do this in hot water, it will form gelatinous clumps that will not dissolve). Add the starch to the broth, stirring constantly for 2 minutes. Turn off the heat and drink when it is warm but not hot. Use this freely throughout the day, preparing more as needed.

---

### Kudzu Apple Juice

Bring a cup of apple juice to a boil; then add 1 teaspoon of kudzu starch diluted in 2 tablespoons of cold water. Stir constantly for 2 minutes; then drink. Pear juice may be substituted; a pinch of cinnamon improves digestion and warms you if you are chilled.

---

- Other teas that can be used effectively for reducing fever, aches, digestive discomfort, restlessness, or irritability during colds include those made with lemon balm, catnip, chamomile, or lime (linden) blossom. You can drink these herbal teas either in a single infusion or with the herbs in combination. Sip them freely as needed.

- If you have an illness accompanied by diarrhea, you must be certain to drink enough fluid. Rehydration Drink (see page 283) is good for this. In addition to remedies already mentioned, you can drink a strong infusion of raspberry leaf tea made with 1 ounce of the dried leaves to 1 quart of water (steep for 20 minutes), taking $^1/_2$ cup every thirty minutes to one hour depending on the severity of the diarrhea. Raspberry leaves are notably astringent, tonifying the intestinal lining and reducing bowel discharge. For extreme diarrhea or dysentery symptoms, you can take 2 "00" capsules of goldenseal powder every four hours until the symptoms abate, but don't take these for more than twenty-four hours.

> CAUTION: *Goldenseal, a uterine stimulant, can cause contractions. If you notice any contractions, discontinue goldenseal immediately. Don't use it at all if you have a history of miscarriage and avoid it during the first trimester.*

# Constipation

This is a very common problem for pregnant women because (1) it is widespread in our society; (2) pregnancy hormones cause decreased bowel activity and tone; (3) the growing baby and womb place pressure on the intestines and rectum, sometimes making bowel movements more difficult; (4) iron deficiency, common during pregnancy, leads to constipation; and (5) commercial iron supplements can cause constipation because they are so hard to assimilate.

Constipation is at the root of many other pregnancy complaints, including indigestion, nausea, headaches, skin problems, and poor mineral absorption. It can be a contributing factor in toxemia and even in a difficult birthing, since an impacted rectum takes up the very room that the baby needs for descent and birth. Constipation is avoidable and, with direct attention, easily remedied.

## General Recommendations

- Get more exercise. A brisk walk each day, especially at the same time, can be a great boost to your digestion and promote regular evacuation. Many yoga exercises are also beneficial. See the bibliography for recommended yoga books.

- Give yourself time each day to sit on the toilet. Relax and wait patiently, breathing deeply and possibly tightening and relaxing your anal muscle a few times to stimulate a bowel movement. The body has regular intervals for elimination, and if you don't go when you get the urge, the urge will pass and the stool will be retained. The longer it sits in there, the harder it will be to eliminate later on. Avoid straining as it will lead to hemorrhoids.

- Squatting is the physiologically natural position for bowel movements; therefore, getting up and squatting on the seat (no kidding!) can facilitate the process. If you can't handle this idea, at least put your feet up on a low stool or on the side of the bathtub while you try to go.

• Recline on your bed or, if possible, in a warm bath. Massage your abdomen deeply in a clockwise direction, starting at the "six o'clock" point and circling back around to it. Do this for ten or fifteen minutes before you return to the toilet.

## Dietary Recommendations

• Eat an abundance of fresh vegetables, particularly various lettuces, kale, and collard greens. Eat raw vegetables with meals and snacks. You should have at least two large portions of raw vegetables each day.

• Eat fresh fruit regularly, at least one to two pieces a day.

• Choose breads, crackers, and pasta made from whole grains. They have a higher fiber content and aid elimination.

• Cut back on cheese, meat, and highly fatty foods.

• Drink a lot of water, about a half gallon daily (herbal teas are also fine). Warm liquids at room temperature improve elimination; cold liquids hinder bowel movements.

• While caffeinated beverages seem to be the most common American drink, they are not healthy for pregnant women or babies; avoid them completely during pregnancy.

• Eating bran for a long time can decrease bowel tone and irritate the intestinal lining. However, bran is an excellent remedy for a bout of constipation. Soaked or stewed prunes are also useful and they can be used on a regular, long-term basis.

• Bran muffins are another nutritious and delicious way to use bran. You can eat them as part of a meal or as a snack.

• Oatmeal, especially when cooked with some raisins, is an excellent laxative and is also highly nutritious. Starting your day with a

---

**Constipation Remedy**

To make a laxative drink from prunes and bran, soak 4 dried, pitted prunes (or 2 prunes and 2 dried black Mission figs) and 1 tablespoon of bran in 1 cup of warm apple juice for 15 minutes. Eat and drink all of the prunes, bran, and juice. This can be done either 1 or 2 times daily, preferably in the morning and evening.

bowl of warm oatmeal is likely to encourage healthy bowel movements.

- Yogurt (live culture) with fruit as a snack or light meal can also help eliminate constipation and populate the intestines with flora necessary for healthy bowel functioning.

## Herbal Recommendations

- The most effective and safest remedy for use by pregnant women is a syrup of dandelion and yellow dock roots in a base of blackstrap molasses. Ironically, this same preparation is used for treating iron-deficiency anemia. Unlike typical iron supplements, which are constipating, the natural remedy is iron-rich and also treats constipation—itself a sign of anemia. These herbs help move the energy of the bowels gently downward without stimulating the uterus.

- Bulk laxatives such as flaxseeds can be used effectively during pregnancy. Soak 1 teaspoon of flaxseeds in $1/2$ cup warmed or cool apple juice until they have absorbed some of the fluid. Eat or drink the contents of the mixture, taking 1 or 2 doses daily as needed.

> **CAUTION:** *Herbal laxatives including senna, buckthorn, aloes, and castor oil can cause labor to begin as they stimulate the bowels. Some may also be harmful to the baby's development, affecting the central nervous system. Therefore, avoid the use of all purgatives during pregnancy.*

---

**Bran Muffins**

*2 cups whole-wheat flour*
*$1^1/_2$ cups bran*
*1 teaspoon baking powder (nonaluminum)*
*1 teaspoon baking soda*
*$1/_4$ teaspoon salt*
*$1/_4$ cup oil (sunflower, walnut, safflower, or canola)*
*$1/_4$ cup honey*
*$1/_4$ cup molasses*
*1 tablespoon tahini or peanut butter, or 1 egg*
*1 cup raisins*
*$1/_2$ cup chopped walnuts*
*1 cup yogurt*
*1 cup water*

Mix all ingredients very well and pour into an oiled muffin tin. Bake at 375°F for 20 minutes or until golden brown and firm.

---

# Cramping

(*See* "Bleeding and Cramping in Early Pregnancy")

# Ectopic Pregnancy

Ectopic pregnancy means a pregnancy where the baby does not lie within the uterine cavity. Most commonly it occurs in a fallopian tube but also may occur elsewhere, including in the abdomen or ovary. Ectopic pregnancies are extremely dangerous, because when they rupture they can lead to sudden, life-threatening hemorrhage and shock. Part of what makes them so dangerous is that the symptoms may be subtle until rupture occurs, and then the situation becomes an emergency. Before this, a woman may not even realize that she is pregnant, let alone that the pregnancy is ectopic.

Certain factors may increase the likelihood that an ectopic pregnancy will occur, including pelvic infections (especially PID, pelvic inflammatory disease), abortions, endometriosis, prior pelvic surgery, use of an IUD (intrauterine device), previous ectopic pregnancies, or any condition that may have caused scarring or adhesions in the pelvic organs.

Possible symptoms alerting you to an ectopic pregnancy include an unusually early, late, missed, or spotty period; abdominal pain that can be dull or intensely sharp; and irregular vaginal bleeding. When there is a rupture, the pain usually becomes severe, gets progressively worse, and most often is located on only one side of the lower abdomen. Other signs may include pain on only one side that may radiate into the arm, shoulder, chest, or upper back; scanty brownish bleeding that is intermittent; and eventually signs of shock, which include dizziness, anxiety, shortness of breath, clamminess of the skin, fainting, and pallor.

> **WARNING:** *Ectopic pregnancy is a life-threatening emergency requiring immediate medical care.*

Usually surgery will be required, and ideally it can be done before the rupture occurs. Most physicians make every effort to repair the tube or ovary, but it may need to be removed; ask whether surgery is the only option.

It is important for you to explore and allow whatever feelings arise because this a frightening medical emergency and it may mean the loss of your baby. National and local support groups dedicated to helping families cope with pregnancy loss can be a great source of comfort and aid during this time.

# Edema

(*See* "Swelling")

# Emotional Swings

Pregnancy is certainly a time of great change for women, both in its physical challenges and in the new responsibilities it brings. It is a time when our bodies are circulating high levels of hormones and when our bodies demand a very good diet. Combine all of these factors and it is not surprising that pregnant women find themselves experiencing highs and lows with great rapidity, even in the course of minutes. Add fatigue, the possibility of an unwanted pregnancy, anxieties about the baby's health, the prospect of motherhood, worries about how to maintain a job and care for a baby, an increasing body weight and a changing body shape in a culture that values thinness, not to mention the general discomforts of pregnancy, and it is even less surprising that pregnant women feel bouts of depression and insecurity. I'm always amazed at how easily I cry over sappy sentimental songs when I'm pregnant, and at how joyful I feel when I see buds opening in the spring and other simple miracles of life.

Pregnancy seems to be a key that unlocks doors to old experiences and feelings, particularly those regarding relationships that have had great impact on us, most notably our relationships with our mothers. For some women, the availability of their mothers as a source of support and information is comforting and valuable, but for others proximity to our mothers can be a source of pain and conflict. For all women, pregnancy causes us to reflect on how we were raised and how we may want to raise our children similarly or differently. Reflecting on childhood can be confusing or painful, but it also offers new opportunities for personal growth. Finding ways to heal painful feelings can be productive, enabling us to move into motherhood with a fresh perspective. Moreover, such reflection may allow you to enjoy extended family support.

How your partner reacts and responds to your pregnancy can influence how you feel about yourself, particularly if you are dependent on your mate for financial (or other) support. Even if you are not financially dependent, if your partner finds your changing body unattractive, for example, you are likely to feel very hurt. If your partner seems disinterested in feeling the baby move, or if he refuses to share in your joy, you may experience rejection, sadness, or a sense of being "in it" alone.

Pregnant women are culturally expected to, and thus "allowed to," have periodic emotional outbursts, be subject to strange whims and cravings, and be somewhat irrational, but we are also expected to be in a state of joyful anticipation about the coming baby—to have a certain pregnancy "glow." Our culture also characterizes feelings of sadness, depression, anger, and anxiety as negative and even as symptoms of emotional problems. As a result, a pregnant woman may feel obligated to keep these

**Audrey's third baby was still breech just a week and a half before it was due. During this time she was experiencing a lot of personal stress—her husband's business wasn't going well, she was overwhelmed by her two children, both under four years old, and she had recently been told some birth horror stories by a neighbor. At a prenatal visit, she opened up and shared all of these worries and had a healthy cry. Within a day, her baby changed to a head-down position and was born after a labor of a few hours. Perhaps this was coincidental—or perhaps letting go of her tensions, which were affecting her pelvic and uterine muscles, provided more room for her baby to change position.**

feelings to herself or dismiss them as "normal emotional outbursts." The problem is that we may be disregarding issues that need some attention. We should tell our mates that we feel rejected when they are disinterested in the baby, or when they do not find our growing bodies attractive. While we may still feel these heightened emotions after such a discussion, we probably will be better able to cope. In addition, when we assume that extreme emotional sensitivity is normal in pregnancy, we may overlook nutritional or other physical factors that can contribute to the unpleasantness of being on an emotional roller coaster.

## General Recommendations

- I cannot overstate the importance of excellent nutrition from both food and herbal sources, as well as adequate rest and exercise. Read chapters 5 through 8 thoroughly for a full discussion of these topics.

- Accepting, not dismissing your feelings is important. This means that you recognize and acknowledge what is bothering you. If you feel worried about birth, you don't have to dwell on gruesome details of rare complications or imagine yourself in some horrible scene from a TV emergency room. You can say to yourself, "Okay, I am afraid about birth." Try to find a source for your fear; ask yourself where this anxiety arises from. Perhaps as a young child you knew someone who had problems or you've heard frightening birth stories. By recognizing the source of your fear, you can separate it from your own personal experience.

- If you are afraid of a particular complication, you can ask your midwife or physician how she deals with it. Becoming more educated often will decrease your anxiety. If your issues relate to other matters, such as relationship problems with your mate, body-image anxieties, or financial worries, try to find constructive ways to address and resolve them. Midwives often help women work through a wide variety of issues, so speaking with your midwife, if you have one, can be helpful and comforting. A close friend or a counselor can also be a good listener and help you get to the bottom of your fears.

- Be true to yourself and deal with your problems to the best of your ability. If you find yourself in a situation that makes you feel bad, it is fair either to change the situation or extricate yourself from it. For example, if other women start to tell you awful stories about birth, it is perfectly reasonable to excuse yourself from the discussion or make it clear that the discussion disturbs you and you don't wish it to continue. You can't always wait for people to read your mind—sometimes you must make your needs known and stand up for yourself.

- Keeping a journal is an excellent way to give voice to your emotions. It can also provide a time of quiet reflection on a regular basis. You can create a nice ritual for yourself: drink a cup of relaxing herbal tea in your favorite cup, listen to soothing music, and write your thoughts, feelings, and impressions. This can be a welcome release from which you emerge refreshed. The act of writing can help you work out and resolve concerns. There are several books available on journal writing, some written specifically for women; inquire at your local bookstore for titles.

- Allow yourself to be human, accepting all the ups and downs we must go through. Don't give yourself the double whammy by feeling bad about feeling bad. Guilt doesn't get you anywhere in this situation. Feel what you feel, and move on—you don't have to psychoanalyze yourself or explain or justify your feelings. How you feel is simply how you feel.

- Try to appreciate your heightened sensitivity. Being attuned to subtle emotional nuances in your interactions with others and to your own emotions can give rise to a deep empathy that will help you understand the subtle messages and feelings that your baby will need you to interpret after birth. When babies' subtle cues are heeded, they frequently have less need to resort to crying to get their message across. Many times crying is a strong way of expressing something that wasn't picked up through more subtle communications. Daily time for reflection and journal writing enhance your consciousness.

- Creative forms of expression can provide a welcome outlet for your emotions. Painting, drawing, sculpting, dancing, or singing can transform inner tensions.

## Dietary Recommendations

- Depression and other difficult emotional states can result from nutritional deficiency as well as lack of exercise. Low blood sugar can cause extreme irritability, sadness, anxiety, or depression. Read chapter 5 on nutrition and be sure you are meeting all of your nutritional requirements.

- Depression can also result from dehydration. Drink plenty of fluids, herbal teas, and fresh fruit and vegetable juices. Insufficient fluid intake can contribute to lower blood volume and indeed a state of depression. Pay attention to your thirst, and try to drink about six to eight glasses of fluid a day.

## Herbal Recommendations

While herbs cannot remove emotional or other problems, they may reduce stress so that you can relax and develop strategies. In addition, herbs can directly help your hormones, act as nerve tonics, and support the functioning of your organs, especially the heart and liver. Herbs will help you so that you don't become bogged down by the increased volume of blood and hormones that you must circulate each day. The following suggestions, in addition to the recommendations discussed above, may help improve your emotional outlook during pregnancy.

- To calm your nerves as well as benefit digestion, drink Calming Tea.

- Oatstraw is another herb that nourishes the nervous system, particularly when taken over an extended time. Take $1/2$ teaspoon tincture of fresh milky oats twice daily. The tincture can be added to Calming Tea.

- Motherwort can be used in small doses, up to 20 drops one to three times daily, after the first trimester. It is a wonderful bitter tonic for the heart, and as its name implies, is a healing herb for mothers. Its Latin name, *Leonorus cardiaca,* means "lion-hearted," implying the herb imparts strength and courage. It is particularly

> ### Calming Tea
> Combine 1 teaspoon chamomile flowers, 1 teaspoon lemon balm, and $1/2$ teaspoon lavender flowers, steep in 1 cup boiling water (covered) for 10 to 15 minutes, strain, and drink warm, with honey if you prefer, as often as you wish throughout pregnancy for stress, indigestion, sleeplessness, and anxiety. You also can take this tea during labor to help you ease discomfort from contractions. A worthwhile additive to your medicine pantry, it is simple to prepare and delicious.

useful when you feel irritable, bothered, or overwhelmed. Take a tincture of this herb (it's too bitter for tea) in doses of 10 to 20 drops up to three times a day for a few days only. Do not exceed three doses daily.

NOTE: *Because motherwort is an emmenagogue, avoid its use in the first trimester.*

- Skullcap nourishes the nerves and brings about gentle relaxation when you feel irritated or restless. While it is not specifically beneficial for depression or weepiness, it is an excellent nerve tonic. Dosage is 1 to 2 cups of tea daily, or 10 to 20 drops of tincture two to four times a day. The herb or the tincture can be added to other teas.

- Passionflower has marked benefits for pregnant women with extreme mood swings, particularly anxiety and irritability. Use as a tincture, 10 to 30 drops up to three times daily.

- Bach Rescue Remedy, now also known as Bach Calming Essence, has brought many people relief from stress and feelings of being overwhelmed. Available at local natural food stores and herb shops, it contains star of Bethlehem, rock rose, impatiens, cherry plum, and clematis. Take 4 drops of the essence, repeating every fifteen minutes for up to one hour, and repeat later on if necessary. It is good for acute stress.

---

**Stress-Free Formula**

1 ounce passionflower tincture
1 ounce skullcap tincture
1 ounce fresh milky oats tincture
$1/2$ ounce chamomile tincture
$1/2$ ounce lavender tincture

Combine all the tinctures and take $1/4$ to 1 teaspoon of the mixture every 15 minutes to 4 hours as needed to promote rest and relief from anxiety. Do not exceed 6 teaspoons daily.

---

- Nettle is an herb that I find effective for moderating mood swings due to adrenal stress and blood sugar swings. When it is taken over time, its nutritive blood-building qualities may combine to reduce irritability, while its mineral content and adrenal-nourishing qualities help to stabilize the blood sugar. Take as a strong infusion, 1 to 3 cups daily.

- Dandelion root helps regulate blood sugar, preventing drastic dips that can cause mild to severe mood swings. It can be taken as a syrup, 1 to 2 tablespoons daily, in a nutritive base of blackstrap molasses; as an infusion, up to 2 cups daily; or as a tincture, 20 drops up to four times a day.

- The general comfort of a warm bath enhanced with a few drops of essential oil of rose or lavender, or a massage with diluted oils of rose, lavender, St. John's wort, and chamomile are very helpful. To promote a more restful sleep and to reduce irritability when you wake, try sleeping on an herbal pillow stuffed with chamomile or lavender blossoms, or sprinkle a few drops of these oils on your pillow or put them in a diffuser next to your bed.

# Fatigue

It is completely normal to need more sleep during pregnancy. Your body is working overtime. As my close friend, also a midwife, says, "It's a time of heavy construction." By the end of your first trimester, you have helped your baby develop all of his or her body parts, and that is an incredible accomplishment! In addition to all this building work, your own body and psyche are undergoing great changes and adjustments.

## General Recommendations

- Getting more sleep now that you are pregnant is important. Your emotions will be steadier, your digestion easier, and you will be less susceptible to infections, constipation, headaches, and morning sickness. Lack of sleep can lead to depression, irritability, and weepiness.

  You may, in fact, find yourself taking naps or dozing off in a chair at eight o'clock in the evening. Learn to listen to your body and your need to rest. Try not to worry about all that you are "not getting done."

- Stress, a job outside of the home, or older children to look after can further increase your fatigue. Women who have had children close together and are still nursing a toddler or keeping up with the needs of a family are particularly prone to exhaustion. This fatigue sometimes will ebb and flow. To minimize this, permit yourself to rest when you can, and prioritize your activities. For example, if housekeeping can wait, rest when you might otherwise be cleaning.

- Exercise, especially in the fresh air, is an excellent way to increase your oxygen intake and improve your circulation, appetite, and bowel function. Your depression will lift and insomnia and restless sleep will lessen. Even a brisk walk at least three times a week can make a tremendous difference in your well-being. A gentle toning exercise such as yoga can help wash away fatigue. Getting a massage can be relaxing and invigorating. If you can't afford a professional massage, have your mate or close friend give you one (or ask your midwife to massage you at prenatal sessions).

- When you need help, be sure to ask for it.

# Dietary Recommendations

- If you find yourself persistently irritable and exhausted, this may be a symptom of a nutritional problem. Frequently this type of deep exhaustion is accompanied by some of the following symptoms: general weakness, pallor, shortness of breath, nausea ranging from mild to severe, dizziness, heart palpitations, and lack of appetite. See "Anemia" above for natural therapies that can help you obtain enough iron in your daily diet. When there is insufficient iron in your diet, your body is not getting enough oxygen and you may feel fatigued.

- Be certain that you are eating regularly and getting enough protein and complex carbohydrates, nutrients that provide your body with a steady source of energy. Excessive reliance on sweet foods (including fresh fruit) without adequate intake of these other nutrients will lead to feelings of fatigue.

# Herbal Recommendations

- Herbs can help you improve your energy by improving your nutrition. However, stimulants—even herbal ones— should not be used during pregnancy. They can give a false sense of energy when what you really need is rest or nourishment. "Superfoods," concentrated food supplements like spirulina (a blue-green algae) and kelp (a dried sea vegetable), can boost your nutrient levels and thus your energy. Unlike stimulants, you can take these daily.

- Take a strong nettle infusion, 2 to 3 cups per day, to nourish the adrenals, regulate blood sugar, improve nutrient intake, and build iron levels.

- Use Iron Tonic Syrup (see page 173) to boost iron levels if fatigue is associated with anemia.

- Use small doses of adaptogenic herbs such as American ginseng, eleuthero, or schisandra to improve adrenal function and restore energy. Combine $1/2$ ounce of each of these tinctures and take $1/2$ teaspoon up to twice daily.

- Take spirulina in pill form, according to the recommended dosage, or up to a tablespoon of the powder daily. It can be taken in smoothies, juice, or capsules.

- Herbal baths can be invigorating, refreshing the mind and spirit and reducing fatigue and depression. Add 3 to 5 drops of an essential oil to your bath. Good choices are peppermint, lemon, orange, sandalwood, and rosemary oils. Splash mildly cool water on your body after the bath and settle in for a peaceful rest. Alternatively, if you don't have time for a full bath, add 2 to 3 drops of oil to a basin of cool water and splash yourself with the invigorating scents—a sure, quick energy pickup!

CAUTION: *Never use essential oils internally.*

# Fibroids, Uterine

Uterine fibroids are benign—that is, noncancerous—growths that may occur on the uterus (subserous myomas) or in it (intramural or submucous myomas). Because a fibroid is an outgrowth of the myometrial, or muscular, layer of the uterus, they are actually encapsulations of your own tissue. They are known to increase in size in the presence of high levels of estrogen, as occurs during pregnancy, or when women are on birth control pills, or in women with high levels of body fat and fat intake. The fact that they are noncancerous and not dangerous is often confusing because they are frequently referred to as "fibroid tumors," and of course the word *tumor* (which simply refers to a growth) conjures up fearful images.

Fibroids occur in up to 30 percent of all females and in nearly half of all women of menopausal age, and are very common in younger women, especially those who have not borne children. Small fibroids are almost always completely painless and asymptomatic; however, fibroids can grow to become quite large, as big as a grapefruit or more! A fibroid is generally described in relation to the size of a pregnant uterus (even in nonpregnant women)—for example, a woman may be said to have a fibroid the size of an eight-week pregnancy.

Large fibroids may cause bleeding, irregular menstruation, and pain; they may prevent conception or cause miscarriage; and they may cause other symptoms such as frequent urination if the uterus becomes quite enlarged and puts pressure on the bladder. A hysterectomy is commonly recommended for women with large fibroids, but this is a very serious surgery with long-term consequences, and one of the most frequently unnecessary surgical procedures performed in the United States. It is also an option most pregnant women would not want to consider. Given the low risks associated with fibroids and the efficacy of dietary and herbal therapies for addressing the problem, and the tendency of fibroids to shrink as estrogen levels go down at menopause, any woman considering a hysterectomy should research the problem, seek second—if not third—opinions, try natural approaches, and determine if the problem is worse than the solution, or vice versa.

Small fibroids generally cause absolutely no difficulty during pregnancy and birth; large fibroids on rare occasion may obstruct the baby's passage out of the uterus, make it difficult to control bleeding immediately after the birth, and sometimes can interfere with the baby's nourishment, as was the case with one pregnant mother I worked with who had a fibroid rapidly growing under her placenta. I note that she successfully curtailed its growth with the following series of recommendations despite her obstetrician's belief that it would become dangerously large.

The following suggestions may be used by any woman with fibroids: all the herbs may safely be used during pregnancy.

Because fibroids grow in the presence of estrogen, the high estrogen levels of pregnancy may precipitate their growth. Therefore, in order to prevent them from growing and interfering with your pregnancy or birth, it is sensible to follow some or all of these recommendations. It will take at least two months before you will notice obvious changes. As estrogen levels decrease after pregnancy, the fibroids will likely decrease in size as well.

## General and Dietary Recommendations

- Milk, eggs, cheese, and butter may contain significant levels of estrogen from the hormones fed to chickens and cows to increase their production of eggs and milk. This exogenous estrogen increases our own levels of estrogen and may stimulate the growth of fibroids. Therefore, try to obtain these foods from organic sources only. Reducing your use of eggs and dairy products, whether or not they are organically produced, is optimal, however, because they tend to lead to mucous congestion and excess fat in the body, both of which can cause fibroid growth.

- Eat a diet rich in whole grains, vegetables, fresh local fruits in season, and high-quality vegetable protein in the form of nuts, seeds, beans, and tofu. Eat animal products occasionally but not as staple parts of the diet. If you are regularly a heavy meat eater, gradually reduce the amount. Drastic changes are not advisable during pregnancy.

- Add sea vegetables to your diet, particularly kelp. Seaweeds are highly regarded for their ability to soften and reduce tumors and growths. In traditional Chinese medicine, foods and herbs of a mildly salty nature are said to do just this. Kelp is also an excellent nutritional supplement. Use kelp on foods or as tea or add it to soups or beans. Or steep a 4-inch long strip of kelp in 1 cup of water for about thirty minutes, and then drink the liquid; or take 2 "00" capsules of kelp powder four times a day.

- A juice made from a combination of freshly juiced apples, carrots, and beets makes an excellent lymphatic cleanser and mineral supplement, nourishes the immune system, and reduces tumors. It has a sweet taste and a lovely pink color. I use predominantly apples and carrots, adding about $1/2$ a beet to an 8-ounce glass of juice. You can adjust the proportions to your taste. Make it fresh each day, and take one 8-ounce glass daily at least five days a week.

- Activities that promote pelvic circulation are beneficial, both physically and psychologically, in reducing blockages and congestion in the pelvis. Yoga, brisk walks, belly dancing, making love—whatever rocks your boat, so to speak—do it at least three times a week for optimal pelvic health. Once or twice a week, you can take a cool (not cold) sitz bath to increase pelvic circulation.

- Visualization, the art of deliberately imagining your desired outcome as something actually happening, can be a useful tool for letting your body know what you want to do. You can imagine your womb filled with warm light, imagine the fibroids actually shrinking, or imagine the wall of your womb as healthy and vibrant. See chapter 8 for more suggestions on creative visualization.

## Herbal Recommendations

- The best way to reduce fibroids is to use a combination of strategies. Basically, you want to strengthen the functioning of your liver so your hormones are effectively moving through your body in appropriate amounts and being transformed and eliminated. In addition, consider using herbs that help promote healthy blood and facilitate bowel elimination. Liver-Strengthening Tea, taken on a regular basis, is very effective for helping your body perform all of these tasks.

- In addition to Liver-Strengthening Tea, take 20 drops of chasteberry tincture two to three times a day.

> **Liver-Strengthening Tea**
>
> Mix equal parts of burdock root, dandelion root, yellow dock root, red clover blossoms, cleavers, and nettle. Steep 1 ounce of this mixture in 1 quart of boiling water for 2 hours. Strain and discard the herbs. Drink 2 cups of this brew daily.

The tincture can be added to the tea. Chasteberry is indicated in the case of uterine fibroids and other gynecological problems.

- Avoid licorice, as it increases estrogen levels.

# Flu

(*See* "Colds, Flu, and Mild Illnesses")

# Headaches

Headaches can stem from a number of causes, most commonly stress, tension, low blood sugar, constipation, dehydration, inadequate protein intake, or dietary insufficiency of other minerals, particularly calcium and iron. Women prone to headaches before pregnancy may continue to have headaches during pregnancy, and women who are unable to nurture themselves adequately may develop headaches.

Severe headaches beginning suddenly after the sixth month of pregnancy can signal toxemia, so check with your midwife or physician and care for yourself accordingly (see "Toxemia" later in this chapter). Untreated, toxemia can become a life-threatening condition. Severe headaches that increase in frequency and pain or that occur in women who are not prone to them (that is, headaches of pathological origin) can be a sign of a serious problem requiring medical assistance. The following discussion does not address headaches of pathological origin.

## General Recommendations

- Stress causes you to contract your muscles, reducing blood flow and making your body function less effectively. Sometimes fatigue can lead to tension headaches, so be sure that you are sleeping enough, and whenever possible, take a nap.

- Creative visualization will be useful. Begin by choosing a comfortable spot in which you can sit or stretch out for as long as you are able, or at least ten minutes. Get comfortable. Close your eyes and allow the tension to melt away, beginning at your feet and slowly working up your body until you reach your head. The different parts of your body should become progressively looser, as if you are floating on water. You can imagine hands massaging you deeply, lightly, or however you prefer. Imagine yourself basking in this relaxed state. Allow your mind to travel then to an environment that comforts, relaxes, and nourishes you. Choose a favorite image—walking on the beach, floating in a luxurious bath, or sinking deeply into a featherbed. When you feel calm and relaxed, open your eyes and slowly come back.

- As you relax, specifically focus on any images that may tell you the cause of the headache or possible remedies. When we enter deep states of relaxation, we are often able to access information that is not immediately available to us in our waking consciousness. You may see images of tension or experience fears about pregnancy or birth. By becoming aware of tension and its source, we can take steps to resolve it. If you want to address pregnancy and birth fears and anxieties, refer to *Pregnant Feelings* by Rahima Baldwin and Terra Palmarini, *Silent Knife* by Nancy Cohen and Lois Estner, and *Birthing Normally* by Gayle Peterson. Relaxation tapes for pregnant women are available, or make your own using the visualization suggestions in chapter 8.

- Constipation is a common cause of headaches. Substances that your body needs to eliminate are reabsorbed. At least one bowel movement daily can relieve headaches as well as prevent other health problems. See "Constipation" earlier in this chapter for more information.

## Dietary Recommendations

- Poor nutrition with resulting hypoglycemia can cause headaches. High-protein, high-carbohydrate snacks can help.

- Dehydration can also cause headaches, so drink enough fluids throughout the day, at least a tall glass of water or a nutritious beverage every few hours. You may feel parched, depressed, or hot if you aren't drinking enough. You may notice that you have some contractions, known to occur when pregnant women become dehydrated. You can reverse all these symptoms by eating and drinking adequately throughout the day.

- Caffeinated beverages (such as coffee and soda) and chocolate can cause headaches. Try to avoid them.

- Iron deficiency may lead you to have headaches, as will protein deficiency.

- You may need to add more calcium and magnesium to your diet. Refer to chapter 5 for dietary recommendations and consider adding a supplement containing 600 to 800 mg of calcium and 300 to 400 mg of magnesium.

# Herbal Recommendations

- Many nervine herbs are effective for soothing tension headaches. Herbs that can be used as teas include chamomile, lemon balm, catnip, lavender, passion-flower, and skullcap. You can take these herbs singly or in a combination of two or three in tea form, taking several cups daily. For more severe headaches, or if you are unable to take tea several times per day, you can use herbal tinctures, $^1/_2$ to 1 teaspoon of tincture, added to an herbal tea or $^1/_4$ cup of warm water. In addition to those herbs previously mentioned, cramp bark, black cohosh, and St. John's wort are effective, especially in combination, for the treatment of tension headaches. After the first trimester, blue vervain and motherwort may also be used.

- Occasionally, mild bitters and herbs that support digestion and liver metabolism can be a helpful adjunct when treating women with recurrent mild headaches. The best herbs for this include dandelion root and leaves, yellow dock root, blue vervain, and burdock root. For convenience, you can take any of these as tinctures, up to $^1/_2$ teaspoon (individually or combined), three to four times daily.

> **Relaxation Tea**
>
> A formula that I enjoy for relaxation during pregnancy contains 1 teaspoon chamomile flowers, 1 teaspoon lemon balm, $^1/_2$ teaspoon lavender flowers, and $^1/_2$ teaspoon fennel seeds. Steep this mixture in 1 cup of boiling water for 10 minutes (covered) and drink hot. You can add milk and honey for flavor. To add calcium, add milk or take 2 calcium lactate capsules with the tea.

# Heartburn

(*See* "Indigestion and Heartburn")

# Hemorrhoids

(*See* "Varicose Veins and Hemorrhoids")

# Herpes

This section discusses Type II, genital herpes, though the recommendations are also applicable to Type I, oral herpes.

Herpes is a viral infection that once contracted stays dormant in the nerves located at the base of the spine. This infection will flare up when triggered by stress, fatigue, and dietary deficiencies. A woman who becomes infected with herpes for the first time during pregnancy, and particularly when she is close to the time of birth, may miscarry, or the baby may develop congenital anomalies or become very sick. It is therefore essential that you know whether your sexual partner has ever been exposed to or had herpes. People think that only promiscuous people, poor people with poor hygienic habits, or drug addicts have sexual diseases. I have met many wealthy, educated people who have had herpes, gonorrhea, crabs, and other sexually transmitted conditions. Most people are embarrassed to admit that they have herpes, but it is very common. A cesarean section is a standard procedure for women in the United States with active herpes at the end of pregnancy.

Women who had herpes before becoming pregnant are at minimal risk for passing the infection on to the baby prenatally because they have developed antibodies to the virus that protect the baby. In fact, it is becoming more common for women to give birth vaginally even with mild herpes as long as it isn't a primary infection. This is a matter of debate among obstetricians: European physicians claim that herpes is a fairly low risk for the baby compared to the higher risk of a cesarean section. But most American doctors are not yet convinced of the safety of vaginal birth with active herpes lesions. See Anne Frye's *Understanding Lab Work in the Childbearing Year* and Nancy Cohen's *Open Season* for discussions of this issue. Obviously, this will be a decision that requires a good deal of thought and the support of your birth attendant. Because of the potential risks, you should investigate the risks and benefits of both vaginal birth and cesarean for you and your baby.

The symptoms of a herpes outbreak usually begin three to five days before the sores appear: flulike feelings, aching in the genital area, tingling or itching where the sores will erupt, emotional irritability, and sometimes painful urination or swollen lymph nodes. The lesions begin as small blisters that turn into small sores that then crust over and heal. There can be one lesion or many, and they can appear on either the external or internal parts of the genitals, including the cervix. The infection is contagious during the entire range of symptoms, so sexual activity should be discontinued at the earliest sign of any symptom until the sores are completely healed and are no longer visible. This can take up to a couple of weeks.

Herpes is quite common. I've worked with a number of women with a history of herpes, including one woman who had two previous cesareans. She went on to have her third baby at home with no lesions present. Most people have a "body barometer," a physical symptom or syndrome that pops up at times of stress. It could be an old injury site that begins to ache, a headache that develops when you have a deadline, or herpes that flares up. These are messages that you are dealing with too much internal pressure. By learning to recognize the early signs of stress, we can learn to slow down. If you anticipate a stressful time coming, you can take measures that prevent an outbreak; and if you do notice prodromal (pre-herpes) symptoms, you can begin to use herbs, address the stress, and improve your diet. You can get to the point where you rarely, if ever, have another herpes outbreak.

If you are troubled by regular herpes outbreaks, it is very important to take an honest look at your beliefs about your body and your sexuality. For example, are your outbreaks an excuse (conscious or otherwise—look deeply) to avoid sexual intimacy with your mate? Are you feeling unclean, unworthy of being loved, of experiencing sexual pleasure? Learning to feel comfortable about yourself sexually can heal herpes.

> Nadine had two prior cesareans for active herpes lesions at the time of birth. With this pregnancy, she chose to eat well, avoiding foods that aggravate herpes and increasing those that prevent it. She chose to follow an herbal program, drinking echinacea and burdock root infusion daily for her third trimester, and she planned for a home birth. She had no outbreaks and gave birth at home, vaginally of course!

## General and Dietary Recommendations

Sexual partners with herpes can also follow the recommendations here.

- Stress reduction will help prevent herpes outbreaks. Make sure you are resting enough, and address any sexual issues that may be causing you anxiety. Refer to the sections on relaxation and creative visualization in chapter 8, and incorporate some of these practices into your life on a regular basis, especially during stressful times. Take up an activity such as yoga or tai chi.

- Learning which foods to emphasize and which to avoid can be a step toward a life without outbreaks.

- Identify the processed foods in your diet and replace them with healthful foods. Eat plenty of fresh fruits and vegetables. Natural foods cookbooks are easy to find at major bookstores and health food stores, and can be a terrific source of cooking inspiration.

Arginine and lysine are two of the many amino acids our bodies require as part of our overall protein intake. However, arginine is known to contribute to herpes outbreaks whereas lysine helps to prevent them. Therefore a diet higher in lysine and lower in arginine is part of a herpes prevention diet.

This list does not imply that you should completely avoid all high-arginine foods, but common sense dictates that those foods not essential for health be avoided, such as chocolate and coffee. Whole grains, for example, should be eaten in moderation with a dietary emphasis on high-lysine foods.

- Some people find that a lysine supplement of 500 mg daily prevents outbreaks. According to Anne Frye, as much as 5,000 mg of lysine during prodromal symptoms may be necessary. If you are close to your due time and sense an outbreak, this higher dosage may be a good idea.

- 1,000 mg of vitamin C daily for prevention of an outbreak, and 2,000 mg daily during an outbreak, can enhance your immunity. Vitamin C is a reputable antiviral remedy.

| **High-Arginine Foods** | **High-Lysine Foods** |
|---|---|
| Reduce these in your diet: | Emphasize these in your diet: |
| *Brown rice* | *Beans* |
| *Carob* | *Beef* |
| *Chocolate, coffee, and caffeinated teas* | *Cheese, milk, and yogurt* |
| *Coconut* | *Chicken* |
| *Eggplants* | *Eggs* |
| *Garbanzo beans (chickpeas)* | *Fresh fish* |
| *Green peppers* | *Fresh vegetables* |
| *Mushrooms* | *Milk* |
| *Nuts* | *Nutritional yeast* |
| *Oats* | *Sprouts* |
| *Raisins* | |
| *Seeds* | |
| *Sugar* | |
| *Tomatoes* | |
| *Wheat* | |

# Herbal Recommendations

For the prevention and treatment of herpes, you can take herbs that nourish, tonify, and calm the nerves. (Remember, the nerves are where the virus actually resides in the body.) These herbs have antiviral capacity internally and topically, strengthening immunity, reducing moist heat in the body, and "purifying the blood," as old-time herbalists would say.

- The primary herbs for reducing stress and tonifying the nervous system are the antiviral nervines lemon balm and St. John's wort. Additionally, chamomile, lavender, passionflower, skullcap, and catnip may be included in a formula. Take tinctures in warm water, directly under the tongue, or add to an herbal tea. Average dosage is 1/2 to 1 teaspoon of any of these (or that amount of a combination), two to three times a day.

- The following remedy has proven consistently effective in my practice for preventing herpes outbreaks during pregnancy. It has immune-enhancing properties as well as antiviral potential and it reduces dampness and heat in the pelvis. Place 1/2 ounce each of echinacea root and burdock root in a quart jar; fill the jar with boiling water, cap tightly, and let steep for 8 hours. Strain and drink, storing the next day's portion in the refrigerator. You can carry this brew with you in a jar or insulated container. Dosage is 2 cups daily, preferably 1/2 cup four times a day. You should take this remedy throughout pregnancy if you have regular outbreaks; otherwise, begin taking it if you notice prodromal symptoms and continue until all symptoms are gone. It will reduce the frequency and duration of outbreaks. For every week you take these herbs, take a three-day break (for example, seven days on, three days off) to avoid sensitization to the herbs and therefore decreased effectiveness. To prevent outbreaks toward the time of birth, take regularly throughout the third trimester (with the recommended breaks).

    Echinacea and burdock can also be taken in tincture form: 30 drops of each taken four times daily in place of the infusion, following the same recommended course as above.

- Other herbs that can safely be added to this infusion (do not substitute any herb for echinacea or burdock) or taken as tinctures include cleavers, chickweed, and yellow dock root; dandelion root; and, for flavor in the infusion, spearmint leaves. Add 1 to 2 tablespoons of the dried herbs to the echinacea-burdock brew at the beginning of steeping.

- Astragalus tincture, 20 to 30 drops three times a day, is a specific immune-system enhancer and can also be added to either the infusion or tincture blends.

- You can effectively treat herpes blisters, reducing discomfort and speeding healing, with several antiviral herbs. A simple combination of licorice root and St. John's wort tinctures can be very effective and can be applied regularly to the sores using a fresh cotton swab. Both of these herbs are specific for the treatment of herpes virus.

- A tincture of calendula oil can be dabbed onto the affected areas with a cotton ball or swab; St. John's wort oil can be dabbed on the affected area during the prodromal phase; propolis tincture can quickly heal oozing sores and reduce pain topically.

- Take sitz baths made with a strong infusion of equal parts of burdock root, echinacea, calendula, comfrey root, and myrrh; steep 2 ounces of dried herbs per quart of water, for four hours.

- In a recent study, significant improvement of symptoms and accelerated scabbing of sores in herpes patients has been shown with the topical application of an extract of lemon balm. Though the preparation was highly concentrated, you may find it beneficial to add this herb to sitz baths and to dab extracts of lemon balm onto the affected area. As it is both relaxing and potentially antiviral, you may want to add a few tablespoons of the dried herb or a handful of the fresh leaves to your burdock and echinacea infusion. To be effective, the study concluded, the treatment must be begun during the early stages of infection.

These recommendations are also applicable for oral (Type I) herpes (cold sores). Herpes is spread through skin contact; careful hygiene is essential if you have either type and are caring for a newborn. Up to six months of age babies are highly susceptible to the herpes virus, with up to a 50 percent fatality rate.

> **CAUTION:** *If a baby shows any signs of illness when there is a family member with either a history of herpes or active herpes, seek immediate medical care for the baby.*

# High Blood Pressure

There are two kinds of high blood pressure: essential hypertension, high blood pressure that preexists pregnancy; and pregnancy-induced hypertension (PIH), which usually shows up after twenty weeks' gestation. The general criteria for the diagnosis of any hypertension is a blood pressure of 140/90 or above, or any rise in systolic pressure (the top number) of 30 points or more and/or a rise in diastolic pressure (the bottom number) of 15 points or more. The rise must be seen in two readings at least six hours apart to be considered conclusive because blood pressure is variable throughout the day and can change according to your mood, environment, and interactions. Therefore, any singular incidents of high blood pressure can be disregarded if you generally have a blood pressure within a normal range.

What I look for in pregnant women is a steadily rising blood pressure over the course of two or more prenatal visits to indicate that the woman is developing what may be problematic hypertension. Of course, physicians, hospitals, and midwives may see women whose health history they do not know and must determine whether those women are at risk for problems associated with high blood pressure.

For example, a woman who shows up at the hospital in labor, or a woman who chooses a midwife very late in pregnancy, can have a blood pressure of 130/80. This can be considered within the normal 140/90 range, but if her blood pressure is normally 100/60, it may be hypertension. The optimal situation, if you are planning to use a care provider for your pregnancy and birth, is that you do so early in the pregnancy to establish your "baseline" vital signs. Only in seeing the whole picture can deviations from your normal pattern become apparent.

Many health-care providers fear high blood pressure in pregnant women because it is one symptom of preeclampsia (toxemia), which has other symptoms: not feeling well; slow growth of the baby; swelling of the ankles, face, and hands; visual disturbance; upper abdominal pain; headaches; kidney, heart, or thyroid problems; and the presence of protein in the urine. While preeclampsia is very serious and needs both thoughtful prevention and careful treatment, not all high blood pressure results in complications. Treatments such as the use of aspirin, diuretics, medications, salt restriction, along with a lack of attention to lifestyle and

> **Beth began experiencing elevated blood pressure—from an initial reading of 106/60 to a steady 128/74. She began a program of motherwort and hawthorn extract, as well as reducing her work load and increasing her fluid intake. Her blood pressure did not continue to rise and stabilized at an average of 124/68.**

diet, leave any true imbalances unresolved and predispose pregnant women to other problems such as hemorrhage and kidney problems. This does not mean that medical treatments should be avoided. It does mean, however, that you should fully explore other approaches beforehand, or that you should use them only in emergencies. Hypertension can be a symptom of kidney infection, kidney disease, and, rarely, tumors, vascular disturbances, nervous-system disorders, hydatidiform moles, and liver disease, all requiring medical diagnosis and treatment (with the exception of a urinary tract infection, which can usually be treated quite successfully with natural therapies). If you are attempting to treat hypertension naturally, it is important to rule out more serious causes that require medical attention. Consult with a midwife or physician to help you determine whether it is safe for you to try a natural approach.

The greatest contributors to high blood pressure are stress, poor nutrition, and lack of exercise. Improvement in these areas will almost always reduce blood pressure if it is high. If the mother has elevated blood pressure but seems otherwise in excellent health, I simply keep tabs on her blood pressure for a few weeks or more (depending upon how far along she is in her pregnancy), and I provide clear instructions on eating well, getting more exercise, and reducing stress. I might suggest herbs that can assist in the reduction of blood pressure. I don't make a big fuss about high blood pressure unless it becomes consistently elevated and doesn't respond to any of my suggestions. In this case, a home birth becomes contraindicated. I've not had this happen, perhaps by luck or perhaps because of the body's wonderful ability to heal itself when it is given support. Of course, if the mother develops symptoms of toxemia or any other complications, a medical evaluation is essential.

The general risks of hypertension in pregnancy are lack of adequate oxygen flow to the baby, the potential for low birth-weight and possible stillbirth, and, because of the force of the blood behind the placenta, the risk of a placental abruption, a situation in which the placenta prematurely separates from the uterine wall, a potentially dangerous situation for mother and baby. It is up to you, along with the educated assistance of your care provider, to determine when high blood pressure seems to be problematic, and to decide whether to try to reduce elevation by attempting to normalize circulation or to use medication to control it. The following suggestions may assist you in preventing high blood pressure if you are prone to it, and in lowering blood pressure should it become elevated.

# General and Dietary Recommendations

- If you are pregnant and have hypertension, you need to evaluate your diet. Keeping a diet diary is the best way to do this (see chapter 5). After completing it, you can ask your midwife to review it for the content, quality, and quantity of the foods you are eating. If you are working with a physician or other practitioner who is not well versed in the nutritional needs of pregnant women from the standpoint of dietary intake, be sure to read the nutritional information in this book or books in the bibliography. Highly processed, refined foods, with their plethora of chemical additives, tax the liver, kidneys, and bowels, placing unnecessary burdens on the whole circulatory system, possibly contributing to hypertension. Preparing homemade foods and salting them to taste, and inviting more natural foods into your diet, especially whole grains, beans, hard cheeses, yogurt, nuts, seeds, and fish, can help prevent and reduce hypertension.

- High salt intake has long been associated with the development of high blood pressure in both pregnant women and the general population. In addition, pregnant women have long been told to reduce their salt intake to prevent water retention. However, a great deal of contemporary research has shown that inadequate salt intake during pregnancy can be dangerous, contributing to the development of both high blood pressure and edema. This is because salt helps keep blood volume adequately expanded, which is essential during pregnancy. Lack of salt causes the blood volume to contract, thus the heart must work harder to circulate less blood volume, and the blood vessels also constrict, leading to higher blood pressure. You do need adequate amounts of salt during pregnancy. The key is what type of salt you are getting. Regular table salt, which is used in most prepackaged foods, fast foods, and as table salt, is high in chlorine as well as stabilizers, and sometimes even sugar, and can contribute to high blood pressure.

  The key is to lightly salt your foods using sea salt, tamari (natural soy sauce), or earth salt, available at health food stores and in many supermarkets. Cut down on oversalted packaged goods and fast foods, and eat freshly prepared vegetables. In the summertime, a you may need to replace extra salt lost through perspiration by salting your food to taste and perhaps even drinking an electrolyte replacement such as Recharge or Third Wind if you've been sweating a great deal.

  A tasty and nutritious salty condiment that my family has used for years is called *gomasio,* a mixture of sesame seeds and salt (*goma* means "sesame"; *sio,* "salt"). It is said that the combination makes salt more usable by the body's cells. To prepare it, simply roast about a cup of raw, unhulled sesame seeds in a skillet on low heat until they begin to "pop" and turn light brown. Stir continuously to avoid burning the seeds. Just before they are done, add 1 tablespoon of sea salt and stir for a minute more. When slightly cool, grind in a blender or in a traditional Japanese mortar and pestle called a *suribachi* (available at many Asian grocery stores) until the mix is mostly ground but not powdered. Gomasio can be sprinkled liberally on grains, beans, cooked vegetables, and salads. It can be kept unrefrigerated for up to two weeks but is best used within a week.

- Be sure you drink enough water throughout the day to help you maintain an expanded blood volume, important for preventing high blood pressure. Frequently, women do not drink enough fluids or drink sodas or coffee, which, even though they contain water, do more harm than good. Caffeinated and sugared fruit beverages do not belong in a healthy pregnancy diet. The way I remember to drink enough of the right kind of fluids throughout the day is to place a full half-gallon jug of water on my table each morning, and drink as close to all of it as I can by that evening. You can use the water to make herbal tea as well, and you can include in that half gallon other fluids such as broths and freshly made fruit or vegetable juices.

- There are several foods that may reduce blood pressure by improving general circulation and kidney function, and by supporting the circulatory system.

- Insufficient intake of essential fatty acids (EFAs) in the diet is also associated with hypertension. It may be improved by using walnut oil and safflower oil added to raw salads and other dishes in place of oils high in saturated fats. EFAs help enlarge blood vessels, thereby reducing high blood pressure. Fatty, deepwater fish such as salmon and tuna are high

---

**Foods for
Blood Pressure Reduction**

Watermelon and cucumbers (two slices of watermelon or one whole cucumber, preferably slightly overripe) and parsley (a few sprigs with a meal, once daily). Buckwheat, the grain, can be eaten for its high rutin content, and vitamin C with bioflavonoids (up to 2,000 mg daily) can be taken during pregnancy. Raw onions and garlic eaten in large amounts each day. Onions can be used chopped in salads and pasta dishes, or sliced on sandwiches. To use raw garlic, mince one clove, put it on a teaspoon with honey, and swallow without chewing by chasing it with water. This technique reduces virtually all side effects associated with eating raw garlic, such as nausea, headache, and garlic breath. You can also use garlic "perles" (encapsulated garlic extracts) available at natural food stores.

in EFAs. You can supplement your diet with 1 tablespoon of raw flaxseed oil added to a daily salad (do not cook the oil as heat destroys the EFAs). Or take two 500 mg capsules of evening primrose or black currant seed oil daily.

- Raw olive oil is associated with low levels of heart disease in Italian women who use it on a daily basis. In Germany, an extract made from the leaves of the olive tree is used to treat essential hypertension. Although the leaves are not appropriate for use during pregnancy, the addition of raw olive oil to the diet on a daily basis may be beneficial for women with high blood pressure (and may work as a preventative). Rather than sautéed vegetables or fried rice, you may want to prepare simple steamed veggies dressed with olive oil and other seasonings, or a rice or pasta salad. One of my favorite meals is a big raw salad with a half cup of garbanzo beans on top, sprinkled with a dash of tamari soy sauce, some olive oil, and Parmesan cheese. You could even add some chopped raw onion or minced raw garlic.

  A practical way to use raw garlic is to keep on hand a batch of garlic oil for seasoning your foods. Simply peel and mince a whole bulb and place it in a jar with 1 cup of olive oil. Let stand on your counter or in the refrigerator for a couple of days before beginning to use it once a day, garlic and all, on top of salad, beans, pasta, or whole wheat bread. A delicious traditional accompaniment to Italian meals is bread spread with olive oil and garlic.

- Daily exercise helps to improve circulatory functioning and therefore is an essential part of any program to reduce high blood pressure. A brisk walk for twenty minutes, working out on a stationary bicycle, swimming, or any exercise that you like that stimulates your circulation is excellent.

- As important as exercise is the time set aside each day for relaxation, stress reduction, meditation, whatever you call it. This is what I alternately call my sacred time, my sanctuary time, my retreat time, or simply taking space. It is a time devoted to unwinding, letting go of worries and worldly concerns, finding a peaceful place within yourself, feeling centered, breathing deeply, and letting go of physical tension. Occasionally, if you are able, include a full body massage from a professional massage therapist, your mate, or a close friend. This deep relaxation experience is particularly effective if it directly follows your exercise time or a yoga session. Your body's restlessness is reduced from the activity you've just done, and your blood circulation and oxygenation are at a peak, which actually promotes deep rest. (Can you remember how well you slept when you played outside all day?) Refer to chapter 8 for further suggestions on relaxation and creative visualization.

- Taking twenty minutes or so to rest on your left side can help reduce blood pressure because it eases the effort of your heart and circulatory system. This is an excellent position during labor if you already have elevated blood pressure.

- Be honest with yourself, your midwife, or other care provider about your anxieties. This is very important, simply because the effort of damping down your anxieties can contribute to high blood pressure. For example, I once worked with a couple who intellectually seemed to want to have a home birth, but who, on a lot of levels, seemed very afraid of birth. Despite my efforts to help them address their anxieties, they insisted that they were comfortable with birth and wanted to have the baby at home. When the woman finally went into labor, a couple of weeks past due, her blood pressure rose dramatically. We chose to go to the hospital for the birth, where her blood pressure normalized upon arrival. When I mentioned this phenomenon to the attending nurse-midwife, the head of a large midwifery teaching program at a well-known university, she confirmed it, remarking that women can and do psychologically create symptoms that land them in the hospital if that is where they truly feel safer. In our culture, where a technologically advanced birth is considered to be the safest, we cannot dismiss high blood pressure as merely a "psychological factor." Blood pressure should be checked at a prenatal visit only after you have had a chance to take your coat off and relax rather than when you first come in. Incidentally, make sure your blood pressure is checked with the appropriate size cuff, as a cuff that is too tight will cause your blood pressure to appear high.

- Funny movies are great for stress reduction. Whoopie Goldberg always gets me laughing and feeling more relaxed! Internal emotional pressure is reflected in high blood pressure, so do things that you enjoy and find ways to let off steam.

## Herbal Recommendations

- When a rise in blood pressure is related to stress and anxiety, herbs may help. These include teas of lemon balm, chamomile, lavender, lime blossom, skullcap, and passionflower. Drink a tea of any of these herbs alone or in combination twice a day to prevent high blood pressure, or sip up to a quart throughout the day to reduce elevated blood pressure. Many of these herbs can also be used as tinctures (although lemon balm and chamomile are best as teas) at a general dosage of $1/2$ to 1 teaspoon taken two to four times a day.

- An excellent herbal combination for the reduction of tension and mild hypertension is equal parts of the tinctures of cramp bark, hawthorn (berries, leaves, and flowers), black cohosh, and motherwort. Cramp bark eases physical stress by reducing muscular and nervous tension; hawthorn is a cardiotonic that dilates peripheral blood vessels and improves cardiac output and reduces strain on the heart, thereby reducing blood pressure; black cohosh relaxes the nerves and the muscles and dilates the peripheral blood vessels; motherwort, a gentle antispasmodic and nervine, reduces muscular tension and emotional stress—it contains bitter glycosides that have hypotensive properties, that is, they help reduce blood pressure. This combination can be taken as a tincture beginning after the first trimester.

> **CAUTION:** *Motherwort has the potential of acting as a uterine tonic and can therefore stimulate contractions. This doesn't usually occur, but it is advisable to wait until after the first trimester to use this herb. Of course, discontinue it if you notice increased contractions before you are due.*

# Indigestion and Heartburn

Indigestion and heartburn (burping, gas, occasional stomach upset) are common in pregnancy for a couple of reasons. The increased level of progesterone that softens smooth muscles also slows digestion and sometimes causes incomplete closure of the valve in the upper portion of the stomach, making stomach acid reflux more likely. This is more common in women who are already prone to digestive complaints. The baby's growing size also puts great upward pressure on the stomach. Sensible eating habits and gently soothing herbs usually reduce these problems, as will foods and herbs that help stimulate digestion. Do not use over-the-counter antacids or baking soda: these are generally contraindicated during pregnancy.

## General Recommendations

- Because the dietary recommendations (given below) are the most important part of this approach, follow all those that are relevant to you.
- If lying down causes heartburn, sleep with extra pillows under your head.

- Deep relaxation exercises (see chapter 8) before bed may also allay nighttime heartburn.

- Physical symptoms are sometimes a manifestation of psychic and emotional imbalance. You might take a look at what's "burning you up" or what you just can't digest in your daily life. Do you feel overwhelmed or angry? This is a good time to deal with any issues that are blocking the free flow of your energy. Writing out issues that are weighing on you is a good way to take stock. You may come up with ways to lighten your burdens.

## Dietary Recommendations

- Oily, heavy, rich, and spicy foods that are hard to digest are major heartburn culprits. Avoid foods that aggravate you, especially at your evening meal.

- Eat small, frequent snacks rather than large meals. A large amount of food consumed at one time can sit in your stomach and disagree with you.

- Have supper at least two hours before you go to bed, and eat a light snack if you are hungry late in the evening. Yogurt is a traditional heartburn remedy.

- To improve digestive activity, try to eat slowly, taking time to enjoy your food thoroughly.

- Some women find that drinking liquids with their meals aggravates them; for others, a glass of water during the meal or a cup of grapefruit juice just before the meal aids digestion. Try it both ways to see what works for you.

- A substance in raw almonds (cyanogenic glycoside) increases the activity of the parasympathetic nervous system, which in turn increases vagal tone (a response of one of your nerves, known as the vagus nerve), slows the heart rate, and improves digestion. A small handful as a snack or after a meal will do the trick. Chew them slowly. Raw cashews may have a similar action.

- A baked potato is sometimes helpful. With a pat of butter or a small amount of cheese and a bit of salt, it makes an excellent snack or small meal.

## *Herbal Recommendations*

- Slippery elm bark is wonderful for relieving heartburn. It is best taken on a regular basis or during a bout of heartburn. The easiest way to use slippery elm is to purchase Thayer Slippery Elm lozenges from a health food store. They are completely safe to use freely during pregnancy, so purchase several packages and keep one in your handbag and one on your bedside table. They have a plain, slightly maple syrup–like flavor, and are amazingly effective for reducing heartburn. Suck 2 to 4 per dose, and take up to three doses daily.

> ### Slippery Elm Lozenges
>
> Take ¼ cup of slippery elm powder and mix with enough honey to make a dough that is neither dry nor sticky. For additional flavor, add 2 to 5 drops of peppermint oil, lemon oil, or vanilla flavoring. Dust a small cutting board with some extra powder. Now roll your dough in this powder to form a long, thin roll (like a snake made out of modeling clay). Next, cut the roll into small pieces the size of a pea or slightly larger. Roll these into little balls and place on a cookie sheet and bake at 250°F for about an hour. When done, these are great to suck on for indigestion (and sore throats).

CAUTION: *Avoid any lozenges that contain coltsfoot or comfrey root while you are pregnant.*

- As an alternative, to make slippery elm tea, stir 1 level teaspoon of the herb into a cup of boiling water or warm milk; add a teaspoon of honey and a pinch of cinnamon. You can also make your own slippery elm lozenges.

- According to Ayurvedic medicine, an ancient Indian system of medicine, there are three "humours," or elemental influences in the body: kapha, the fluid substance; pitta, fire; and vata, wind. It is said that too much vata in the intestines causes nervous difficulties. Interestingly, herbs that can be used to reduce "wind" in Ayurvedic terms can also reduce general digestive complaints. Prepare and drink Digestion Tea after a meal, or take it before bedtime to ease your digestion.

> ### Digestion Tea
>
> In a teapot, place 1 teaspoon each of catnip or lemon balm, meadowsweet, chamomile, spearmint, fennel or anise seeds, and organic orange or tangerine peel. Pour 2 cups of boiling water over the herbs, cover the pot, and let it steep for 15 minutes. Strain, sweeten with 1 teaspoon of honey, and drink warm.

- Dandelion is an excellent bitter tonic that pregnant women can use for indigestion. Take 20 drops of tincture four times a day or when you are having a spell of heartburn.

- Kudzu root tea seems to reduce stomach acidity.

- Activated charcoal is a great emergency remedy for severe heartburn. It absorbs and eliminates poisons and is effective in relieving stomach acidity. Take two activated charcoal tablets if you have a bad case of heartburn. Repeat only on occasion, when absolutely necessary.

---

**Kudzu Root Tea**

To prepare, bring 1 cup of water to a boil in a small saucepan and then decrease the heat. Meanwhile, dissolve 2 teaspoons of kudzu starch in 2 tablespoons of cold water. Add the starch to the simmering water and stir continuously for 2 minutes. Kudzu has a completely bland taste, so you may wish to add 2 teaspoons of soy sauce, a bouillon cube, or honey to taste. Drink while still warm.

---

# Insomnia and Anxiety

Insomnia is a common problem during pregnancy. It can be difficult to go to sleep, and if we have to get up to urinate or if the baby's movements wake us up, we may find it hard to go back to sleep. This section will provide you with suggestions for treating insomnia as well as techniques you can use to relieve your anxieties.

## General Recommendations

- Try to give yourself a wind-down time in the evenings before you go to bed. If you are pushing yourself all day, your body cannot be expected to suddenly switch gears. Instead, induce your body and mind into a quieter state by slowing down your activity level in the evening, reducing stimulating influences (television, phone calls, the newspaper). Read a pleasant book, take a bath or a walk, read poetry or a story to your children. By slowing down, you will be closer to the relaxed state needed for sleep.

- Regular exercise increases the body's calcium utilization, which in turn helps with relaxation. You will greatly increase your ability to sleep if you practice mild aerobic exercise at least three times per week, for twenty minutes each time.

## Dietary Recommendations

- One of the most common reasons for insomnia is hunger. You may feel restless, hypersensitive to touch, and slightly nauseated. Perhaps you may even have a vague sense of hunger but are too tired to fix a snack. If this is the case, your problem may be simple to resolve: eat a high-protein snack before bed, especially one that is also calcium rich. For some women (myself included), you may occasionally need to eat again when you wake in the middle of the night. You can ask your mate to get up and get a snack for you. Or you can anticipate hunger and keep a snack beside your bed. A cup of yogurt, a banana, a handful of almonds, melted cheese on toast, or a cup of soup—really anything that strikes your fancy is fine. One late evening during my fourth pregnancy, I couldn't come up with an appetizing snack, so I called a friend for an idea. She came up with a super snack (it probably sounds like a gastronomic disaster to anyone who isn't pregnant) from *The Moosewood Cookbook* by Mollie Katzen: slice up an apple and some walnuts, grab a few raisins, and put them all on a piece of whole-wheat bread; then put Cheddar cheese on top of the whole deal and melt it under the broiler. Believe it or not, it really hit the spot. If it's nutritious and it strikes your fancy, go ahead. Just avoid foods that give you indigestion. See *What to Eat When You're Expecting* by Arlene Eisenberg, H.E. Murkoff, and S.E. Hathaway, listed in the bibliography.

- Calcium helps insomnia and also gets the muscles to relax. A deficit of calcium can induce anxiety and tension. Adding high-calcium foods to your diet (such as almonds, dark greens, broccoli, hard cheese, yogurt, kelp, beans, carrot juice, oats, beets, fish, and blackstrap molasses) can help. High-calcium herbs can also help; these include nettle, oatstraw, red raspberry leaves, chamomile, and dandelion greens prepared as infusions. Drinking cow's milk is not an optimal way to obtain calcium because it is high in fat and is hard to digest, but a cup of warm milk before bed with a pinch of cinnamon added is very relaxing. A calcium lactate supplement (preferably a calcium-magnesium blend to maintain the proper 2 to 1 ratio of

> Stacy was having insomnia, nightmares, occasional heart palpitations, and feelings of being overheated. She began taking tinctures of motherwort and skullcap in lemon balm tea several times each day. Within a week, her nightmares and palpitations had ceased, and her feelings of being overheated subsided. She was no longer experiencing insomnia.

these minerals in your body) is best taken before bed as calcium is most readily absorbed by the body while you sleep. You can take approximately 600 to 800 mg of calcium and 300 to 400 mg of magnesium a day.

- Caffeinated foods, coffee, chocolate, and soda can interfere with calcium absorption because they bind to calcium receptor sites in the body. Plants that are high in oxalic acid, such as beets and spinach, should be eaten in moderation, not more than once or twice weekly.

# Herbal Recommendations

- Herbal nervines are relaxing to the nervous system and mildly sedating; some are calcium rich. They can be used to help you sleep. Chronic insomnia may indicate underlying worries and nutritional deficiencies, so you should address these possibilities by improving your diet and exploring your concerns even while using nervines.

- Chamomile is a prime example of a nervine that is calcium rich and aids digestion. You can take it regularly to bring about a peaceful feeling.

> **Chamomile Tea**
>
> To prepare, steep 1 tablespoon of chamomile blossoms in 1 cup boiling water for 10 to 15 minutes; cover the cup while steeping to preserve the volatile oils.

- Passionflower is a highly reliable herb to safely promote sleep during pregnancy.

- Milky oat tincture is another nutrient-rich herb that you can use on a regular basis. Used over time, it will help reduce nervous tension. It is best prepared as an infusion rather than as a tea.

- Skullcap, a gentle nerve tonic, promotes restfulness, stress reduction, and sleep. I prefer to use it in tincture form, about 15 drops at a time, but it can be prepared as a tea or in infusions. You can take it up to four times a day during periods of acute stress or twice before bedtime with a fifteen-minute interval. Skullcap tincture can be added to chamomile tea.

- Lavender blossoms promote a sense of calm. They make a mildly bitter tea that is best steeped for a short time and then sweetened with 1 teaspoon of honey. Use 2 teaspoons of the herb to 1 cup boiling water and steep with a cover on the cup for 10 minutes. My own favorite is to use equal parts of lavender and chamomile blossoms to make a tea, add 10 drops of skullcap tincture, and drink hot.

- Other relaxing herbs include lime (linden) blossom, lemon balm, catnip, motherwort, St. John's wort, and valerian.

- Herbal baths help you sleep. Create a nightly bedtime ritual: a cup of your favorite relaxing tea to drink, quiet music, perhaps a candle, and a warm bath. To the bath, add 1 quart of lavender or chamomile infusion or 5 to 10 drops of lavender essential oil. Soak for a while, feeling the baby's movements in your womb, and consciously relaxing your muscles. Let the water ease your tension away. (Take care not to fall asleep in the bath, and take fire-safety precautions if you use a candle.)

- For more relaxation techniques to reduce anxiety, refer to chapter 8.

## Itchiness and Skin Troubles

Many women notice that their skin improves during pregnancy. However, you may notice some itchiness. The skin stretches over the belly, breasts, and thighs; extra sweating and decreased bowel functioning causes the skin to work harder in eliminating toxins. The liver, which must now process an increased hormonal load, may be overworked and cause the skin to itch. With a natural diet and herbs, you can prevent as well as reduce skin discomfort during pregnancy. Itching can also be related to stress. Itching can be a signal that something is "getting under your skin." Take a look at whether you are manifesting stress as a skin problem.

> **WARNING:** *If itching is persistent or progressively worsening, seek medical evaluation. Although rare, it can be a sign of liver disorders specific to pregnancy.*

### General Recommendations

- Clean your skin with a mild natural soap or just a warm cloth with no soap. Be certain that the soap you use has no additives and no strong perfume. A loofah sponge or a soft body brush can stimulate circulation and clean away dead cells, leaving your skin cleaner and softer.

- Daily exercise gets your circulation moving, bringing a healthy glow to your skin. As your circulation improves, so will your bowel functioning, reducing the burden of elimination on your skin, and the resultant itching.

## Dietary Recommendations

- Eat plenty of fresh fruit and vegetables daily, as well as whole grains, nuts, seeds, and beans. Eliminate processed foods and reduce your intake of saturated fats, butter, and fried foods.

- Drink a lot of water. About a half gallon a day is ideal for most pregnant women.

- You will have to work on promoting healthy bowel functioning as part of clearing up skin complaints. See "Constipation" earlier in this chapter.

- Make sure you have adequate essential fatty acids in your diet. Supplement with 1,500 mg of evening primrose oil daily and, in addition, take a high-quality fish oil supplement according to dosage recommendations on the package. EFAs can improve skin health by improving moisture and reducing inflammation.

## Herbal Recommendations

- For itching skin, prepare the following infusion using bulk herbs or, if unpalatable, herbal tinctures (the infusion is more effective for skin itching than the tincture):

    1 to 2 ounces each of echinacea root, burdock root, licorice root, and dandelion root (omit the licorice if there is hypertension). Steep 1 ounce total of the herbs in 1 quart of boiling water for 4 hours. Strain and take $^1/_2$ cup twice daily. For tincture, combine the above in liquid measure amounts, and take 1 teaspoon twice daily. Discontinue when the condition is improved.

- Rub cocoa butter on your body each day to reduce itching. Cocoa butter is also purported to prevent stretch marks, though to some degree these do seem either hereditary (in my practice, women of Italian descent seem to have the fewest) or related to the length of the torso (women with longer torsos seem to develop fewer). You can also use coconut oil, or the following blend that one of my clients came up with: to a base of almond oil add a few drops each of essential oils of lavender, rose, and tangerine, and rub on your belly each day.

- Calendula oil can be used to reduce itching and irritation.

- Slippery elm bark powder or marshmallow root powder can be sprinkled in the creases, such as on the "ledge" between your breasts and belly, to reduce chafing or rashes from heat and increased sweating.

- You can reduce stress-related itching with the use of nervine herbs as discussed in this chapter under the topics "Emotional Swings," "Fatigue," "High Blood Pressure," and "Insomnia and Anxiety."

## Ketones in Urine

(*See* "Urine Testing for Protein, Sugar, or Ketones")

## Late-Pregnancy Bleeding

(*See* "Bleeding, Late-Pregnancy")

## Leg Cramps

Leg cramps usually indicate that you need more minerals than you are getting: the muscles spasm because of inadequate calcium or magnesium, or from inadequate oxygenation caused by lack of iron. In addition, lack of exercise not only contributes to leg cramps but also decreases your body's mineral absorption. Overly vigorous exercise during pregnancy can also cause cramping. Leg cramps tend to be most annoying at night. Improve your mineral intake, get appropriate amounts of exercise, and learn to release tension in your muscles consciously. Not all women will experience obvious cramps but instead may have a vague, uncomfortable, restless, fidgety, pulling, or aching feeling in their legs. These are all symptoms of the same condition.

> Neesa was having severe leg cramps during the night. She began taking a calcium and magnesium supplement and within a few days the cramps ceased. She continued the supplement throughout her pregnancy and had no further problems with cramps.

*General Recommendations*

- When you get a leg cramp, stand up and place your feet flat and firmly against the floor, as if you are pushing your heels into the ground; then massage the cramped area vigorously and firmly. Another method is to flex your foot gently by holding onto it, curling your toes up toward your knee, and massaging your calf. This can be done while either standing or lying down. If you have varicose veins in that area, don't massage it.

- Avoid pointing your toes during pregnancy—it can start a cramp.
- Exercise daily by walking and doing leg exercises such as leg lifts and lunges. If at all possible, swim or exercise your legs in a pool of water.
- Elevate your legs periodically, preferably for twenty minutes a day, to improve circulation. You can put your feet up on a chair or lie down and put them up on two pillows.

## Dietary Recommendations

- Be sure you are getting enough calcium and magnesium in your diet (see chapter 5). These herbs can increase dietary calcium intake: nettle, dandelion leaf, oatstraw, chamomile, and all seaweeds, but especially kelp and hijiki. If your cramping is severe, add a calcium-magnesium supplement to your diet in a 2 to 1 ratio, that is, 600 to 800 mg calcium to 300 to 400 mg magnesium.
- Lack of salt can cause muscle cramps, so salt your food to taste with sea salt, and replenish salt lost through perspiration in hot weather or after exercise. Also take care to drink enough fluids.
- Vitamin E is also said to reduce cramping. Take 200 IU daily unless you have a heart condition or high blood pressure, in which case you should begin with 50 IU daily and gradually, over the course of a couple of months, work your way up to 200 IU daily. Foods high in vitamin E include whole grains, sunflower seeds, cold-pressed oils, eggs, molasses, wheat germ, and organ meats (obtained from organic sources only). Cooking destroys the vitamin E in foods, and eating cooked foods increases your body's need for vitamin E, so try to eat some foods daily that are rich in vitamin E and uncooked—for example, sunflower seeds and olive oil in a raw salad.
- Vitamin C deficiency may also be associated with leg cramps. You can take up to 2,000 mg in a supplement in addition to your food sources of this nutrient.

## Herbal Recommendations

- Include calcium-rich herbs as mentioned above as part of your daily diet. I've included two recipes for high-calcium brews.
- Herbal foot baths can relieve muscular tension. Soak your feet (and calves, if possible) in a very warm bath to which you add 5 drops of wintergreen oil, 2 drops

of camphor oil, and 2 tablespoons of ginger juice. (Grate about a 2-inch section of fresh ginger root and squeeze until the juice comes from it.)

- Foot and leg massage promotes muscular relaxation, improved circulation, and the release of nutrients stored in the muscles, all of which make it useful as prevention and first aid for leg cramps. The optimal time for a deep foot and leg massage is at bedtime, but it can be given anytime. Use massage oil that contains arnica, St. John's wort, and chamomile, or use a Chinese herbal liniment such as Dit Dat Jiao, an old remedy used for martial arts injuries (credit for this recipe goes to Michael and Lesley Tierra).

- Black haw or cramp bark tincture can be taken to reduce leg spasms. Take $1/4$ to $1/2$ teaspoon of either herb as needed, up to four times a day. In addition, drink teas or use tinctures made from any of these herbs: chamomile, lemon balm, catnip, lavender, and skullcap.

> NOTE: *Persistent leg pain, especially when accompanied by local heat or varicosities (swelling), can be due to phlebitis and merits the attention of an experienced health practitioner. If you suspect this problem, do not massage the area.*

---

### High-Calcium Tea

Mix 1 ounce each of nettle and red raspberry leaf with $1/2$ ounce of alfalfa and $1/8$ ounce of slippery elm. Prepare an infusion, adding $1/4$ ounce of the mix to 1 pint of boiling water, and steep for 1 hour. Sweeten to taste.

---

### Calcium Vinegar

Another high-calcium preparation that you can make at home is herbal vinegar. Take 1 ounce each of nettles, red raspberry leaf, and alfalfa and place in a quart-sized jar. Add 1 small bunch of chopped fresh dandelion leaves (available at most farmers' markets). For flavor, add a sprig of fresh rosemary and 2 to 4 cloves of chopped fresh garlic. Add 2 cups of apple cider vinegar, making sure that the vinegar reaches at least one inch above the herbs to prevent spoilage. Let sit for 2 weeks, shaking the jar once each day. At the end of the 2 weeks, strain, bottle, and refrigerate. Use on salads as a dressing, 1 tablespoon per day.

---

### Dit Dat Jiao

*6 parts angelica root*
*6 parts comfrey root*
*4 parts cinnamon bark*
*4 parts valerian root*
*3 parts hyssop*
*3 parts safflower petals*
*3 parts calendula blossoms*

Place the herbs in a wide-mouth jar and cover with 80- to 100-proof liquor (I use vodka) until the liquid rises two inches over the herbs. Cover the jar, store in a warm, dark place, and shake the jar daily for 2 weeks. Strain and bottle for use. This liniment is absolutely for external use only and should be labeled clearly. It warms the skin, dissolves clots and congestion, stimulates circulation, soothes, and heals. Be aware that it may stain fabrics.

# Minor Illnesses

(*See* "Colds, Flu, and Mild Illnesses")

# Miscarriage

Miscarriages, pregnancies that end spontaneously, usually before twenty-eight weeks' gestation, occur in about 20 percent of all pregnancies in the United States. As cited in *The Encyclopedia of Childbearing* by Barbara Katz-Rothman, each year in the United States between 600,000 and 800,000 women miscarry. Many women miscarry very early in pregnancy, without ever realizing they were pregnant, having what appears to be a heavy period. Miscarriage rates are highest for young teenagers and middle-aged women (especially when pregnancy has been accomplished with the use of reproductive technologies), and they are more common in early pregnancy than after the first trimester. For women who want to be pregnant, particularly those with a history of repeated miscarriage, losing the pregnancy and the baby is a devastating experience. Many women fear that something is wrong with them as women or that they did something to harm the baby. Because of our culture's refusal to talk about miscarriage, few women know what to do or what to expect when it happens.

If you are experiencing cramping and/or bleeding because of a threatened miscarriage, you can do a number of things to prevent the miscarriage from becoming inevitable if the baby is healthy. The recommendations that follow are in no way harmful to the baby if the baby is otherwise healthy. As blunt as this may sound, miscarriage is nature's way of preventing unhealthy babies from being carried full term. This is painful for the woman to accept, but it may spare the baby a life full of adversity. Our bodies have a wisdom of their own. It is important to realize that attempts to prevent miscarriage will not be effective if the baby is not healthy.

Other causes of miscarriage include hormonal imbalances, cervical looseness (called an "incompetent cervix" in the medical world—I detest this term), infections, and nutritional deficiencies. Many of these conditions can be improved naturally.

## *Preventing a Threatened Miscarriage*

A miscarriage is threatened when you experience spotting, bleeding, or cramping, often with a low backache. These symptoms may begin abruptly or slowly and will usually persist for hours or even days. You may experience some spotting or bleeding and that is the end of the whole episode, or the symptoms may be so severe you will fear you are going to lose the baby. At this time the cervix will be closed, but an internal exam is best avoided, as it is unnecessarily intrusive and may stimulate the uterus further. Chances are you will still feel pregnant, with continuing breast tenderness and nausea, but you may feel anxious and question whether you are really feeling these signs or you just want to feel them. Most often, if you still feel pregnant, then you are. While I am opposed to the routine use of the doppler (an electronic device used to hear the fetal heartbeat), in this situation it can be very reassuring. Usually at about ten to twelve weeks, the baby's heartbeat can be heard with the doppler. A midwife can do this test at home. Of course, if the doppler is tried earlier, the heartbeat may not yet be audible and this could unnecessarily discourage the mother. An ultrasound can also confirm the baby's wellness or indicate otherwise.

## General Recommendations

- You may have to come to terms with whether in your heart of hearts you really want to be pregnant or whether you or your partner have fears, anxieties, or ambivalence about having a baby. We can influence our receptivity to a baby in our wombs. In no way does this mean that all miscarriages are a result of ambivalence, because the baby's health certainly influences its ability to maintain life. But your desire to continue the pregnancy will support your efforts.

- On a spiritual level, you can communicate your desire to have the baby, also giving the baby permission to go if he or she needs to. Both partners can place their hands on the mother's belly, directly over the womb, and speak to the baby, either aloud or silently. Let your hearts flow with your feelings of love for the baby and for each other, particularly if there is strain between you. Your bond as a couple can strengthen the bond between you and the baby and can aid your efforts to arrest a miscarriage. This can be a strong time of healing.

- As part of making clear your intention for the baby to stay, you can set up a small pregnancy altar in your home on the top of a dresser or bed table or even on a sunny windowsill. You can go to this special place to send loving thoughts to your baby and visualize your womb surrounded with protection. On this altar, place objects that remind you of healthy babies, healthy pregnant mothers, and families: pictures, small statues or figurines, a healthy plant, a stone egg, candles, or anything else that arises from your imagination.

Marley had been hav-
ing aching in her
bones all night, had
dark puffy circles
under her eyes, and
had vomited in the
morning. She had no
appetite, severe leg
cramps, pelvic pres-
sure, aching in her
lower back beneath
her ribs, and a tem-
perature (oral) of
99.2°F. She was thirty
weeks pregnant (third
baby) and was having
mild, irregular con-
tractions. She began
taking echinacea at a
high dose, along with
an infusion of uva-
ursi, increased fluids,
vitamin C, and cran-
berry juice. Within
twenty-four hours, all
symptoms subsided,
and there was no
recurrence. Marley
gave birth at home at
forty weeks' gestation.

- Treat yourself with the utmost love and care. This is a trying experience that may also challenge your faith in your body. Try to love your body and don't blame yourself for miscarrying.

- If you are having contractions or bleeding or spotting, get off your feet and rest. Try to get up only if you need to use the bathroom. Take time to visualize the baby as healthy, your placenta as strongly connected to your uterus, and your body providing love and nourishment to the baby. Avoid lifting heavy objects and abstain from sexual activity until all signs of miscarriage have been gone for a week. Think positively and use relaxation techniques to help you rest and to reduce anxiety-ridden thoughts.

- Warm baths (not hot) can reduce uterine irritability and bring some relief to low backache. A warm bath is also a great place for relaxing and having a good cry to release pent-up feelings.

## Dietary Recommendations

- For the prevention of miscarriage, it is very important that you avoid all cold-natured and cold-temperature foods, including foods that have just come out of the refrigerator; cold or iced beverages; fruit and veg-etable juices; all tropical fruits, including citrus (unless you live in an environment where they are grown locally); and all foods out of season, including fresh salads when locally grown produce is not available. I've seen a consistent connection between the intake of "cold" foods and the onset of threatened miscarriage. In traditional Chinese medicine, there is a notion of cold as a downward-moving, heavy force, so perhaps it is not unreasonable to think that such substances could cause an excess of downward flow in the pelvic region. As a practical matter, it takes a certain degree of warmth in the womb, not unlike incubating eggs until they hatch, to create the conditions necessary for the optimal health of a baby. Cold-natured substances may cause warmth needed in the womb to fluctuate, destabilizing the environment.

- It follows that it is preferable to eat foods of a warmer and nourishing nature, such as soups. Miso soup, prepared from a protein-rich paste of aged soybeans, is excellent, as are chicken soup and bean soups. Also, emphasize whole-grain stews and hot cereals, root vegetables, and dark greens until your symptoms have been gone for at least a week. Warm tea or water at room temperature can be taken as a beverage.

- Vitamin E (alpha-tocopherol) has been said to strengthen the placental attachment to the uterus, thereby reducing spotting and the likelihood of miscarriage. It should be taken in doses of up to 800 IU each day for up to three weeks. However, prolonged use may result in the placenta becoming abnormally attached to the uterine wall, a complication in itself. Therefore, do not exceed this dosage, and do not take vitamin E for longer than three weeks. If you have heart disease, do not exceed 50 IU per day without discussing it with your physician.

- Vitamin C plus a bioflavonoid complex—that is, along with the whole group of vitamins that naturally occur with vitamin C in foods—strengthens the capillary bed of the uterine lining, reducing the likelihood of miscarriage. You can take up to 1,000 mg daily, including the amount that is in your prenatal multiple vitamin. High doses of vitamin C—in excess of 2,000 mg—can cause a miscarriage, so do not exceed the recommended amount.

- Be certain that you are getting adequate protein, carbohydrates, vitamins, minerals, and fluids. Thoroughly read the section on nutrition in chapter 5.

## Herbal Recommendations

- Miscarriage Prevention Tea (see page 232) seems to be so effective in preventing miscarriage that midwives across the nation recommend it in one formulation or another. Variations on the theme follow here.

- Partridge berry tones the uterus while also causing uterine relaxation, reducing cramps and contractions. It also supports the nervous system, perhaps helping to reduce the anxiety and apprehension associated with a threatened miscarriage.

- Cramp bark and black haw have very similar actions on the uterine muscles, relaxing them and reducing the severity of contractions. They also have some relaxing effects upon the nervous system, making them appropriate choices in a formula for preventing miscarriage. One herb may be substituted for the other, or the two may be used together.

- False unicorn root contains steroidal saponins, precursors or building blocks of our sex hormones. For this reason, it is an excellent hormonal balancer as well as a specific uterine tonic, making it applicable for threatened miscarriages. It may be particularly helpful to women whose progesterone levels are low, but it can be taken by anyone who is bleeding and cramping in the first trimester. Because it is an endangered plant, it should be used only when absolutely necessary, and for environmental conservation should only be purchased from cultivated, not wild harvested, stock.

- Chasteberry helps to increase progesterone levels so that the pregnancy can be sustained, most probably by causing the pituitary gland to increase the progesterone levels so necessary for the maintenance of pregnancy.

- Lobelia, a strong sedating herb, is used in this formula specifically for reducing uterine contractions, and also for calming the nerves. In high doses, however, it is potentially toxic. It is important to avoid exposing the developing baby to excessive doses of this herb. In the amount in this formula, you are unlikely to experience side effects. If you do notice nausea, strange feelings, scratchy throat, or low blood pressure, immediately reduce the amount of lobelia in your formula by half or omit it completely.

- Ginger root is added for its mildly stimulating and warming properties, and also for the taste it imparts to the infusion, which is not particularly delicious.

---

### Miscarriage Prevention Tea

Mix 1 ounce each of partridge berry, cramp bark or black haw, false unicorn root, and wild yam, as well as $1/4$ ounce of lobelia and $1/8$ ounce of dried ginger root (you may have to break the root into small pieces so it mixes evenly throughout the blend). Take a total of 1 ounce of the mixture and place it into a quart-sized jar. Completely fill the jar with boiling water, cover the jar, and let the tea steep for 4 hours. (If you need it quickly, you can begin to drink it after 2 hours.) After steeping, strain the liquid and drink between $1/4$ and $1/2$ cup every 2 hours. If you are cramping a lot, you can drink this brew by taking a mouthful every 15 minutes.

- In my practice, I mix these herbs in tincture form. This is the most convenient form for the taking the herbs consistently, and it eliminates the problem of taste as the tea is less than a delicious beverage. Combine the tinctures as follows:

> 1 ounce cramp bark or black haw (interchangeable)
> 1 ounce chasteberry
> 1 ounce wild yam
> $1/2$ ounce partridge berry
> $1/4$ ounce lobelia
> $1/8$ ounce ginger

Mix all of the tinctures together. This combined tincture can be taken $1/2$ to 1 teaspoon twice daily for preventative care in women with a history of miscarriage. If symptoms of miscarriage begin (cramping, spotting), the dose should be increased commensurate with the severity and frequency of contractions, in a dosage range and frequency from $1/2$ to 1 teaspoon every 15 minutes to every 2 hours until symptoms have abated.

If you have a history of miscarriage, use this formula for at least two weeks past the latest weeks of pregnancy when a previous miscarriage occurred (that is, if a previous miscarriage occurred at eight weeks' gestation, stay on the formula until ten weeks' gestation). For current symptoms of miscarriage, continue on the formula for one week past the end of the symptoms, using a more moderate dose of $1/2$ to 1 teaspoon two to three times daily.

## When Miscarriage Continues

Not every miscarriage can be stopped. My heart goes out to those of you whose baby is unable to stay with you right now. It is my hope that you will find peace and inner strength in this experience and not blame yourself.

When a miscarriage is inevitable, the bleeding and cramping will not stop until all the products of conception (the tissue that was the developing fetus, the placenta, and the uterine lining that is shed) pass from your body. If the pregnancy ends in the first couple of weeks, it will seem like a normal to heavy period. The further advanced the pregnancy, the more noticeable will be the signs of miscarriage and the more effort you will need to make to clear everything out. Inevitable miscarriage can be suspected when cramping becomes more intense and inconsistent, and the bleeding becomes heavier, to the point of soaking through your clothing or pads. At this time, the cervix will usually be dilating, will be shorter than usual, or will be slightly bulging. It is not necessary for you to check your cervix—I offer this information to those who are familiar with how their cervix feels.

How you choose to handle a miscarriage is a very personal decision. Most women who allow nature to take its course and who receive support through the process will miscarry with no complications. However, miscarriage should not be taken lightly, carrying as it does risks of hemorrhage and infection. The follow-up procedure at the hospital is generally a dilation and curettage, which carries the risk of damaging the womb, or a vacuum suction. Any time you enter the hospital, you are exposed to a host of pathogenic germs unlikely to be encountered in most homes. Also, certain exams and interventions are routine in hospitals. Each woman and each situation must be evaluated on an individual basis and with an open mind, common sense, and a healthy dose of caution.

Your vitality and coherence as well as how long and how much you've been bleeding are good indications of how you are doing. If you feel very weak, strange, or spaced out, or have been cramping heavily (experiencing strong pain, much more than a normal period) and bleeding steadily for more than two hours without emptying the contents of your womb, then going to the hospital is probably warranted. If you are having a lot of cramping but are not bleeding heavily, you can probably continue to take a wait-and-see attitude until you complete the miscarriage or unless bleeding becomes heavy.

> **WARNING:** *If at anytime you become spaced out, fuzzy, incoherent, unusually anxious, sleepy, clammy, or begin to look pale, you need to get to the hospital immediately. These can be signs of shock, which is life threatening.*

If everything seems normal and you choose to stay at home, or if you are unable to reach medical services, the following information will often help to complete a miscarriage at home. Again, if at any time you notice the above signs, seek emergency medical care.

A miscarriage is similar to any birth in that the uterus, in the effort to empty its contents, goes through contractions that build in intensity until it completes the process. However, a normal miscarriage tends to have more continuous bleeding than a normal birth. Women who are miscarrying have not yet experienced the blood volume expansion that usually occurs at about twenty weeks, and therefore are not protected against blood loss. The amount of bleeding in a miscarriage can vary from mild to severe, and depending upon a woman's health reserves, she can become very weak from blood loss.

Therefore, if you are miscarrying, you should not remain alone. Always have with you someone who can get you to the hospital—and stay in close contact with someone who is knowledgeable about the process, such as a midwife or nurse-practitioner.

At some point during the process, you will pass the tissue that was the fetus as well as the placenta and the sac of membranes that surrounded the fetus. Since you will also be passing clots, you will want to save any such matter for a closer look, in order to determine if you have in fact emptied your womb. A womb not fully cleared out predisposes you to continued bleeding, cramps, and the risk of serious infection. You can look at the tissue yourself (it can be fished out of the toilet if necessary) and try to determine if you see any tissue that looks like a small sac (ranging from about the size of the bowl of a teaspoon to the bowl of a tablespoon, depending upon how early in the first trimester you are). It will be milky white or clear, with some light pink tinges. Clots are more like gelled masses of blood, with some stringiness from the clotting factors that cause the blood to bind. You may find other matter as well, such as small vesicles that look like grapes—a sign that a baby never developed after conception. (This requires medical attention.) Saving any material that you pass for analysis by your midwife or physician can help you and them determine whether the miscarriage was complete.

A miscarriage may build up for several days or even weeks before it actually is complete, with cramping and spotting building in intensity. The actual miscarriage, with regular cramping and heavier bleeding, usually takes place within a couple of hours. After the tissue has been passed, cramping and bleeding will subside, though you may have some more contracting and will definitely bleed some afterward. This will be about the length of time of a regular period, about five days. Heavy bleeding at any time (soaking a pad within thirty minutes is very heavy bleeding) or bleeding persisting for more than five days may mean that pieces of tissue are retained in the uterus. Until the womb is emptied, it cannot completely clamp down, hence the continued cramping is an effort to do so, and the bleeding is a sign that something is preventing this from happening.

> **WARNING:** *Retained tissue can cause serious, life-threatening infection. If natural treatment recommendations (below) for completing a miscarriage are not effective in the first days after the miscarriage, or if at any time your temperature becomes elevated or you notice a foul-smelling vaginal discharge, you should seek immediate medical help.*

In some cases a D & C (dilation and curettage) is the best recourse. Sometimes a physician can simply prescribe Methergine (an ergot-rye fungus derivative), used historically by midwives but now available only by prescription. An antibiotic may be warranted if infection is present.

## General Recommendations

- Have an experienced or a very responsible person with you at all times until your miscarriage is definitely completed. A miscarriage is completed when bleeding and cramping stop and the uterus has passed the products of conception.

- Take it very easy throughout the miscarriage, but do not go to sleep if you are bleeding—drowsiness can be a signal of shock.

- Drink fluids regularly, a cup of liquid every one to two hours, to keep your blood volume expanded. Rehydration Drink (see page 283) can keep your electrolytes and minerals in balance, as can such drinks as Recharge, Third Wind, and Gatorade. Remember to urinate regularly; a full bladder can aggravate cramping and prevent effective emptying of the uterus.

- Keep yourself warm and comfortable.

- Visualize your cramps effectively emptying your womb. Surround your uterus with light, and imagine the placental tissue releasing from your uterine wall and from your body.

- Have somebody massage your feet or your lower back, especially applying firm pressure to the area over your sacrum. A hot-water bottle applied to this area can also be comforting.

- As painful as this is for you emotionally and physically, try to remember that your body knows how to do this job. Listen to what your body is telling you.

## Herbal Recommendations

Herbs can be used to encourage complete emptying of the uterus, prevent hemorrhage and infection, help reduce anxiety during the process, and promote healing afterward. Before using herbs, it is essential to have definitive confirmation that the baby is no longer alive. You'd be amazed at how much women can bleed and cramp and still have a completely healthy pregnancy. Get ultrasound confirmation before using these herbs. Further, these herbs are not recommended for deliberately stimulating an herbal abortion—they do not work well if there is a viable fetus and can be toxic to a healthy baby.

- Perhaps the most widely recommended herbs for facilitating a miscarriage are blue and black cohosh. Additionally, cotton root bark is excellent and reliable for safely, gently, and effectively promoting contractions. Combined, these three herbs help regulate uterine contractions, reducing spastic muscle contraction and promoting an effective labor. Black cohosh is also an effective nervine, reducing anxiety as well as physical tension. During a miscarriage, tinctures are the most effective and convenient form for taking these herbs.

  To use: combine 1 ounce each of cotton root and black cohosh tinctures, and $^1/_2$ ounce blue cohosh tincture.

  Day 1: Take 1 teaspoon of the above combination every 4 hours. Discontinue.
  Day 2: Take 1 teaspoon of the above combination every hour for 4 hours. Then take $^1/_2$ teaspoon of the tincture every 30 minutes for 4 hours. Discontinue.

  Uterine contractions will usually ensue by the end of the second day, if they have not already. They sometimes ensue several hours after the herbs have been discontinued, so don't be discouraged if they do not occur immediately.

  If after two days of using the herbs no contractions begin, skip a day and then resume, following all of day 2 one more time.

- A combination of bayberry bark, shepherd's purse, and witch hazel in the form of tinctures or infusion can be taken to prevent or offset heavy bleeding after a miscarriage. Combine equal parts of the tinctures and take $^1/_2$ teaspoon every hour if there is mild to moderate bleeding.

  NOTE: *Herbal remedies may help prevent excessive bleeding but are not a substitute for medical care during hemorrhage. If there is heavy bleeding, obtain medical care immediately.*

- Beth root is another excellent herb for promoting uterine contractions and reducing bleeding. It may be added in equal parts to the above formula, or it can be taken on its own, $^1/_4$ to $^1/_2$ teaspoon of tincture every two hours to promote contraction or as often as every fifteen minutes during the acute stage of the miscarriage if there is bleeding.

- You can sip a tea of basil or of cinnamon throughout and after the miscarriage to promote contractions and prevent excessive bleeding. Steep 1 teaspoon of either herb in 1 cup of boiling water (cover while steeping) for 10 minutes.

- If the miscarriage is proceeding efficiently and the main problem seems to be anxiety, sip tea of chamomile and lavender blossoms (2 teaspoons of herbs combined in equal parts to 1 cup boiling water, steeped covered for 10 minutes).

## After a Miscarriage

When the miscarriage is complete, your immediate concerns are infection and bleeding. Much healing needs to occur in the first weeks, then a longer-term physical healing over the following months, and, for some women, an emotional healing that can take years. When you miscarry, your body must make a hormonal adjustment from a pregnant to a nonpregnant state, and you must make an adjustment in your view of yourself. It is important that you give yourself the time to treat yourself gently during the transition. Essentially, you have gone through a birth without getting a baby.

During the first few days after your miscarriage, you can expect to bleed as if you have your period, and you may pass some small clots.

> **WARNING:** *If after four or five days you are still bleeding, or if at any time you are soaking a medium-sized sanitary pad in thirty minutes, you must seek immediate medical attention. Also, if you are passing large clots, have a lot of cramping, or notice any foul-smelling discharge, you probably have retained tissue and possibly have an infection, and need prompt medical attention.*

## General, Dietary, and Herbal Recommendations

After a miscarriage, it is advisable to use herbs that work to prevent infection, facilitate the discharge of retained tissue, and promote the healing of your uterus. A general program for the first three days after miscarriage is as follows:

- Check your temperature three to four times each day. It should be normal (close to or at 98.6°F).

- Get plenty of rest, eat nourishing foods such as hearty soups and stews, and drink plenty of fluids. If you have lost a considerable amount of blood, refer to "Anemia" above.

- Take 2,000 mg of vitamin C over the course of each day as a preventative measure against infection.

- Take 1 teaspoon of echinacea tincture four times daily to stimulate your immune response and as a preventative against infection. Other herbs that can be used in conjunction with echinacea to prevent infection include calendula tincture (10 drops with each dose of echinacea) or goldenseal tincture (10 drops with each dose of echinacea) or capsules (2 "00" capsules four times daily). Both calendula and goldenseal also promote uterine contractions and act as astringents to prevent hemorrhage.

- Angelica has a reputation for helping to clear the uterus of any retained fragments and is also a warming uterine tonic. Take 15 to 20 drops three times daily to ensure complete uterine emptying, and increase that dosage to as frequently as every two hours if you are having cramps and are passing clots. Ground ivy is another tincture with this reputation, and, though I've not used it for these purposes, herbalist Susun Weed recommends it highly for retained placenta after birth. Do not use it to prevent miscarriage, but if you are still cramping and passing clots, take 20 to 30 drops of fresh ground ivy tincture every two to three hours.

- Change your menstrual pad every couple of hours to avoid infection from bacteria in the pad. Be sure to wipe from front to back after you have a bowel movement to prevent rectal bacteria from entering the vulva and causing infection.

- Refrain from all sexual activity until the bleeding has completely stopped. If anyone needs to examine you (your midwife or doctor) make sure that he or she does so with sterile hands. Do not take a bath (you can shower) for the first few days.

- It is essential that you seek a trusted person to help you work out your grief, disappointment, and guilt.

- While you cannot use any substances, including herbs, to heal your grief, a few herbs can help you steady your emotions. If you are unable to rest, you can drink warm teas of chamomile and lavender combined, adding, if you wish, up to 20 drops of motherwort, hops, or skullcap tincture (or a combination of these to equal $1/2$ to 1 teaspoon total). You can also take these as tinctures up to three times a day. Other herbs that support the nerves and promote gentle relaxation include oatstraw, rosemary, lemon balm, catnip, and valerian.

> **Women's Nourishment Tea**
>
> Mix together $1/2$ ounce each of red raspberry leaf, nettle leaf, strawberry leaf, dandelion root, spearmint leaf, skullcap, and $1/8$ ounce of ginger root. Store this dry mixture in an airtight jar or plastic bag. To prepare the tea, place $1/2$ ounce of the mixture in a jar, add 2 cups boiling water, and let it steep for 2 hours. Strain and drink $1/4$ to $1/2$ cup of this brew 3 to 4 times a day for 6 weeks after the miscarriage.

After the first week, you will probably begin to feel more like your prepregnant self, with all signs of pregnancy gone, particularly if the miscarriage was early. Herbs that nourish the female reproductive system, including those that help to regulate the hormones and the menstrual cycle, can be used to assist you in this transition: red clover leaves and blossoms, red raspberry leaves, chasteberry, false unicorn root, wild yam, calendula, dong quai, ginseng, and licorice. A small amount of ginger root or cinnamon bark can be added to infusions to facilitate the actions of the herbs, while warming your pelvic region and promoting healthy circulation.

Chinese herb formulas such as Tang Gui and peony can be used to restore strength and build the blood if there has been much blood loss. Recommendations for anemia can be followed, particularly taking beef stew and using Iron Tonic Syrup (see page 173), if there is weakness from blood loss.

This is naturally a painful time for many women, especially if this was your first pregnancy or if you have a history of miscarriage. People who are unaware that you miscarried may ask how the pregnancy is going. You will have to adjust your view of the future, which recently included the expectation of a baby. Miscarriage can also add stress to your relationship with your mate. At the time most women miscarry, the pregnancy may not have felt "real" to the father. He may not take your emotional response to the miscarriage seriously, saying that you can simply try again. For many women, these responses are, in the least, insensitive. The idea of trying again and possibly experiencing such disappointment again is unbearable. For the sake of the relationship, the dad needs to be deeply sensitive to and supportive of his partner. He must listen to you and offer love without dismissing your pain. If you are both deeply grieved and disappointed, this can be a time of holding each other closely and reaffirming your commitment to being a family. If this miscarriage makes the relationship more difficult or intensifies or makes more apparent the stresses you were already having, you may want to consult a professional to help both of you work through the crisis together.

## *Preventing Future Miscarriages*

After having miscarried once, many women are eager to conceive, yet fearful of miscarrying again. In the vast majority of cases, repeated miscarriage is not likely, but it is best to wait until you've had at least three regular periods in a row before you conceive again. By doing so, you allow your uterus to regenerate fully at the implantation site and replenish your blood supply if you bled a lot during the miscarriage. The delay will allow you to experience your next pregnancy as a fresh experience. It really is better not to try to fill the void of your lost pregnancy with another one, but to heal your loss and then embrace your new experience. Books and support groups can assist you in integrating your miscarriage into the experience of your life.

Whether or not you went into your previous pregnancy well prepared, now is a time for getting yourself into excellent health. Creating a pregnancy altar, for example, can give you a place to affirm your desire to have a healthy pregnancy and a healthy baby. The work of creating a gift for your baby, such as a quilt, can give you a concrete way to manifest your intention.

If you don't have children, this is a time to be completely honest about whether you want to become a mother right now. If you already have children, be honest about whether you want another child. Discussing these issues openly with your partner can clear the air and help you make the decision.

If you decide that you do want to become pregnant again, you can use herbs to support the pregnancy and prevent miscarriage. These are basically the same herbs used to prevent a threatened miscarriage and may be taken both before you conceive (begin taking them up to a month before you try) and then into your first trimester, preferably until two or three weeks after the time of your last miscarriage or throughout the whole first trimester. This is the basic formula: 1 ounce each of wild yam, partridge berry, and false unicorn root; $1/2$ ounce of cramp bark or black haw; $1/4$ ounce of red raspberry leaf. Combine all of these herbs and store in an airtight jar or plastic bag. Place 4 to 6 tablespoons of the mixture in a quart jar, fill with boiling water, and steep until the tea is cool enough to drink. Strain out the herbs and drink $1/4$ cup four times daily. (If you begin to miscarry, refer to "Preventing a Threatened Miscarriage" earlier in this section.) If you find it difficult to prepare or carry these herbs with you each day, use tinctures. Mix together (in a small bottle with a dropper) equal parts of wild yam, partridge berry, false unicorn, and cramp bark, and take 20 drops two to four times daily, the frequency depending upon your miscarriage history. If you've had more than one miscarriage, take the herbs four times daily. Also, if you have such a history, begin taking these herbs for up to two months prior to conception, and consider seeking an experienced doctor of traditional Chinese herbal medicine and acupuncture. The combination of both approaches can be very effective for preventing miscarriage and strengthening you for a healthy pregnancy.

# Morning Sickness

Women experience different degrees of morning sickness ranging from no problem at all, to very mild discomfort, to nearly constant nausea and vomiting during the first trimester or longer. I once heard it said that the reason it is called "morning sickness" is because it starts in the morning and lasts all day. Actually, morning sickness can occur at any time of the day or night. Generally, this nausea begins around six weeks into pregnancy and persists until the fourteenth week. It is triggered by different factors:

- Empty stomach, hunger, low blood sugar (hypoglycemia)
- Strong smells (fumes, food cooking)
- Hormonal surges and imbalances
- Normal pregnancy-related changes in the digestive system
- Oily foods
- Very sweet, sugary foods (which for some women may include fruits)
- Vitamin or mineral deficiencies
- Lack of exercise
- Fatigue
- Stress
- Constipation
- Ambivalence or anxiety about pregnancy

Nausea that persists much longer than the fourteenth week is usually related to insufficient nutritional intake, unresolved emotional issues, or, rarely, a health problem. If you are experiencing persistent nausea past your first trimester, please seek the help of an experienced health-care practitioner who is knowledgeable about the nutritional needs of pregnant women.

There is much speculation as to what actually causes morning sickness and why some women experience it while others don't. Theories include hormonal fluctuations, emotional reactions to pregnancy, nutritional factors, and biological mechanisms that cause women to reject substances that may cause the babies harm. It has been suggested that women who do experience morning sickness have a greater likelihood of a healthy pregnancy and a healthy baby and a decreased incidence of miscarriage. But as yet, no one has come to a definitive conclusion. Medical attempts to reduce morning sickness through medication have not proven safe for the fetus. The only advice I can give is to avoid eating stuff that prompts nausea, and at the same time improve your eating habits.

Pregnancy-related nausea is not dangerous, but if you are vomiting excessively, you (and the baby) run the risk of dehydration and severe malnutrition. The condition occasionally requires hospitalization and rehydration with intravenous fluids. (See "Vomiting, Severe" later in this chapter for a further discussion of severe nausea and vomiting during pregnancy.)

## General Recommendations

- Normal physiological changes of early pregnancy, such as increased levels of estrogen and progesterone, hormones that maintain pregnancy, cause body tissue to become soft and more engorged, and promote such changes as breast enlargement and milk production. They also cause the entire digestive system to slow down and become "softer." The processing of these hormones (equivalent to one hundred birth control pills a day) in addition to these changes can lead to nausea. Moreover, the softening and slowing down of the digestive tract increases the likelihood of constipation, which aggravates nausea; and the incredible amount of work being done by the body causes first-trimester fatigue, which can reduce the likelihood of your eating well, also instigating nausea. By staying well rested, eating well, and taking other precautions to prevent constipation, you can minimize nausea.

Nancy was very nauseated all of the time and was unable to find appetizing, easy-to-digest foods that satisfied her hunger. She'd been a vegetarian for many years, but I had a strong feeling that chicken might settle her stomach and satisfy her. I asked her if she'd consider eating chicken soup, and at this point she was ready to do just about anything. Her husband prepared her a pot of chicken vegetable soup. The chicken broth was immensely satisfying; she ate the meat and vegetables, and began to feel much better. Occasionally, such flexibility can make a tremendous difference in morning sickness.

- Avoid smells that nauseate you. Don't walk near busy roads if exhaust nauseates you; ask someone to fill your gas tank; let your partner, friends, or relatives help you in the kitchen; and don't prepare those foods that are distasteful to you (by smell, sight, or taste). Often just the smell of a particular food (or a few foods) will completely turn the stomach of a pregnant woman.

- Lack of cardiovascular stimulation—exercise—can contribute to nausea because greater levels of acids and carbon dioxide will build up in the blood. A brisk walk in fresh air or some form of exercise daily can reduce the severity of nausea. Regular exercise also reduces fatigue and prevents constipation. Eating a snack about a half hour before you plan to be active will help prevent nausea or low blood sugar. It is also essential that you eat well after exercising to replenish lost calories, particularly if the exercise is strenuous. If exercising triggers nausea, try regular massage, a form of passive exercise.

- You can reduce nausea by getting plenty of rest, using relaxing herbs, and asking for help with your responsibilities if you are fatigued. Perhaps you can think of at least one or two people who will watch your older kids or help with household chores.

- Ambivalence about the pregnancy can cause internal tension that may exacerbate feelings of nausea, and vice versa. Even women who are completely thrilled to be pregnant may have misgivings. It is important to acknowledge and accept your feelings rather than feel guilt for these emotions. Worrying that you are harming your baby with your negative thoughts only adds to your tension. Talk to friends, other pregnant women, or a midwife or counselor; use a journal as an outlet for your concerns. It is perfectly normal to go through a time of uncertainty—children are a great responsibility. Perhaps there are steps you can take to enjoy your pregnancy. If your ambivalence is triggered by the nausea, know that this too shall pass and you will soon begin to enjoy your pregnant body much more.

- Nei guan patches or bracelets (for example, Sea Bands), special devices available from acupuncturists and at many health food stores that put pressure on acupuncture point PC-6, have been clearly demonstrated in clinical studies to reduce nausea associated with pregnancy. They are completely safe and therefore worth the try.

# Dietary Recommendations

- Eat small, frequent snacks that contain complex carbohydrates and protein. A simple snack of a cheese sandwich on whole-wheat toast will quell hunger, prevent blood sugar from dropping with ensuing nausea, and is quick and easy to prepare. Other suggestions are tofu sandwiches, bean or chicken noodle soup, pasta dishes, yogurt with granola, peanut butter on toast with a topping you enjoy, hummus on toast, chips, crackers, or vegetable sticks. Eating snacks about every two hours is less likely to trigger nausea and vomiting than a few large meals a day; in doing so, you will prevent your stomach from becoming empty. Eating a snack such as crackers or toast when you first wake in the morning can reduce the nausea caused by stomach acids in an empty stomach. Some women find that a grapefruit or a small cup of fruit juice just before a meal gets the digestive juices going just enough to help food go down. Breakfast, or its lack, can set the tone for your entire day, so be sure not to skimp on it.

- Many women wake in the night and find themselves unable to return to sleep. This is frequently due to unrecognized hunger; the baby takes nourishment from you even while you sleep, causing you to become hungry at odd hours. Try eating a snack before bed and, if necessary, in the middle of the night. This may seem odd, but you'll find yourself sleeping more restfully. Yogurt makes an excellent before-bed or middle-of-the-night snack, as does toast, a banana, a handful of almonds, or any food that you enjoy and that digests easily.

- Always carry nutritious food with you whenever you go out. Skipping food for as little as two hours during early pregnancy can cause you to feel extremely nauseated and depleted. Hypoglycemia—low blood sugar—can trigger not only nausea but also dizziness, headaches, hot flashes followed by cold sweats, anxiety, and fainting. A mix of nuts and seeds, a container of yogurt, or even small containers of food can keep you feeling well. Don't tide yourself over with caffeinated beverages or candy bars—you won't be providing yourself or your baby with any nutrients, and you'll still end up feeling nauseated in the long run. There is no need to feel embarrassed about eating in public wherever you are, even if no one else is eating.

- Many pregnant women find that drinking fluids aggravates nausea, but actually dehydration causes worse problems. You need to drink plenty of liquids throughout the day. If you are vomiting, you are losing fluids; you must replenish them. Water with a squeeze of lemon, natural grape juice, grapefruit or orange juice, or carbonated water with a squeeze of lemon are all choices that may be palatable and settle your stomach. Avoid coffee, soda, and other caffeinated or sugar-laden drinks. Taking sips of liquids throughout the day may be easier than drinking glassfuls at a time.

- Oily foods are hard to digest. Sweet foods may lead to a quick blood sugar drop after their initial energy boost, leaving you feeling nauseated and drained. Choose foods that are prepared by steaming, water-sautéing, or baking; choose foods that contain complex carbohydrates. These will sustain your energy level in a more balanced way and are also easier to digest, helping you avoid nausea. See chapter 5 for a discussion on nutrition.

- Nutritional deficiencies—too little iron, vitamin B-complex, magnesium, or calcium—as well as too little protein or complex carbohydrates can cause morning sickness. Perhaps you didn't really notice these deficiencies until your body had the increased nutritional demands of pregnancy. Consider taking a vitamin and mineral supplement designed for pregnant and lactating women. See chapter 5 for more information.

   Unfortunately, supplements may aggravate nausea in the first trimester. If this is the case, avoid taking supplements on an empty stomach; instead, try taking them while eating. Some women have found that taking between 50 and 200 mg of vitamin $B_6$ daily can alleviate nausea because it helps regulate blood sugar levels. This is safe. Once you have gotten past the nausea stage, you should take vitamin B-complex, not just $B_6$ by itself. Another remedy is to take 50 mg of vitamin K once daily, and 250 mg of vitamin C twice daily.

## Herbal Recommendations

During my pregnancies, I would try something for nausea and that would work for a few days. But I would quickly become tired of a certain herb and keep changing. Play around with different approaches to see what works for you.

- Ginger is by far the best-studied herb for the treatment of nausea and vomiting in pregnancy, having been demonstrated effective in numerous clinical trials. It can improve sluggish digestion and gently warms the digestive tract. It is pleasant tasting when sweetened lightly with honey. Steep 1 teaspoon of freshly grated ginger root in 1 cup of boiling water for 10 minutes and sip throughout the day, not exceeding 2 full cups daily. Or take 2 "00" capsules of powdered ginger every few hours, but do not exceed 10 capsules per day.

Sucking ginger-flavored hard candies or crystallized ginger can also be help-ful. Look for these in a health food store.

> **CAUTION:** *Ginger is considered an emmenagogue, that is, it can stimulate menstrual flow in large amounts. Therefore, excessive use (more than one to two grams a day) is not recommended. Do not use if you have a history of miscarriage, and do not exceed the dosages mentioned above.*

- Dandelion root is one of my favorite herbs. A bitter, it promotes digestion, calms and strengthens the stomach, improves the appetite, and supports the liver, which must work overtime during pregnancy to process the increased quantity of hormones surging through you. All of these functions of dandelion root plus its safety during pregnancy make it an excellent choice for morning sickness either alone or in combination with other herbs, such as ginger root. To prepare an infusion, use 4 to 6 tablespoons of the dried roots or twice that amount of the fresh roots in 1 quart of boiling water, and steep for 4 hours. Strain and take mouthfuls at a time, up to 2 cups daily. Or take 30 drops of tinc-ture three or four times a day.

- Chamomile tea is another of my personal favorites. It relaxes the stomach, reduces acidic feelings, supports the liver, and improves appetite. It also reduces anxiety and tension. Prepare by steeping 1 tablespoon of the herb in 1 cup of boiling water for 10 to 15 minutes. Cover while steeping to retain the volatile oils in the blossoms. You can sip it throughout the day or drink up to 2 cups daily.

- Many herbs in the mint family, including peppermint, spearmint, catnip, and lemon balm, will reduce digestive upsets. To prepare any of these teas, steep a heaping teaspoon of the dried leaves or 2 teaspoons of fresh leaves in 1 cup of boiling water (steep with the cover on to retain volatile oils) for 15 minutes. Occasionally women find that strong mint teas actually aggravate nausea. This is probably due to the nature of the plant, which causes a strong rising up of the body's energy, and the oil, which relaxes the sphincter between the stomach and the esophagus. Most women find the scent of peppermint beneficial, how-ever. You can place 1 or 2 drops of peppermint oil on a small piece of cloth and smell it periodically, or, if you have access to the fresh plant, crush a few leaves between your fingers and smell it as needed. I always found this to be helpful on long car rides, which terribly aggravated my nausea during pregnancy.

- Wild yam is an herb that reduces irritation and irritability in the hollow organs, including the stomach and the uterus. It is an excellent herb for reducing nausea, relieving vomiting, and relieving spasms in the stomach. The dosage is up to 30 drops, 4 to 6 times daily. Combined with dandelion root (30 drops of each), it has proven very effective for reduction of nausea and vomiting.

Other remedies that can be useful for morning sickness include

- Ginger ale or carbonated lemon water, plain or to which you add 20 drops each of ginger root tincture and dandelion root tincture.
- Umeboshi (sour plum) candies, available at natural food stores (the sweet-and-sour taste of umeboshi can allay nausea).
- A warm bath to which you add essential oils such as lavender and rose or a few drops of sandalwood.

In addition, some women gain relief from Chinese herbs and acupuncture or acupressure treatment. For information on Chinese therapeutics for pregnancy, you may wish to consult *The Path of Pregnancy* by Bob Flaws, listed in the bibliography.

# Protein in Urine

(*See* "Urine Testing for Protein, Sugar, or Ketones")

# Sciatica

(*See* "Backaches and Sciatica")

# Skin Troubles

(*See* "Itchiness and Skin Troubles")

# Stretch Marks

Silvery jewelry draped on the belly of Woman, adorning her and reflecting her ability to grow and change—this is how I view stretch marks. Some women develop stretch marks; others don't. Various factors may be involved: heredity, nutrition, tissue strength, the elasticity of your skin. There are no definitive answers.

Most women do not want stretch marks any more than they want sagging breasts. Our society tells us that flat bellies, perky breasts, and tight flesh are sexy and beautiful. Unfortunately, these characteristics are present in young women who have not borne children. They are associated with a sexual ideal that few women actually approach even before childbearing. The body after childbearing is typically not considered beautiful in our culture, although in others, for example the Mbuti pygmies of Africa, pendulous breasts are respected because they reflect the fact that a woman has nourished her community through her very flesh. In fact, the more a woman's breasts sag, the greater her status in the community. It is time that we, as active participants in our culture, take pride in our individual form, shape, and markings, and help change society with our values.

Women are often advised to massage their bellies with cocoa butter or other oils to prevent stretch marks. This is all well and good. It may be effective, but it is not loving yourself to rub your belly with the intention of preventing stretch marks. To love yourself, rub your belly and breasts with awe at the amazing accommodation your body is giving to your growing baby. Babies can feel this attention and they love it! Praise and admire yourself, and you will be rewarded with self-respect, whether or not you develop stretch marks.

Oils and herbs that are nourishing for the skin include cocoa butter, pure almond oil or wheat germ oil, shea butter, and herbal oils made with chamomile, orange, lavender, calendula, rose petals, and comfrey. You can make a wonderful belly and breast massage oil by mixing a few handfuls of any of these herbs in a pint jar with 2 cups of an oil of your choice. If you wish to use cocoa butter, use half oil and half cocoa butter, and carefully cook the mixture over a double boiler for twenty to thirty minutes because cocoa butter is hard at room temperature. Cover the jar tightly and let sit on a sunny windowsill for one week. Strain the oil into another jar, and it is ready for use. You can add a few drops of an essential oil for fragrance, if you wish, and 400 IU of vitamin E as a preservative and skin nutrient. See appendix I, Herbal Preparations, for further instructions on making herbal oils.

# Sugar in Urine

(*See* "Urine Testing for Protein, Sugar, or Ketones")

# Swelling

Mild swelling of the feet and ankles is considered normal as pregnancy advances and may actually signal that blood volume has expanded enough to meet the needs of the pregnancy. Some women do not swell at all, and as long as they've gained weight adequately, have plenty of amniotic fluid, and anemia is not a problem, that is also fine.

I pay attention to the severity and constancy of the swelling. "Healthy" swelling is usually mild, occurs mainly in the feet and ankles, and tends to come and go—appearing more after you've been on your feet a lot or at the end of the day, and going down a good deal after you rest and in the morning when you've just awakened. Swelling that is present all the time, swelling that leaves an impression on your leg a few seconds after you press on it, or swelling that particularly occurs in your face and hands that is visible the first thing in the morning may be signs of toxemia. This section addresses only normal physiological swelling, but you can use these suggestions in conjunction with other therapies for more specific conditions.

## General Recommendations

- Elevate your feet for twenty minutes, three to four times each day. Put them on pillows to get them above the level of your heart to improve circulation. The weight of your uterus on your blood vessels impedes venous return, causing blood and fluid to collect in your lower body. Allowing this circulation to freely return to your heart not only reduces swelling but also can be invigorating and lift depression.

- Lying on your left side while you sleep or rest can also improve circulatory function, thereby lessening swelling.

- Exercise for thirty minutes a day. Pelvic rocks, leg lifts, and gentle yoga can enhance circulation and reduce swelling. See the bibliography for books on yoga and exercise during pregnancy.

## Dietary Recommendations

- Be certain that your diet contains plentiful amounts of high-quality protein and adequate salt plus all the other nutrients you need. Inadequate intake of protein and salt is linked to toxemia. Without this adequate intake, your cells cannot retain fluid, and you will have swelling from the seepage of fluid into the interstitial spaces (the spaces between the cells). Pregnancy is a time to eat foods salted to taste. Be certain to compensate for salt lost in perspiration either in hot weather or after exercise, and use only sea salt, available at natural food stores.

## Herbal Recommendations

- Soak your feet in a warm bath, using $^1/_2$ cup of Epsom salts in a basin, or 1 cup in the bathtub, high enough to cover your feet. To the Epsom-salted water, you can add lavender flowers, rose petals, sprigs of rosemary, or drops of wintergreen oil.
- Get a regular foot massage. Arnica oil rubbed into swollen areas reduces soreness and aching in muscles and joints. Your mate or friend can easily give you a foot massage as you sit together. Perhaps have your partner rub your feet before you go to sleep at night. (Lie on your left side to enhance effectiveness.)
- Drink a nettle and dandelion leaf infusion, 1 to 2 cups daily, or take $^1/_2$ teaspoon of each of these tinctures twice a day to improve general circulation, help the kidneys remove and retain the appropriate amounts of fluids for your body, and improve your overall nutritional status.

If you have persistent swelling, speak with your care provider for further suggestions. Do not accept diuretics and salt-restricted diets as your solution as they are almost always inappropriate for pregnant women. Consult books by Anne Frye and Gail and Tom Brewer (see bibliography) for further discussion of the problems associated with these treatments.

# Toxemia

I would like to thank midwife and author Anne Frye for her remarkable work to educate and enlighten midwives and other related health professionals on the key issues underlying toxemia and on the very real ways we may address and prevent this serious health problem with excellent prenatal care. I am also indebted to her commitment to restore healing and empowerment to all women whether pregnant or in their work as midwives, and her gracious permission to incorporate her research into this section.

Toxemia, formally called "metabolic toxemia of pregnancy," or "preeclampsia," is a serious condition, the consequences of which include placental insufficiency (insufficient nutrients get to the baby, resulting in undernourishment and low birth weight), placental abruption (the placenta separates prematurely, which predisposes the mother to hemorrhage and is often fatal for the baby), premature birth, complicated births, and, if untreated, eclampsia, a complicated stage of the disease that can lead to seizures and liver damage for the mother, and even her death. In short, it is not a condition to be ignored or taken lightly.

The causes of toxemia have been related to a few factors, including heredity, faulty implantation of the placenta, and poor nutrition.

Toxemia is usually diagnosed when three main symptoms—high blood pressure, swelling, and protein in the mother's urine—occur together. Women can have one or two of these signs and may or may not be at risk. In fact, women who exhibit only one or two of the symptoms may be at risk for toxemia, but it may be overlooked as a possibility in part because toxemia symptoms often do not become apparent until the third trimester. Other symptoms may indicate toxemia: severe and persistent nausea past the first trimester, poor appetite, headaches, poor weight gain, upper abdominal pain, blurry vision or seeing flashing lights before your eyes, feeling "lousy," and persistent hypoglycemia.

If your baby seems small for its gestational age and you have symptoms of toxemia, you certainly should consult your health-care provider. It is always wise to determine the origins of your symptoms. If you are eating an excellent diet and feel otherwise healthy and vibrant, and the baby is growing steadily, you are unlikely to have or develop toxemia.

Any woman who is having trouble obtaining high-quality nutrients (meaning adequate protein, carbohydrates, vitamins, minerals, fluids, and salt) is at risk for toxemia. Pregnant teenagers, poor women, underweight women, and exercise-conscious women are at higher risk. If you fit into any of these categories, you should eat well and discuss any eating problems with your midwife or obstetrician.

While all of this may seem rather grim, the good news is that the incidents of toxemia appear to decrease in those who receive excellent prenatal care, both the care you give to yourself and the care you receive from others.

The guidelines in this section are for the prevention of preeclampsia, and therefore you would be wise to read them carefully before you exhibit symptoms.

WARNING: *Should toxemia develop, begin following these suggestions immediately and get medical help.*

# Dietary Recommendations

- Inadequate nutrition is the common denominator in toxemia. Read the information on nutrition in chapter 5, and follow the suggestions for creating an ideal diet diary.

- Make sure you get between 60 and 100 grams of protein per day. (See chapter 5 for a full discussion of protein and nutritional sources.) Protein is essential for healthy cell functioning and proper kidney functioning. It is also essential to help the body maintain fluid in the cells. Women who get enough protein rarely develop toxemia.

- Complex carbohydrates are essential for energy, blood sugar stability, and healthy weight gain. Eat whole-grain foods at all meals and as part of snacks during pregnancy.

- You must obtain enough salt to maintain the blood volume you and your baby need. Salt-restricted diets can actually lead to toxemia. You need extra salt as well as extra protein and carbohydrates if you exercise regularly.

- Vitamins and minerals are also essential. You should get them from organic foods and herbs, and take nutritional supplements when necessary.

- Junk foods are an express ticket to poor health. They keep you from eating nutritious foods because their high sugar or fat content causes you to feel full. Teach yourself about healthy eating. Your health and your baby's health depend upon it!

- Healthy absorption of nutrients is as important as healthy eating. Regular constipation or frequent diarrhea is a sign that your intestinal health needs direct attention. See "Constipation" earlier in this chapter. For diarrhea, mix equal parts of slippery elm bark powder, marshmallow root powder, licorice root powder, and cinnamon powder. Place in "00" capsules and take 2 capsules three times a day, preferably just before meals. Try this for one week and discontinue when your bowels are no longer loose.

- An excellent nutritional supplement for pregnant women is spirulina. This superfood is a blue-green algae with high protein, vitamin, and mineral content.

---

### Spirulina Smoothie

In a blender, combine 1 cup of naturally sweetened vanilla yogurt; 1 tablespoon of spirulina; 1 or 2 bananas; 1 tablespoon of peanut, almond, or sesame butter; and if in season, a handful of blueberries or strawberries. Blend well at a high speed and enjoy.

---

It is harvested from lakes where it occurs naturally. The dosage is 2 tablespoons of powder or 15 to 30 tablets (depending on the particular brand you choose) daily. Powdered spirulina can be added to smoothies to disguise the taste. (It will turn your smoothie an interesting shade of green!) Spirulina Smoothie is a nutritious recipe even kids will drink.

## Herbal Recommendations

- The liver and kidneys are the two organ systems most likely to need support for preventing toxemia. Weakness of these organs seems to play a role in the development of toxemia, and these organs are likely to be further damaged if it arises. Liver and Kidney Wellness Formula can be taken daily for toxemia prevention and for restoring health if you seem at risk for this condition (take 2 cups daily).

- Nettle infusion can be taken as well. Drink 2 cups as a beverage in addition to the above formula. Dandelion greens, which are highly nutritious and beneficial to health, can be added to the diet as a lively tasting green, steamed or used in salads.

---

### Liver and Kidney Wellness Formula

Mix together the following tinctures: $1/2$ ounce each of nettle leaf, schisandra, American ginseng, dandelion root, and burdock root; and $1/4$ ounce each of passionflower and linden. Take 1 teaspoon one to two times daily as a general tonic for the kidneys, liver, and nervous systems.

---

## Urinary Incontinence

Involuntary leaking urine (urinary incontinence) can happen when you sneeze, cough, jump, or perform any physical exertion. It can vary in amounts ranging from a small dribble to a deluge wetting your pants. It is a common problem in America. Women who have already borne children are particularly susceptible to developing incontinence because the muscles of the pelvic floor stretch during birth. Further pregnancies will aggravate this tendency because pregnancy increases urination and because the uterus places a great deal of pressure on the bladder. Incontinence is not inevitable, however. In fact, it is quite preventable. In addition to urinary dribbling, you can also prevent uterine, bladder, and rectal prolapse (see the bibliography for an article I wrote on this subject), maintain long-term pelvic health, and improve your sexual experience.

The levator ani is a muscle group, commonly known as the pelvic floor, that forms a sling extending from the back of the pelvis to the front and supports all the pelvic organs and structures, including the uterus, bladder, vagina, urethra, and rectum. When the muscles forming this sling become weakened, they are less able to support these organs, and signs and symptoms of weakness begin to appear, one of the earliest and most common being urinary incontinence. At the first sign of this, do pelvic floor exercises to improve the tone of your muscles. If you wait until you have severe incontinence or prolapse of your organs, you will have to work much harder to improve tone.

Pelvic floor exercises, generally referred to as "Kegel exercises" after the physician who originally popularized them, are a nonsurgical method of healing urinary incontinence. Chapter 7 offers specific exercises that are beneficial for the prevention and healing of pelvic floor weakness, including incontinence. Follow these exercises each day. With commitment, you will see improvement after a few weeks, even if you begin during pregnancy.

I have no internal recommendations for incontinence, although you may wish to try a sitz bath with astringent herbs such as witch hazel and nettle to help tighten the outer muscles and tonify your tissues.

# Urinary Tract Infections (UTIs)

The urinary tract consists of the kidneys, ureters, bladder, and urethra. Growing a baby places an additional load on these organs. Hormonal changes that soften the ureters, along with the weight of the womb upon them and the bladder, increase the likelihood of stasis, or stagnation, in your bladder or ureters, which breeds bacteria that can lead to infection.

Bladder infections (cystitis) can nearly always be treated at home with natural remedies. Beginning treatment at the earliest symptoms is optimal. Symptoms include extrafrequent urination (it's normally somewhat frequent during pregnancy), often accompanied by burning or pain ranging from subtle to severe; low abdominal tenderness just above the pubic bone; recurrent Braxton-Hicks contractions (the contractions normally occurring during pregnancy that you may or may not have noticed); flulike feelings; and, in some cases, vaginal bleeding ranging from mild to severe. A kidney infection (pyelonephritis) is evidenced by fever, chills, backache, and a worsening of the previously mentioned bladder infection.

> **WARNING:** *Left untreated, a bladder infection can easily become a kidney infection. Kidney infections can place the mother's health in danger, so the care of an experienced health professional should be sought immediately.*

Persistent UTIs can increase the risk of premature labor. You should always be screened for this if you are having a lot of premature uterine contractions or have a history of premature labor. If you experience persistent urinary tract infections, you will want to do more than address each individual bout; you will need to tonify your urinary organs and also improve your overall immunity. You may also want to have a vaginal culture for possible beta-strep infection, a bacteria that many women carry around with no symptoms and that can lead to UTIs, premature labor, and neonatal infection. A high blood sugar level can also predispose you to UTIs, as can recent overconsumption of highly sweetened foods; see "Sugar in the Urine" below. You may not have sugar in your urine, but the dietary and herbal recommendations in that section will likely be useful. Consultation with a Chinese herbalist may provide help in preventing these repeated infections.

Refer also to "Vaginal Infections" below for recommendations. Because the urethra (the entrance to the bladder) is located just above the entrance to the vagina and not far from the rectal opening, bacteria can easily spread to the bladder.

Many times women who have chronic urinary tract infections have underlying anger that seems to correlate with UTI recurrences. I've always gotten a chuckle out of the common expression for anger—"pissed off"—realizing that language arises from our subconscious mind as much as from our literal or analytic minds. Language can be revealing. Look within yourself about anger you may have, and if this registers, take the steps that will help you address and express your anger or resentment so you can resolve your problems without internalizing them as illnesses.

## General, Dietary, and Herbal Recommendations

The following program has repeatedly assisted pregnant women in clearing up UTIs. It must be followed diligently.

- Dramatically reduce your intake of all sugars—sugar breeds bacteria.

- Be sure to urinate as soon as you feel the urge, and empty your bladder thoroughly. When you hold urine too long, it can serve as a breeding ground for bacteria. Too many women are accustomed to putting off urinating until they can no longer wait. This is an unnecessary and health-defeating habit based on not listening to our bodies and making external tasks more important than the body's needs. When you've got to go, go!

- Take echinacea root tincture, 1 drop per every 2 pounds of body weight every four hours until symptoms are gone, then 20 drops three times a day for a few more days to prevent recurrence. Echinacea is antimicrobial, it is an immune-system tonic, and it reduces inflammation.

- Cranberry juice, an old wives' remedy for UTIs, has been clinically demonstrated to be effective as an antimicrobial agent in the treatment of bladder infections, preventing pathogenic bacteria from adhering to the wall of the bladder. Eight ounces of unsweetened cranberry juice, or diluted cranberry juice concentrate, should be taken every four hours, along with four 8-ounce glasses of water each day, for a total of 64 ounces of fluid. This will dilute your urine, so that it is less burning. It also dilutes and flushes out the infecting organisms.

  One way my family enjoys cranberries is to combine ¹/₂ cup of frozen cranberries in the blender with 1 cup unsweetened apple juice and 2 cups water. We also put cranberries and fresh apples through our juicer for a refreshing, mildly tart drink very high in vitamin C. Take this high dosage for three to five days; then, when the infection is gone, continue to drink cranberry juice once a day for at least a few days.

- Take 500 mg of vitamin C four times each day for three to five days. Vitamin C encourages acidification of the urine, helping to kill bacteria and is also a reputable resource for helping the body resist and overcome infection.

- Uva-ursi is a leathery-leafed bush that provides a medicine known to act on urinary tract infections,

> Suzanne was experiencing insomnia, frequent urination, nausea, low backache, mild discomfort in her lower abdomen, and a slightly elevated pulse. She followed dietary and herbal protocols for the treatment of a urinary tract infection, and also began to take a relaxing nervine tea in the evening, including chamomile, lavender, and skullcap. Within two weeks, all symptoms of the UTI had cleared up and she was sleeping restfully.

working specifically as an antimicrobial and gentle diuretic. It is a highly effective remedy for cystitis. It can also be used for mild kidney involvement, but any signs of pyelonephritis require medical attention. Uva-ursi contains a chemical constituent called "arbutin" that transforms into another chemical called "hydroquinone." Hydroquinone is considered toxic and thus uva-ursi should not be used during the first trimester unless under the supervision of a highly qualified practitioner, and should only be used for short durations (five days or less). Unlike standard antibiotics, the use of uva-ursi for UTIs does not lead to recurrent bladder infections, nor does it lead to problems with yeast infections as so often happens with prescription antibiotics.

To prepare uva-ursi, place $\frac{1}{4}$ cup of the leaves in a quart jar along with $\frac{1}{4}$ cup of marshmallow root (an herb that is soothing to the urinary tract) and fill the jar with boiling water. Some herbalists say that this herb is more effective when steeped in cold water, and you can certainly do this, but I've found that hot water makes an effective remedy. Either way, remedies directed to the urinary system are most efficient when drunk at room temperature or slightly cool—hot herbal teas encourage perspiration, whereas cool teas encourage urination. Let steep for 2 hours, strain, and use. The dosage is $\frac{1}{4}$ cup every four hours for subtle signs of a UTI, $\frac{1}{2}$ cup every four hours for obvious symptoms, and 1 cup every four hours for a raging UTI. Do this until symptoms abate, decreasing the dosage as symptoms subside, but continuing to take 1 cup a day for five days at the maximum. For chronic UTIs, the effectiveness of the uva-ursi may be enhanced by taking 2 "00" capsules of baking soda three times daily.

- Wild yam is a urinary tract antispasmodic, reducing pain and inflammation. Take $\frac{1}{2}$ teaspoon of tincture, two to four times daily, along with other herbal treatments if there is bladder pain, spasm, or associated uterine contractions accompanying the infection.

## Urine Testing for Protein, Sugar, or Ketones

These are not complaints specific to pregnancy, but this section is included here because urine tests for these substances are an almost universal, routine part of the prenatal exam and every woman should know what they reveal.

In urinalysis, chemically coated test strips are dipped in a sample of urine. (That's why a midwife or a nurse in a physician's office will ask you to urinate in a cup.) After thirty to sixty seconds, the colors on the strip will change according to the reaction of each chemical with substances in your urine. Most commonly looked for are protein, sugar, and ketones, as well as a few other substances such as leukocytes and nitrites, both of which can indicate a urinary tract infection. In my practice, I usually have mothers check their own urine at their prenatal visits rather than handing it over to a technician. I want to give the women a better opportunity to understand the results. This section explains the significance of the three main substances I have mentioned and provides recommendations should you come up with "positive" test results.

Urinalysis is a simple, noninvasive method for evaluating kidney functioning as well as dietary intake of carbohydrates and proteins. It can be an excellent tool for detecting an imbalance before a disorder arises. At this point, an emphasis on excellent nutrition and natural therapies can strengthen the mother, thereby averting a later health problem. Nevertheless, these tests are no substitute for the common sense and intuitive awareness you should bring to your observation of your health. This advice should hold for your health-care practitioner, too. If an imbalance shows up, it should lead to further investigation and to a decision as to what care would be beneficial.

During pregnancy our bodies are working much harder—we are literally eating and eliminating for two. This places an increased load on the kidneys, which control blood volume and remove wastes from the blood. According to the philosophy of traditional Chinese medicine, the kidneys play an important role in fertility, conception, pregnancy, and longevity; therefore, the child's healthy development, as well as the mother's continued wellness, will be influenced by the healthy functioning of the kidneys.

## Protein in the Urine

Usually the urine of a healthy pregnant woman will not contain protein. If, however, urinalysis indicates the presence of protein, it's possible that the protein is actually from vaginal discharge mixed into the urine. This is not uncommon. Protein occurring in conjunction with dark, concentrated urine indicates that the mother is not drinking enough fluids. Pregnant women need to drink close to two quarts of fluid a day to keep their blood volume expanded, their kidneys from becoming taxed, their bowels from becoming constipated, and, of course, the baby adequately surrounded by amniotic fluid. Adequate fluid intake even helps prevent depression.

A urinary tract infection may also cause the presence of protein in urine. Usually there will be nitrites (a by-product of the breakdown of bacteria in the urinary tract) and leukocytes (white blood cells) as well. Often the mother will have symptoms such as lower back or lower abdominal pain, contractions, flulike feelings (chills, achiness, mild depression, or fatigue), soreness beneath the back ribs, frequent and possibly burning urination, and occasionally even vaginal bleeding. A urinary tract infection is usually highly responsive to natural remedies (see page 262), but kidney infections often require medical attention.

Other possible contributors to the presence of protein in urine are heavy physical activity, long periods of standing up, carrying twins, severe high blood pressure, and toxemia. If you must do heavy physical labor during pregnancy, it is very important to wear some form of abdominal support and to be certain you are eating enough. If at all possible, you should cut back on heavy work. If you are carrying more than one baby, you must also be certain to eat adequate amounts of protein and carbohydrates, and you may also want to wear a body support designed for pregnant women. (Such supports are available at maternity shops and via the Internet from maternity clothing companies.) The symptoms of toxemia are high blood pressure, swelling, and protein in the urine (usually an amount of "plus 2"), but these signs in themselves do not necessarily indicate preeclampsia or toxemia. However, one can have toxemia without classic signs. Where toxemia is not the problem, herbal remedies may improve kidney functioning and reduce excessive swelling and the amount of protein in your urine.

## Sugar in the Urine

The greatest medical concern regarding the presence of sugar in the urine (glucosuria) of a pregnant woman is that it is an indicator of diabetes. There is an enormous amount of debate in the medical and midwifery communities over this condition, which is linked with high levels of blood sugar, very large babies and the attendant risks of birthing larger babies, and "unexplained" fetal deaths. Nevertheless, it is perfectly normal for pregnant women to have a lower kidney threshold that allows more sugar to be spilled in the urine. Sugar in the urine leads many health-care practitioners to insist upon testing blood glucose levels. But this test does not necessarily mean that a woman is diabetic. In fact, even a slightly high result from a blood sugar test (glucose tolerance tests or one-, two-, or three-hour postprandial or after-meal testing) does not always imply diabetes. A common cause of glucosuria is the recent consumption of foods with a high sugar content, even those containing natural sugars like fruits and juices, and even sweet, high-carbohydrate items like granola or pancakes with syrup. Consequently, a practitioner is left with the question of how to interpret the sugar in the urine, and what to do about it if it is consistently present, especially if it is high.

In my own clinical experience, I have seen mothers who have had consistently high levels of glucose in their urine (up to "plus 4" at three successive prenatal visits) but who reduced their levels of urinary glucose to zero simply by making dietary changes. All these women, when tested in a medical setting for blood glucose levels, had normal levels according to a one- or two-hour postprandial test—after eating a high-sugar meal, their blood levels were tested after either one or two hours—and had normal pregnancies and babies with no unusual difficulties at the birth. This is not to say that health-care practitioners should ignore the possibility of gestational diabetes. However, greater attention may need to be paid to factors that influence its development, and therefore factors that can prevent it. Of course, if you find that you consistently see high glucose levels despite preventative measures, and the baby seems exceptionally large, you may choose to investigate further with a nonfasting blood glucose test, particularly if you have evidence of regular yeast or urinary tract infections that are also unresponsive to treatment or reoccur despite dietary and other measures. Other common symptoms of diabetes include frequent thirst and lack of weight gain or actual weight loss in spite of a voracious appetite.

> **Ruby was having high levels of glucose appearing in her urine test ("plus 3" sugar) at several consecutive prenatals. Prior to her fourth visit, she agreed to eliminate most sugars from her diet, including fruit and natural sweeteners, and she daily took a strong infusion of nettles. Within one week, her urinary sugar levels were completely normal; not a trace of sugar was present.**

There is overwhelming evidence that the use of routine glucose testing for pregnant women is an unnecessarily invasive procedure that is best reserved for situations in which the need for the test is clearly indicated. Fasting or loading up on concentrated amounts of sugar, as in a glucose tolerance test, is not good for a pregnant woman. Speak with your midwife or physician about alternatives if a blood test seems necessary to rule out gestational diabetes. Request that a first morning blood sugar be drawn or a one-hour postprandial be done early in the morning after you consume a high-carbohydrate meal (like a large amount of pancakes with maple syrup for breakfast). These methods put the least nutritional stress on both you and the baby. I encourage you to read the sections on gestational diabetes in Anne Frye's books *Understanding Lab Work in the Childbearing Year* and *Holistic Midwifery* and bring the well-researched, thoroughly documented information in her books to the attention of your care provider. In addition, you may want to try the nutritional and herbal suggestions later in this section, which can be effective in preventing gestational diabetes and will strengthen your kidneys and improve your general wellness.

## Ketones in the Urine

The body of a well-nourished pregnant woman is supplied with energy by the regular intake of a high-carbohydrate and protein-rich diet. When the intake of food becomes inadequate, the body must burn fat to supply energy until food sources again become available. Ketones are a product of the metabolism of fat and occur when the body suffers nutritional deprivation. This may be the result of fasting or inadequate nutritional intake, or a great deal of physical energy being expended and not replenished, such as during vigorous exercise and labor. If you have ketones in your urine (ketonuria), you are not eating enough or you are not eating frequently enough. This condition is often signaled by symptoms of hypoglycemia (low blood sugar): extreme and sudden hunger accompanied by shakiness, nausea, cold sweat, feelings of faintness, slurred speech, a vague sense of dread, and extreme exhaustion. After you eat, you may feel the need to rest or even sleep. If these symptoms continue, serious health problems can emerge for both you and the baby.

The treatment, quite logically, is to eat more high-quality foods, eat more often, and drink plenty of fluids! The exception is when ketones and glucose are occurring together, which is an indication of diabetes. Although this condition may also be nutritionally related, it does require further consideration and testing. In either case, it is essential that you focus on learning more about your nutritional needs during pregnancy and take steps to improve your diet—not just what you eat but how much and how often. In addition to the suggestions given below, see chapter 5 and refer to the bibliography for books on prenatal nutrition.

## General, Dietary, and Herbal Recommendations

- If you have only a trace of any of the above substances on just one test, then really nothing needs to be done other than to consider the possible causes. For example, if you have a lot of vaginal discharge, you may have a trace of protein show on the "pee stick" (as they are fondly called). If you ate a sweet breakfast or drank a large cup of juice before an early morning visit, that could easily account for sugar in your urine. Similarly, if you worked out or skipped a meal before your urine check, that is the likely explanation for ketones. In this case, you need to eat extra food before and after your workout to compensate for the extra burning of calories so you don't develop ketonuria.

- A trace of protein occurring on a regular basis could be due to an abundance of vaginal discharge, a urinary or vaginal infection (see appropriate sections in this book), or weakened kidneys.

- If sugar is consistently present in your urine, you will want to work on your diet and observe whether the changes you make have influenced its level. To do this, you need to reduce your consumption of sugar in all forms for three days. This includes eliminating fruits and fruit juices, bakery-type products, and any products containing sweeteners—anything that is sweet or readily breaks down into simple sugars. Your diet should consist of whole grains, preferably rice, millet, and other grains; high-protein foods such as beans, nuts and seeds, hard cheese, fish, and poultry (organic whenever possible to avoid contaminants); and plenty of fresh vegetables. After three days, recheck your urine. If there is just a trace of sugar or none at all, you can most likely avoid further testing and continue on this type of diet with the addition of one or two pieces of fresh fruit daily. You can periodically check your urine to see if it is affected by the intake of sugary foods and if it is negative when these are again eliminated from your diet. If the dipstick still shows a high sugar result in spite of your dietary efforts, a blood test may be warranted. Refer to the suggestions below for herbs that can be used along with dietary changes to improve kidney functioning and regulate blood sugar.

- Perhaps the most effective and yet gentlest herbal ally for nourishing and strengthening the kidneys during pregnancy is the humble nettle plant. This herb is reputed to restore health to damaged kidneys, improve the kidney filtration process, tonify the kidneys, regulate blood sugar, ease fatigue, improve the functioning of the adrenal glands and the thyroid, reduce stress, and provide a rich banquet of minerals. Taken daily, nettle can reduce both protein and sugar in the urine, reduce swelling and varicosities, and alleviate low backache, urinary tract infections, circles under the eyes, damp feet, and other signs of compromised kidneys. A preventative dosage is 1 cup of nettle infusion daily, and a therapeutic dosage is up to a quart daily. I prepare a dark green nettle brew—à la Susun Weed, who told me she makes her nettle infusion so strong that the spoon stands up by itself in the cup—by steeping a handful of nettle herb in a quart of boiling water. (More than once I've been asked, "What's that green stuff you're drinking, Aviva?") I leave the herbs in the jar rather than straining them out, and I just sip off the top as the leaves gradually sink to the bottom over the course of the day. This drink has a flavor similar to a liquid chlorophyll supplement. For a milder brew, you can steep $^1/_4$ cup of nettle leaf in a quart of water for 30 minutes or up to 2 hours, and then strain out the herbs and drink the infusion. It will keep in the refrigerator overnight and is delicious with the addition of a dash of tamari soy sauce or umeboshi plum vinegar, a salty and sour Japanese seasoning available at health food stores. Nettle may also be obtained in freeze-dried form, which some claim to be highly effective (see resources).

# Vaginal Infections

Engorgement of the vulva with increased blood circulation and hormonal changes that alter the balance of vaginal acidity cause vaginal infections and heavy mucous discharges, a common complaint of pregnant women.

Drugs, such as metronidazole, used to treat common vaginal infections such as candida (yeast) are often not safe for developing babies, so you would be wise to avoid them.

Some vaginal infections, such as chlamydia and beta-strep, can be asymptomatic (or at least some women may be unaware of the symptoms) yet pose a health threat to a baby born vaginally in the presence of these organisms. For example, chlamydia can lead to respiratory infections and blindness in newborns. While this is rare, you may choose to have vaginal cultures taken during your pregnancy to see if you have any such infections and discuss the findings with your midwife or another care provider. It may or may not be necessary to take precautionary steps before or during labor to prevent transmission of an infection to the baby, or you may be informed of specific symptoms to look for in your baby after birth.

> **WARNING:** *If you suspect that you have gonorrhea or syphilis, especially evidenced by vaginal or vulvar lesions or discharge, or if you have had a positive test for either of these infections, seek medical treatment as soon as possible—before the birth of your baby. The risks of these diseases outweigh the risks of treatment.*

## General and Dietary Recommendations

- Drink plenty of fluids, especially water. Lemon juice and herbal teas are also good.

- Wear cotton underwear or none at all. Synthetic fibers trap moisture in the crotch area and provide an excellent breeding medium for many organisms. You may even need to change cotton underwear by midafternoon if it gets damp from discharge or sweat.

- Wear loose-fitting cotton clothing; try not to wear pantyhose, especially those without a cotton panel in the crotch.

- Avoid all concentrated sugars, including honey, maple syrup, and corn syrup.

- Avoid caffeine, including coffee, caffeinated sodas, chocolate, and black tea.

- Don't use bubble bath, bath oils, bath salts, or strongly perfumed soaps in your bath or around your vulva.

- Use white, unscented toilet paper.

- Don't use any "feminine hygiene" or douche products.

- Practice excellent personal hygiene: Wipe from front to back after a bowel movement. Rinse your vaginal area with water (no soap) during the day, then pat dry, to reduce the likelihood of bacterial or fungal growth.

- Bacteria spread readily in heat and moisture. Dry yourself gently but thoroughly after bathing or swimming. Change out of wet swim clothes soon after swimming. Change undergarments and launder (with a mild detergent) frequently. Use 1 cup of white vinegar in the rinse cycle of your washer to remove soap residue, acidify garments, and disinfect and remove any remaining body fluids.

- Don't scratch your crotch. Scratching will further irritate the area and spread the infection.

- Avoid intercourse during the worst symptoms or if painful. Your partner may also need to be treated to prevent reinfecting you. Men can harbor asymptomatic infections that you then pass back and forth, and your attempts at eliminating the infection will be ineffectual.

- Use some form of natural lubrication during intercourse, such as almond or coconut oil. Urinate after sex and thoroughly rinse yourself off with warm water.

- Take 500 to 1,000 mg of vitamin C complex (with bioflavonoids) daily as a preventative or when infections occur.

- Eat plenty of live-culture plain yogurt each day to both prevent and treat vaginal infections. This is especially good when you are under stress or when you must take antibiotics. (Let your doctor know if you are prone to yeast infections before you take antibiotics.)

- Cut back on simple carbohydrates (starches and sugars, including processed flour and fruits and fruit juices).

- Eat nutritious meals that emphasize whole grains, vegetables, and high-quality protein foods. Reduce the amount of sweets in your diet while you are treating vaginal infections. Eliminate sweets altogether if you are prone to such infections. This includes reducing the amount of fruit you eat (get your vitamins and minerals from extra vegetables) and using rice, oats, millet, and other whole grains in place of yeasted breads whenever possible. These dietary changes alone can often clear up a yeast infection.

- Reduce stress in your life as much as possible. Get adequate rest. Infections thrive when your body is run-down.

## Yeast Infections

*Candida albicans* is the fungal organism that causes what is commonly known as a yeast infection. All women have this organism in their bodies, but various circumstances, such as the increased vaginal discharge that accompanies pregnancy (especially if you wear clothes that prevent adequate aeration of your vulva), changes in vaginal pH, increased consumption of carbohydrates, and stress and fatigue, can lead to the overgrowth of yeast. Symptoms of a yeast infection are itching and redness of the genitals; white, thick, yeasty-smelling discharge that may look curdy like cottage cheese (but might be slight); burning of the vulva; and painful intercourse. There may be frequent urination or even an attendant bladder infection caused by irritation of the urethra. Symptoms range from mild to severe, with itching and burning being the most noticeable.

If you have no history of yeast infection, the problem will likely clear up with no treatment at all as soon as the baby is born and can simply be kept under control with simple dietary and herbal treatments. If you have a history of yeast infections, continue treatment after birth if they persist. Occasionally, a woman who has a yeast infection may pass it on to the baby during birth. The baby may then develop oral thrush, which can cause digestive distress, and in turn pass it on to the mother's nipples, causing her mild to extreme discomfort and difficulty with breastfeeding. Therefore, you should at least try to minimize all yeast infections with natural remedies before the birth. For treatment of thrush in babies and on the breasts, refer to my book *Naturally Healthy Babies and Children*.

Treatment of a yeast infection includes close adherence to all the general and dietary guidelines above, as well as the following internal remedies and your choice of external applications.

### INTERNAL REMEDIES

- Chickweed, burdock root, dandelion root, and echinacea are among my favorite herbs for cooling and soothing all manner of damp, inflammatory conditions. They are perfectly safe for use during pregnancy. They may be used singly or in combination, as infusions or tinctures, short or long term. To prepare an infusion, place 1 ounce of any of these herbs, or a mix of equal parts, into a quart-size jar. Fill the jar with boiling water, cover, and steep for 2 hours. Drink 2 cups daily as needed. Or, if you prefer, take a total of 20 to 40 drops of any single tincture or combination two to three times daily depending upon the infection's severity.

- Drink 1 tablespoon of apple cider vinegar in water once or twice a day. It can help prevent and reduce yeast infections while adding extra B vitamins to your diet. Cranberries and cranberry juice also acidify the urine, preventing bladder infections, which often occur in the presence of vaginal yeast infections.

- If your yeast infection seems related to your use of antibiotics, or if you also have gas regularly, your intestinal flora may have been overly reduced by the use of antibiotics, which can allow yeast to overgrow in your system. Eat $1/2$ cup of live-culture yogurt daily to help restore your intestinal flora.

### EXTERNAL REMEDIES

Choose a few of these suggestions to see what works best for you. Note that all of these remedies are for external use only.

- Live-culture, plain, unsweetened yogurt is perhaps one of the most effective remedies for treating yeast infections. Applied directly to the vulva it reduces inflammation, restores your pH balance, and also restores your normal vaginal flora while destroying the yeast. The best method I know for applying the yogurt is as follows:

    1. An hour before you are ready to apply the yogurt, put about $1/4$ cup of it in a dish and let it come to room temperature. This is merely a comfort measure, but it is well worth it—very cold yogurt applied to your bottom will certainly cause you to catch your breath! Use a separate dish so you don't inadvertently contaminate the entire yogurt container.

2. Insert your index finger into your vagina and gently scoop out all the yeast you can. (This is best done in the shower.) Yeast likes to thrive on the vaginal walls and in the area up around the cervix. Do not attempt to scrape it out; merely get out what you can so that the lactobacillus and acidophilus cultures in the yogurt stand a better chance of overcoming the yeast.

3. Wash your hands thoroughly; then put 1 to 2 tablespoons of the yogurt onto your index and middle fingers. Smear this up inside your vagina.

4. Now apply the remaining yogurt to your vulva, the external genitals, getting it well into the creases.

5. Repeat this twice a day during an acute yeast infection, and a couple of times a week if you are prone to yeast outbreaks.

- Apple cider vinegar makes a great rinse for the vulva and works like yogurt. Mix $^1/_4$ cup vinegar in $^3/_4$ cup of warm water and apply as you did the yogurt. Vinegar can sting considerably, especially if your flesh is raw or if you have been scratching, so it is best applied in a tub of warm water.

- One traditional remedy for yeast infections is to peel a clove of garlic very carefully so as not to nick it at all. Dip the clove in olive oil and insert vaginally. Remove after several hours or in the morning if you've put it in before bed, which is ideal, as it stays in more easily if you are lying down. Repeat with a fresh clove each night for several days in a row. It may occasionally cause burning, but garlic is highly regarded for its antifungal properties. This treatment is not always effective.

- A combination of calendula, lavender, and thyme can be made into an infusion that can be used as an antifungal rinse for your vulva (not a douche). To make the infusion, mix 1 ounce of the herb mixture per 4 cups of water; boil for 20 minutes, and then strain. Rinse once a day during an active yeast infection.

- Acidophilus, a live culture, can be used in capsules as a nightly suppository or in liquid form as a wash. You can also smear the liquid up inside of yourself as you did with yogurt. Acidophilus can acidify an overly alkaline vaginal environment and decrease the yeast population, although some women find that acidophilus aggravates the irritation, possibly because the vaginal environment is already overly acidic. In this case, a baking soda rinse—2 tablespoons per cup of warm water—can be applied to your vulva and smeared inside of the birth canal.

- Slippery elm bark powder, marshmallow root powder, and comfrey root powder soothe irritated and inflamed tissue. Sprinkle the powder on your irritated vulva or rinse yourself with a tea of any of these (or a mixture of them), getting some up inside of yourself with your fingers. To prepare a tea, mix 1 tablespoon of herbal powder with 1 cup hot water, stirring well. You can also prepare an infusion with the whole dried herbs by boiling 4 to 6 tablespoons of the herbs in 4 cups of water for 20 minutes.

- The juice of the aloe vera plant is exceptionally cooling and soothing and mildly antiseptic as well. It can be scraped from the inside of fresh leaves or purchased at natural food stores in the form of aloe vera gel and applied. In the case of an extremely irritated vulva, you can spread some of the gel onto a cloth menstrual pad and wear it throughout the day.

- A poultice or tea of fresh chickweed is a marvelous healing and anti-inflammatory application for a yeast infection. Chickweed is readily available as a wild herb, easy to recognize, and safe to use. It's one of my favorite healing herbs. Refer to a field guide for identification of this plant.

- A healing salve can be applied to your sore vulva as a comforting ointment. To prepare, refer to appendix I, Herbal Preparations. Include chickweed, plantain, and calendula in your salve.

- Yeast-Gard is a prepackaged homeopathic suppository that many pregnant women find highly effective for the treatment of persistent, difficult yeast infections. It is available at many regular drugstores and even at some supermarkets. Health food stores also carry it.

- You can also create your own boluses (suppositories) for persistent yeast infections. While it takes a little effort, they are well worth it, highly effective, and you can make a large supply at a time that keeps indefinitely in the refrigerator if well wrapped. Boluses are effective for soothing inflamed vaginal membranes and are mildly antifungal. Because it is safer not to douche during pregnancy, an herbal bolus is an excellent way to apply herbs up in the vagina. By varying the herbs, you can use boluses after birth to heal hemorrhoids.

    To prepare a supply, you will need ½ cup of coconut oil or a combination of coconut oil and cocoa butter in equal parts (these oils become hard when cold, holding their shape, but then soften when warmed), and approximately ½ cup of powdered herbs. A good reliable combination includes equal parts of goldenseal powder, echinacea powder, and slippery elm powder. Melt the oil in a small pot over low heat, but do not boil. When the oil is melted, turn off the stove. To this mixture add 2 teaspoons of calendula oil and 7 drops each of lavender essential oil and thyme essential oil.

Add the herbal powders and stir thoroughly until the mixture forms a thick, sticky dough. Add additional powder if necessary. Now put some slippery elm powder onto a cutting board and place your "dough" on it. Roll the dough into the shape of a long, thin log (like the clay "snakes" you made in kindergarten) about as thick as your index finger. Cut the roll into pieces $1^1/_2$ to 2 inches in length, wrap in foil, and put into the refrigerator. They will be ready to use in a couple of hours.

To use, place one bolus up into your vagina each night before bed. The bolus will melt and can be a bit messy, so wear underwear with a pad or sleep on a towel. Repeat for a week.

## Trichomonas

This infection, caused by a single-celled protozoa, often causes a yellow-green, foamy, fishy, foul-smelling discharge that usually burns and itches. The smell and color will be the main indication that you are dealing with "trich," though it can occasionally be present without these symptoms. It is usually spread through sexual contact, but can be contracted from hot tubs, sitting on moist towels belonging to someone with trich, or even toilet seats. Trich can inhabit the penis without causing any symptoms to the man, but will cause symptoms when spread to you, so male partners should also be treated.

Trich is considered difficult to cure, so your efforts to eliminate it must be very persistent. Medications for trich are strong and should be used only as a last resort. Flagyl (metronidazole), the most commonly used drug for treating vaginal infections, is not safe for pregnant women or babies though it is regularly prescribed during pregnancy. The brochure included in the package cautions against use during pregnancy. If you absolutely must use a medication for a vaginal infection, ask your doctor for an alternative.

> **WARNING:** *I am personally and strongly against the use of Flagyl for anyone who is pregnant. It is potentially carcinogenic, may damage the liver, and can affect the central nervous system.*

### TREATING TRICHOMONAS

- To treat trichomonas, you must completely abstain from sex until the treatment is complete and the infection totally cleared up. This may take a month.

- Treatment of men: During this time, your partner should also be receiving treatment. An excellent internal remedy for men is the following combination of herbs, which reduces what in traditional Chinese medicine is known as "damp heat" and eliminates infection. Mix together $^1/_4$ ounce each of echinacea root, yellow dock root, gentian root, goldenseal, dandelion root, and marshmallow root. Prepare an infusion by boiling 1 ounce total of the mix in 5 cups of water for 30 minutes. Strain and drink $^1/_4$ to $^1/_2$ cup three times a day for ten days. Store the prepared tea in the refrigerator for no more than two days. Or take 60 drops of echinacea tincture, 30 drops of goldenseal tincture, and 20 drops of myrrh or calendula tincture four times a day for four weeks. Wash the penis twice daily with a solution of $^1/_4$ cup apple cider vinegar and $^3/_4$ cup water or thyme infusion. During this regimen, men can also take two cloves of garlic each day or the equivalent amount of garlic perles. To take raw garlic, chop it finely, put it into a teaspoon of honey, and, if you can, swallow without chewing, and chase with water. This will prevent nausea, headache, and bad breath, which sometimes occur with raw garlic.

- Because trichomonas requires an alkaline environment in which to thrive, your goal is to create an acidic vaginal environment. To do this, you need to rinse yourself twice daily with apple cider vinegar—a solution of $^1/_4$ cup vinegar to $^1/_2$ cup water. Adding 2 teaspoons each of echinacea and calendula tinctures to the wash or replacing the water with $^1/_2$ cup of thyme tea can help reduce the infection. All of these herbs have antibacterial and antifungal properties, making them excellent for use in all cases of vaginal infection.

- It may be advisable to use a mild douche if you are dealing with trich. Use 2 tablespoons of apple cider vinegar and 1 teaspoon each of echinacea, usnea, and calendula tinctures per 2 cups of water. Repeat every day for ten days for maximum effectiveness.

> **WARNING:** *Because there is the risk of a fluid embolism from air being forced into the uterus, it is absolutely essential that you apply the douche very slowly, gently, and low in the vagina.*

- Anne Frye recommends the following for treating trich: Douche daily (2 tablespoons white vinegar and 1 tablespoon activated charcoal powder to 1 quart water) for one week, every other day the next week, and twice weekly for the next two weeks. At the same time, place two to three garlic cloves in the vagina every three hours for the first three days of treatment, then once a day overnight for the next four days. During the third week, use garlic suppositories every other day, then twice during the fourth week. As garlic is a bactericidal, take yogurt in conjunction with its use. After treatment is completed, place 1 to 2 teaspoons of yogurt into your vagina (use your index and middle finger or a vaginal applicator) daily for a week to prevent a secondary yeast infection.

- Drink water with lemon, or with 1 tablespoon of apple cider vinegar and 1 teaspoon of honey, or with cranberry juice concentrate, every three hours throughout the day. Take 2,000 mg of vitamin C daily and 60 drops of echinacea tincture four times a day for up to four weeks.

- A final resort for eliminating trich is to insert 2 "00" capsules of boric acid (a pharmacy grade that is pure—check at the drugstore) into the vagina up near the cervix each night for seven days. Midwives across the United States use this home remedy with no obvious long-term side effects; however, it can cause temporary, but nonetheless mildly painful, burning sensations in the vagina. If you find it too uncomfortable, sit in a tub of water and discontinue the use of this remedy.

**CAUTION:** *Never take boric acid by mouth—it is toxic!*

## Vaginitis, Nonspecific

Most of the other vaginal infections are lumped together under the term "nonspecific vaginitis." They are not venereal diseases or caused by one of the organisms already mentioned. The microbes are not specifically identified. They can be treated by following all of the general guidelines for vaginal infections as well as the suggestions for treating trichomonas.

## Beta-Strep Infection (Beta-Hemolytic Streptococcus, Beta-strep, or Group B strep)

Anywhere from 15 to 40 percent of all healthy women at any given time will be carriers of the organism known as beta-hemolytic streptococcus—or in short, beta-strep or group B strep. This organism, which is different from group A strep (which causes sore throats, for example), is also found on the bodies of more than 40 percent of all newborns. Of these newborns, only 1 percent will become ill from this bacteria. Given the prevalence of this germ with the relatively low incidence of related disease, one might wonder why physicians and midwives would be concerned about its presence in a woman's vaginal canal prenatally. The reason is that the rate of complications (including paralysis from meningitis, kidney damage, and sight and hearing loss) and mortality to the baby is very high. It is estimated that as many as two thousand babies in the United States die each year as a result of beta-strep infection.

Because it is simple to determine the presence of vaginal beta-strep with a vaginal culture, many doctors and midwives will request that you have a culture done at around twenty-six to thirty weeks pregnancy. If beta-strep is found, then your birth will be handled differently. It is recognized that the risk of beta-strep infection for the baby grows in the presence of prolonged rupture of membranes—that is, the longer your bag of waters has been broken, the greater the risk. The greatest risk is considered to occur when the waters have been ruptured for over twenty-four hours; therefore, part of the management of your labor will be to get your baby to be born before twenty-four hours has passed, even if this necessitates a cesarean. The other aspect of labor management is to place the mother on antibiotics either prior to her due date, at the time the membranes rupture, or when the mother commences labor. Different doctors, hospitals, and midwives will all vary slightly in the length of time they allow a woman to labor before becoming aggressive in speeding along the birth, and their schedule for prescribing antibiotics may also vary.

There are advantages and disadvantages of routine prenatal screening for beta-strep, and there are possibilities for natural treatments that exist beyond waiting until a woman is due to begin labor to address the potential for infection. There are also practical and natural approaches to facilitating labor and monitoring the baby during labor and in the immediate postpartum so that aggressive methods are rarely required. Here I will discuss the advantages and disadvantages of routine prenatal screening, as well as natural treatments you might wish to try if you do have vaginal beta-strep.

The primary advantages of prenatal testing for beta-strep are that if the organism is present you can approach your labor in a way that considers the optimal health of the baby. You can also do things prenatally that reduce the amount of the organisms, reducing the likelihood of your baby contracting the organism and becoming ill. The main disadvantage is that the standard accepted medical procedures for "managing" pregnant and laboring women with beta-strep can be unnecessarily invasive, especially considering the fact that this organism is a natural part of the vaginal flora for so many women, the vast majority of whom will have babies who don't become infected.

All practitioners who assist pregnant women face a double bind with beta-strep: because of its prevalence and potential risk it is too dangerous to ignore, but because of the prevalence of the organism and relatively low incidence of problems, it is excessive to assume the worst for all women. Therefore, the best approach may be to identity those women with the greatest risk and to provide natural prenatal treatment that is natural to reduce the presence of the organisms.

> **WARNING:** *Any newborn showing signs of infection should receive immediate medical care.*

Women who are at the greatest risk for having an active beta-strep infection that could be passed on to the baby include those with a history of urinary tract infections, with persistent yeast infections, who go into labor before thirty-seven weeks, whose bag of waters ruptures prematurely, whose membranes rupture before contractions begin, who had a fever before or during labor, who previously had a strep-infected baby, and who had a high beta-strep count earlier in the pregnancy. Not all these factors prove the presence of beta-strep; however, if these symptoms have occurred and the presence of beta-strep is confirmed, you should try to reduce the bacterial count starting at about thirty-two weeks. If you have been positive for beta-strep, the baby should be monitored carefully in the first few days after birth.

# General Recommendations

- A positive attitude toward your body, your sexuality, and your pregnancy, along with excellent nutrition, can go a long way in promoting the strength of your immune system, and preventing and reducing any infections.

- Visualize your vaginal canal as pink and healthy, a nourishing place that your baby will pass through on his or her birth journey.

- Any vaginal infection, such as yeast, that causes tissue irritation can allow other organisms (such as beta-strep) to attack the damaged tissue. Therefore, follow all of the General Recommendations for vaginal organisms found at the beginning of this section.

- Be informed (read, research, ask questions, and consult your inner wisdom) about the risks, interventions, and issues surrounding beta-strep. Be sure that you understand whether you've had this test performed and what your care provider's protocols are. Some midwives, for example, might not be aware of beta-strep, while others might immediately transport you to the hospital if your waters have been broken for longer than eighteen hours.

- Don't allow yourself to panic when a health-care provider is nervous about beta-strep. Remember, while the risk to a small percentage of babies is high, the overall incidence of this infection compared to the incidence of its presence is very low. Do your best to reduce risk factors, but continue to trust your inner guidance regarding yourself and your baby.

- Refer to other relevant topics in this book if you are experiencing factors associated with beta-strep, for example, urinary tract infections.

## Dietary Recommendations

- Overall, an excellent diet will keep you healthy and prevent organisms from proliferating in your vaginal canal. Refer to chapter 5, Nutrition during Pregnancy, for a full discussion of this important aspect of your prenatal health.

- A prenatal vitamin and mineral supplement can provide nutrients that may be missing in your diet and can aid your body in creating a healthy environment that prevents a growth of unwanted organisms.

- As beta-strep infections may often occur in conjunction with persistent yeast infections, addressing the dietary factors that cause yeast to proliferate may assist you in reducing beta-strep.

## Herbal Recommendations

Ideally, you will begin treatment at about thirty-two weeks, on confirmation of the presence of beta-strep in a vaginal culture, a urine sample that showed beta-strep, or a rectal sample. (Some doctors will do both a vaginal and rectal swab.) Treatment will include taking herbs orally that strengthen your immune system and applying herbs vaginally that will restore your healthy vaginal flora, that will enable your body to reduce bacterial overgrowth, and also that will directly fight the bacteria. As you enter the last few weeks of pregnancy, from thirty-seven weeks onward (since your baby is unlikely to be premature), most midwives will be willing to assist you at home if this is your plan. In the hospital, your baby will also be considered close to full term and will not be treated as premature in most circumstances. At thirty-seven weeks, you can therefore begin to use certain herbs both orally and vaginally that are sometimes considered labor stimulants, but are nonetheless effective for reducing bacterial infections.

- At thirty-two weeks, begin to take a supplement of 500 mg of vitamin C, and 1 cup of burdock root and echinacea root infusion. To prepare the infusion, steep ¹/₂ ounce of each of these herbs in 4 cups of boiling water for 2 hours. Strain and take the above dose, storing the rest in the refrigerator for the next day.

- Eat a lot of fresh garlic every day.

- Take ¹/₂ teaspoon each of echinacea and astragalus tinctures twice daily. You can also get dried astragalus in the herb department of your health food store and cook two strips into a pot of rice or soup two to three times per week. Remove the strips when done cooking and eat the rice or soup. Astragalus is an immune system tonic well known in the Chinese pharmacopoeia, but also grows in America.

> ### Garlic Remedies
> - Chop a clove of fresh garlic and mix with a teaspoon of honey. Swallow this without chewing it. This can be done several times a day, preferably with a meal.
> - Make a garlic elixir by blending ¹/₂ cup of honey, ¹/₄ cup of apple cider vinegar, and half a bulb of fresh garlic in your blender until liquidy. Take ¹/₂ teaspoon up to twice a day. Adjust the taste as necessary with more or less of the honey or vinegar.
> - Chop fresh garlic onto a salad, or mix with olive oil to use as a dressing or dip French bread into this as a condiment.
> - Take garlic perles according to the dosage on the brand you purchase.

- Beginning at thirty-two weeks and continuing until the end of your pregnancy (warning: discontinue if you have broken waters!), take regular sitz baths (a bath filled to the height of your hips is sufficient for this) and rinse your vaginal and perineal area with a clean "peri-bottle" (available at a pharmacy or through Cascade Health Care Products—see resources) of the following herbal infusion and essential oil mixture. This will help to restore vaginal flora while reducing vaginal bacterial counts. Infuse equal parts of thyme, calendula, rosemary, and yarrow, 6 tablespoons of the herbal mix per quart of water, and steep for 30 minutes. Strain into a clean jar and add ¹/₄ cup of sea salt and 10 drops of lavender essential oil. If you are taking a sitz bath, add the entire jar to the tub; if you are using a peri-bottle, fill the bottle and save the remainder as a refill. You can bathe as often as once daily, and can cleanse your vulva with the peri-bottle solution after each time you urinate. Spreading your labia apart with your fingers makes the peri-rinse more effective.

- After thirty-seven weeks (and if your waters are not broken), you can begin to insert one capsule of goldenseal into your upper vaginal canal each night before bed. Goldenseal is a natural antibiotic. You can ask your midwife or other care provider to show you how to do this if you are uncomfortable trying it on your own, but all you need to do is push the capsule inside of your birth canal as far as you can reach. The capsule will dissolve, releasing the goldenseal. You may want to sleep in an old shirt and put a towel under you to protect the sheets should the goldenseal leak out.

- After thirty-seven weeks, if your care provider agrees, you can use the above peri-bottle and sitz bath rinse as a very gentle douche. It is imperative that the douche be low and gentle, as a forceful douche can cause an embolism in the mother, which can be fatal. If you are uncomfortable with douching, spread your labia wide open, and irrigate your whole vulvar and perineal area quite thoroughly.

Remember that a healthy diet and a healthy sexuality—both your sense of yourself as a sexual being, and your relationship with your partner—are also important in preventing and healing vaginal infections. No amount of herbal remedies can compensate for these aspects of your life. Please give thought to these ideas and find ways to nourish your body as well as finding clarity, joy, and love in your sexual experience. Also, always remember that in healing any infection you are working to restore your body's natural balance and defenses, not just attacking organisms.

## Varicose Veins and Hemorrhoids

Varicose veins occur when the valves that keep blood flowing one way through the vessels become weak, allowing blood to pool up in the veins and causing the veins to become lax and distended. This weakness of the valves may be due to diet, lack of exercise, or heredity. The hormonal changes of pregnancy can contribute to laxity of the valves. Pregnancy also predisposes women to congestion of blood in the lower body because the pressure from the heavy uterus reduces venous return from the legs and pelvis. Varicosities most commonly occur in the legs and feet, the vulva (vulvar varicosities), and the anus (hemorrhoids). They generally become more pronounced as pregnancy advances. Vulvar varicosities may or may not be noticeable until labor, but women usually notice large ones during pregnancy. A gentle birth and hot compresses applied to the distended veins usually prevent trauma to them. Occasionally, bleeding or a hematoma (an internal pooling of blood from a broken blood vessel) can result and may require medical care. Hemorrhoids usually become enlarged at the birth with the mom's pushing and may

Jody had severe leg and vulvar varicose veins that had become very difficult during her second pregnancy. Now in her third pregnancy, the varicosities were becoming a problem, and were looking extremely red and inflamed. She began a therapeutic dietary and herbal program to include foods high in bioflavonoids and rutin, nettle infusion and hawthorn tincture, and regular periods of rest as well as daily inversion on a slant board. Externally she applied compresses of witch hazel extract from the pharmacy. The inflammation completely subsided and while the varicosities were still obviously visible throughout the pregnancy, they remained unproblematic, and Jody gave birth at home with no difficulty.

persist for a few days postpartum. Again, gentle pushing whenever possible will reduce their severity. Constipation during pregnancy aggravates hemorrhoids and should be treated because it can cause other health problems as well.

Natural remedies regularly taken and applied can effectively prevent and reduce varicose veins.

## General Recommendations

- Follow all dietary and exercise suggestions, and use appropriate herbal remedies.

- Exercise can vastly improve circulation and must be a vital component in both the prevention and treatment of varicosities. By increasing your circulatory rate you are effectively removing stagnation in your blood vessels and directly reducing blood congestion, a primary factor in varicosities.

- Take a brisk walk for thirty minutes each day or ride a stationary bicycle for approximately that length of time. Swimming is also an excellent form of exercise—as you swim, feel the water massaging your legs.

- Yoga postures and commonly known exercises such as leg lifts, lunges, and, if you can do them, shoulder stands can successfully strengthen your circulatory system and encourage venous return.

- Vigorous pelvic tilting vastly improves pelvic circulation and venous return. This can be done for five to ten minutes daily. Stand with your feet shoulder-width apart, hands on your hips. Slowly tip your pelvis forward, then backward, gradually increasing your speed until you are swinging your hips forward and backward vigorously. You can also roll and rock your hips and make "figure eights" in belly-dancer fashion.

- Dance, dance, dance! Open to your creative flow as you exercise your legs, pelvis, heart, and spirit.

- In addition to exercising daily, you will want to spend at least twenty minutes, twice a day, with your feet elevated higher than the level of your heart. Putting your legs and feet up on two pillows as you recline is usually sufficient. If you are sitting at a desk, put your feet up on it!

- Don't sit in one place for any length of time because it encourages insufficient pelvic and leg circulation. Get up and walk around about once an hour for ten minutes to improve blood flow. You should do this on long car trips in your third trimester of pregnancy even if you don't have varicosities.

- Use support stockings if you have severe varicosities. If you put them on in the morning when you first get up from bed, they will be easier to get on and the most effective. You can dust a bit of slippery elm powder on your legs to help them slide on.

> **CAUTION:** *Never massage varicose veins. Massage can dislodge clotted blood and lead to an embolism, a very dangerous situation. If you see signs of phlebitis (swelling, heat, pain, infection around the veins), seek the care of an experienced midwife or physician.*

- Visualizing your varicosities reducing in size may help you produce this result. Imagine your life flowing smoothly as you imagine the blood flowing smoothly through your veins. Let obstructions dissolve, and let yourself feel strong.

- Look at the emotional support you have. Are you getting the support you need, or are you afraid you won't have it after the birth? Allow yourself to ask for the help and support you need, and let go of the notion that you must be a superwoman.

## Dietary Recommendations

- A diet rich in healthful foods, especially a variety of whole grains, high-quality protein, and vegetables, will supply the nutrients you need for the maintenance of a healthy circulatory system.

- Vitamin C with bioflavonoids is vital for maintaining strength in the walls of blood vessels. Foods high in vitamin C include all citrus fruits, rose hips, dark green leafy vegetables, cherries, alfalfa sprouts, strawberries, cantaloupe, broccoli, tomatoes, and green peppers. In addition, a daily supplement of up to 2,000 mg of vitamin C with bioflavonoids can add to the integrity of the circulatory system. Bioflavonoids (vitamin P) are brightly colored substances that often appear in foods in conjunction with vitamin C. Sources of bioflavonoids include lemons, grapes, plums, black currants, grapefruit, apricots, buckwheat, cherries, blackberries, and rose hips. In citrus fruits, they are more abundant in the inner skin (the white, pithy part) than in the juice. One of the main purposes of this vitamin is to increase the strength of the capillaries. One of the bioflavonoids, rutin, is specifically used to treat hemorrhoids and varicose veins, and is best taken in conjunction with vitamin C and a bioflavonoid complex. The best way to obtain rutin is to eat foods with a high bioflavonoid content.

- Vitamin E is also reputed to have a beneficial action on the vascular system. It apparently works by dilating the blood vessels, thus directly facilitating the blood flow. Between 200 and 600 IU is considered a safe daily dosage during pregnancy, but do not exceed this amount.

  > CAUTION: *If you have heart or blood pressure problems, begin at 50 IU daily and work up to about 400 IU over a three-month period, gradually increasing the dosage each week. Also, if you have such problems, speak with your midwife or physician before taking this supplement.*

- Vitamin B complex is also necessary for healthy veins. Brewer's yeast, fortified nutritional yeast, whole grains, and organ meats contain substantial levels of B vitamins. B vitamins are also produced in our intestines to some degree when we have healthy intestinal flora. Alcohol, sugar, and antibiotics can damage intestinal flora, while an active-culture yogurt, eaten in small amounts on a regular basis, can help replenish and restore intestinal flora.

- I cannot overemphasize the importance of including dark leafy green vegetables in the diet on a daily basis. Salad greens like romaine, green or red leaf, and butter lettuce, as well as greens like kale, collards, mustard greens, dandelion greens, and turnip greens that are tastier cooked, all promote health and vibrancy and are particularly important for a healthy circulatory system.

## Herbal Recommendations

This section is divided into two parts: herbs to be used internally and herbs to be used externally.

### HERBS FOR INTERNAL USE

- The humble but highly nourishing nettle is by far the best herb for pregnant women with varicose veins. Because of its high mineral content and its ability to tonify the blood vessels, nettle makes a wonderful supplement and astringent brew for varicose veins. Women with severe varicosities may find that the blood vessels don't disappear completely, but will not develop into painful and swollen veins. Prepare an infusion using 1 ounce of herb to 1 quart of water, and steep for 2 hours. Drink between 1 cup and 1 quart daily depending upon the extent and severity of the varicosities.

- Other herbs that may be used for the vascular system include garlic, onions, oatstraw, calendula, hawthorn berries, motherwort, and dong quai. These should be used under the guidance of an experienced herbalist. Garlic and onions can be eaten as foods (see garlic oil on page 215 under "High Blood Pressure"), and garlic can safely be taken in perles during pregnancy. (Kwai and Kyolic are both reputable brands.) You can add oatstraw to your nettle infusion (use about two-thirds nettle and one-third oatstraw), as well as 1 tablespoon of calendula.

- Kelp is a food-herb so high in trace minerals that it should be included in any program designed to strengthen the blood vessels. You can take 2 "00" capsules of kelp powder up to four times daily, or use kelp in food or as a tea.

- A deficiency of essential fatty acids may exacerbate varicose veins, so you may want to take 500 mg of one of these oils once a day: evening primrose oil, flaxseed oil, black currant oil, borage oil.

### HERBS FOR EXTERNAL USE

- The primary aim of external therapies is to tonify the tissue and vessels and to maintain healthy circulation in the problem area while gently reducing obstructions in the blood vessels. To do this, you will want to alternate the following applications at least once, but preferably twice, each day.

> **CAUTION:** *You must not massage varicose veins. Massage could lead to the dislodging of a clot, which may result in a dangerous embolism.*

*Astringent herbal application:* Use witch hazel extract from the pharmacy or make your own (see appendix I, Herbal Preparations). Soak a cloth in the extract, wring it out (save the liquid for future use), and wrap the affected areas with the cloth. In the case of vulvar and anal varicosities, apply the cloth as a compress. Leave it on for twenty minutes each time, up to three times a day, whenever it is convenient for you. For an even more effective astringent, prepare your own infusion of these herbs in equal parts: witch hazel, bayberry bark, white oak bark, and calendula blossoms. Simmer a total of 2 ounces of this mix over a low heat (in a covered pot) for 30 minutes. Apply when cool enough to tolerate. This will keep refrigerated about three days if well strained.

***Circulation-promoting herbal application:*** Dit Dat Jiao liniment, a Chinese herbal liniment intended for martial arts injuries, makes an excellent application for varicose veins. It reduces inflammation and bruising, and by promoting healthy circulation in the areas to which it is applied, helps to reduce and prevent blood clot formation. It can be gently rubbed into affected areas (but not on hemorrhoids) twice a day. It is most suitable for varicosities of the legs and feet. The recipe for this easy-to-make and worthwhile liniment is found on page 227. It has many applications beyond pregnancy, including for bruises and injuries in which the skin is unbroken and for all muscle aches and tight muscles.

# Vomiting, Severe *(Hyperemesis gravidarum)*

This is a condition in which you are vomiting excessively and unable to keep much of anything down, causing you to lose vital nutrients and fluids and to become physically exhausted and emotionally drained. If severe, it can become a life-threatening, medical emergency in which you become clinically dehydrated with a mineral and electrolyte imbalance; it can also contribute to miscarriage. Treatment requires hospitalization, usually intravenous fluids to replace fluids, electrolytes, and nutrients, as well as medication to control vomiting.

You must seek medical treatment for this condition, but you may be able to mitigate its severity with home treatment, preventing the problem from becoming serious. The following combination of therapies may help you avoid serious illness. It may take a few days to notice complete improvement, but you should see significant improvement within the first twenty-four hours. If you find no relief from these suggestions or if your condition worsens, seek medical care immediately.

## General Recommendations

Follow all of the general recommendations under "Morning Sickness" in this chapter.

## Dietary Recommendations

- Each time you throw up, drink a small amount of fluid. In addition, do this throughout the day. Even a quarter cup of liquid every fifteen to thirty minutes can help replace vital fluids. Also, try to eat a small portion of food after you vomit, to prevent clinical starvation.

- To keep your electrolytes in balance, drink Third Wind, Gatorade, or Recharge. Or, preferably, prepare the following drink by the quart and sip it throughout the day, up to every five minutes. Even if you vomit it up, you will still get some, and over the course of a few hours it will often decrease the frequency of vomiting. This preparation, called "Rehydration Drink," is used worldwide as a remedy to prevent and offset dehydration and electrolyte imbalance, even in cases of severe vomiting and diarrhea in impoverished countries. It consists of 1 quart water, the juice of 1 lemon, 1 to 2 tablespoons honey, $^1/_4$ teaspoon salt, and $^1/_4$ teaspoon baking soda. You can replace the water and lemon with a half quart each of water and orange juice, if you prefer.

- If you are vomiting and unable to keep nourishment down, a nutritive enema is an effective method for infusing nutrients and fluids that can't be tolerated by mouth. This is an excellent technique that I've seen work several times. It can prevent the need for intravenous fluids in a hospital. To prepare the enema, mix 2 tablespoons of blackstrap molasses in 2 cups of warm spring water, and put the solution into your enema bag or bottle. Lying on your left side or on your hands and knees with your chest near the floor, slowly take the enema. If you are quite dehydrated, you may actually retain all the fluid; it will have been absorbed. This can be done up to twice a day during the acute phase of vomiting.

## Herbal Recommendations

- Take wild yam tincture by the dropperful, up to every two hours throughout the day, and, in addition, sip ginger tea throughout the day. Try a few of the other herbal suggestions as well.

- A remarkably effective treatment for vomiting is to apply a warm salty pack to your stomach (not over your belly—just directly over your stomach). To do this, heat $^1/_2$ cup of sea salt in a skillet for 3 minutes. Put the salt into a pillowcase—it will be very hot. Fold the pillowcase (or other suitable sack) into a small square or rectangular "pad" and apply. If it is too hot, wrap the pad in a towel before applying. This Japanese treatment sends penetrating warmth into the stomach, decreasing spasms and cold, and reducing the frequency of vomiting. Do it when you feel a bout of vomiting coming on, or if you have been vomiting repeatedly.

# Herbal Preparations

Preparing your own herbal products is both rewarding and cost-efficient. This section provides you with all of the information you need to begin this venture. In the resources section later in the book, you will find companies that supply herbs and other products, such as jars, oils, and even decorative labels, that are useful in herbal product making. While you do not need fancy equipment or supplies for making or packaging most herbal products, get yourself a sturdy notebook for recording your recipes, successes, and failures, and be prepared to have friends, relatives, and even neighbors putting in requests for that special liniment or salve that you have created!

## Herb Gathering

Whether you plan to grow your own herbs, gather them from the wild, or purchase them, you are certain to find the process of making your own medicines fun and rewarding. In the long run, putting up a batch of iron tonic or belly massage oil that will last for months is less costly than buying vitamins or lotions. Although you may still need to buy packaged preparations, I think you will find yourself relying more and more on your home remedies. Making your own herbal preparations is empowering, giving you a new understanding of herbs.

## From the Wild

Whenever possible, use herbs harvested from the wild in the area where you live. An uncultivated plant has more vitality than a cultivated one, just as wild animals retain more of their natural qualities than those living in zoos or in houses. Instruction in plant identification and harvesting is beyond the range of this book, but I encourage you to learn to identify a few local medicinals to enhance your connection with the plant world.

> **WARNING:** *If you are going to use local wild plants, be absolutely certain that your plant identification is accurate. Mistakes can be fatal. Seek out the advice of experienced botanists at local nature centers. Never pick plants that grow near roads, under power lines, or in any areas exposed to chemicals including fertilizers, pesticides, or toxic wastes. Choose healthy plants in clean, unpolluted areas.*

Don't pick all of the plants in one location. Leave enough growing to repopulate the area. Avoid endangered or rare plant species. Always offer your thanks to the plants and ask for their blessing and assistance in healing.

## In Your Garden

Herb cultivation is a very broad field, one in which I am by no means an expert. I do know, however, that I experience the greatest joy when I am sitting in a garden filled with healing plants. Many herbs are not only useful but also beautiful, particularly when they are in bloom. Then the bees and butterflies will flock to your garden, and you will feel a new, profound connection to the plant world.

When you grow your own herbs, you will develop a greater understanding of them. You will see how they change through the seasons and what conditions cause them to thrive, and you learn to recognize their scent and appearance.

The initial investment in seeds or starter plants can vary. A small garden well cared for can provide you with enough herbs to make small amounts of a few remedies. A large garden could potentially provide you with all the herbs you could want and some to spare for friends or for sale. Many herbs are prolific, so even a small plant, tended well, will yield a plentiful harvest over time. Perennials return year after year, so if your budget is limited, go with these instead of annuals. Not at all herbs grow in every climate or location, so consult books and local gardening stores to determine exactly what can be raised where you live.

# Purchasing Herbs

It is preferable to obtain organic, wild-crafted plants or at least organically culti-vated plants. Preparations such as capsules and tinctures should likewise be prepared from organic herbs. Many inorganic herbs are fumigated with fungicides and insecticides during storage, and some are even irradiated. Check your sources. All herbs and herb products should have a fresh smell, and their color should resemble that of the fresh plant. Herb freshness will affect the potency and there-fore the effectiveness of your treatments. A moldy, dusty odor indicates that the herbs are not fresh. Look closely for insects; one infested batch of herbs can let tons of bugs loose in your home. They can then get into other herbs in your pantry as well as your food.

# Preparing Herbs

Seeing different herbs turn water, alcohol, and oils into lovely shades of gold, red, orange, green, and brown is nothing short of magic. Preparing one's own remedies adds a special potency to the medicines: that of love and care.

Common supplies are required for making everything from teas to salves in your kitchen: glass jars of varying sizes with lids, glass or stainless steel pots, a sharp knife, a small funnel, a mesh strainer, a vegetable grater, measuring spoons, and a cutting board. Water, vegetable oil, vodka, and beeswax complete the list once you have the herbs you need.

Some preparations cannot be made easily at home. These include essential oils, which require special equipment for extraction, and herbs that must be powdered finely with a special grinder. If you wish, try experimenting with a coffee grinder to see if you achieve a powder that is satisfactory.

If you plan to use your own preparations as primary medicines, you will want to look through this book and plan ahead. Tinctures take weeks to prepare, for example, so you will need to have these on hand, since if you need a tincture today you can't wait. Keep in mind that most herbal preparations such as oils and tinc-tures will keep for up to a few years (oils must be kept refrigerated), so if you prepare small batches of medicines at a time, you will find that little gets wasted.

Throughout this book I've made every effort to give specific measurements for preparations in the form of teaspoonfuls, tablespoonfuls, and ounces. For conven-ience, I sometimes have listed recipe ingredients in parts. You can translate these to any measure you are using. For example, if you are using tablespoons, 1 part would be 1 tablespoon, 2 parts would be 2 tablespoons, and a half part would be about $^1/_2$ tablespoon.

Choosing an appropriate measurement for these recipes allows you to determine the amount of preparation you want to make.

## Forms of Preparation

Water, alcohol, and oil are the most common bases used. ("Menstruum" is another word for a base or solvent.) Some herbalists also use vinegar but since it is not suitable for all herbs, I reserve it for steeping fresh culinary herbs.

### WATER BASES

The Earth, plants, and our bodies are primarily made of water, so our bodies accept water-based solutions easily. These include teas, infusions, decoctions, and syrups. Infusions and decoctions are used for baths, washes, and compresses as well as internal use.

*Tea* is the most basic herbal preparation. To make a tea, steep 1 teaspoon to 1 tablespoon of a dried herb in 1 cup boiling water for up to 20 minutes. Herbs with a lot of volatile oil content are easily extracted this way and so should be covered during steeping to prevent loss of their oils. Peppermint, catnip, lemon balm, chamomile, fresh ginger, lavender, and seeds such as fennel and anise are in this category.

*Infusions* are medicinal-strength teas. More herb material is steeped longer in slightly more water than is usual for a tea. The result is a darker, stronger-tasting, more potent brew. Pint- and quart-size canning (Mason) jars are the best vessels in which to make infusions.

To make an infusion, steep 4 to 6 tablespoons of chopped, dried herb or twice that of chopped, fresh herb in either a quart or pint jar filled with boiling water for anywhere from $^1/_2$ hour to 8 hours. The steeping time and the amount of water correspond to the intended strength of the remedy and also depend upon the part of the plant being used. The general recommendations are as follows:

ROOTS: Use 1 ounce dried root to 1 pint of boiling water; steep for 8 hours.

BARK: Prepare as for roots.

LEAVES: In general, when using delicate leaves or those rich in essential oils, use 1 ounce of dried leaves or 2 ounces of fresh leaves to 1 quart of water and steep for 1 to 2 hours. Thick leaves (such as uva-ursi) require steeping for up to 6 hours. Leaves used for nutritional purposes (such as nettle) should be steeped for up to 8 hours.

FLOWERS: As these are delicate, steep 1 ounce of dried flowers in 1 quart of boiling water for a maximum of 1 hour.

SEEDS: In general, you first gently crush the seeds with a mortar and pestle and then steep them for up to $\frac{1}{2}$ hour. Usually $\frac{1}{4}$ to $\frac{1}{2}$ ounce of seeds per pint of water is sufficient.

Generally the dosage of an infusion ranges from $\frac{1}{4}$ to 1 cup, two to four times daily. Sometimes an infusion is sipped throughout the day.

*Decoctions* are concentrated infusions. This makes for a strong brew that is taken in smaller dosages. A decoction is an excellent way to take herbs when it is difficult to tolerate large amounts of a strong-tasting preparation. The method is especially suited for nutrient roots such as yellow dock and dandelion because you can get concentrated doses of minerals without having to drink cupfuls of beverage. Leaves, flowers, and seeds are rarely decocted as their constituents can be damaged by boiling.

To prepare a decoction, make an infusion and steep it for up to eight hours. Strain the liquid into a saucepan (discarding the used plant material), and simmer it until it is reduced to one-quarter to one-half of the original amount. Take care not to boil off all the liquid. Reducing a pint of liquid by one-half (down to a cup) takes approximately an hour. Pour into a glass jar, let cool to room temperature, and then refrigerate.

When unsweetened, decoctions last in the refrigerator for up to three days. Two tablespoons of honey per $\frac{1}{2}$ cup of liquid or about 2 tablespoons of brandy per cup of liquid can extend the life of a decoction for up to three months when kept refrigerated.

Dosage is usually 1 teaspoon to 1 tablespoon, two to four times daily.

*Syrups* are easy to make from a decoction. Syrups have two main advantages over decoctions: you will more readily take a small amount of a sweet-flavored medicine than any amount of an unpalatable one; and the large amount of sweetener in the syrup preserves the preparation so that you can keep it in the refrigerator for a longer time than a sweetened decoction. Simply sweeten your decoction by adding an equal amount (by weight) of sweetener. One cup of a decoction is 8 ounces, so a decoction of this amount would require 8 ounces of sweetener. I use $\frac{1}{4}$ to $\frac{1}{2}$ cup of honey per cup of liquid and find this adequate; honey is considered to be twice as sweet as sugar. Add the sweetener to your hot decoction, bring to the boiling point while stirring, and then immediately pour into clean jars. Cool to room temperature, label, and refrigerate. Dosage is similar to a decoction but of course will vary from herb to herb.

*Herbal baths* are a rejuvenating ritual and are useful for all sorts of complaints: sore muscles, injured skin, exhaustion, irritability, congestion, and fever, to name a few. Be very careful to avoid burns from overly hot water.

A foot bath is given in a basin of water wide enough for the feet and deep enough to reach at least above the ankles. Add a quart of herbal infusion to enough hot water to fill the basin.

A sitz bath requires a quart of decoction or a couple of quarts of infusion placed in a shallow tub with enough water to reach hip level.

A full bath can be made two ways. You can fill a cotton cloth or sock with at least an ounce of herbs and fasten the closed cloth to the faucet so bathwater runs through it while the tub is filling. Squeeze the sack now and then to wring out the tea. This will make a mild but pleasant herbal bath. You can also prepare a couple of quarts of herbal infusion or decoction and then strain these into the tub.

If you keep the door to the bathroom closed, the aroma of the herbs and any volatile oils will fill the air, adding to the relaxing effect of the bath. Herb baths are a nourishing gift to yourself during pregnancy. Floating herb flowers directly in the tub makes for a fun bath, but use a screen of some sort to keep the plant material from clogging the drain.

*Poultices and compresses* are ways of applying herbs externally to specific areas of the body. You can quickly make a poultice by mashing, bruising, or even chewing fresh herbs into a pulpy mass and applying it to the affected area. You can also make one by mashing fresh or dried herbs (dried herbs need to be moistened with warm water first), and spreading the material on a thin cotton cloth, which is then applied to the area. A hot-water bottle can be placed over the herbs or cloth to retain the warmth. Poultices are used for stings, bites, localized infections, wounds, boils, abscesses, swellings, and tumors.

To make a compress, soak a cloth in a hot infusion or decoction, wring out the excess liquid, and apply the cloth to the area. Replace the compress when it cools by dipping again into the hot infusion or decoction. As with a poultice, a hot-water bottle placed over the preparation retains heat.

*Washes* are just what they sound like: you wash the area with an infusion or decoction. For example, you might want to use an eyewash for conjunctivitis or a wash for a skin infection such as ringworm. Washes are an effective and simple external remedy.

### ALCOHOL BASES

Alcohol is used for making tinctures, which are concentrated alcohol extracts of herbs. It is a valuable menstruum because certain plant substances can be extracted only by alcohol. Tinctures are concentrated, quick acting, and convenient (they can easily be transported in a small bottle), and they have a shelf life of many years. Because they are so concentrated, only a few drops are needed, making them particularly convenient for those who can't easily prepare infusions or decoctions. They are not, however, used when the nutritional aspects of herbs are being sought. For this, one should use teas, infusions, decoctions, and syrups.

The amount of alcohol ingested when taking tinctures is fairly insignificant, but if you are concerned, many tinctures can now be purchased in a glycerin base, which has no alcohol and a slightly sweet taste.

Making tinctures at home is fun and much less expensive than buying them. Because tinctures made with fresh plant material are superior to those made from dried herbs, obtain fresh herbs for your homemade tinctures. The best alcohol to use is 100-proof vodka, which is 50 percent alcohol and 50 percent water. Grain alcohol (almost 200 proof) or brandy can also be used. Brandy is nice for use in tinctures that will be given to very young kids because it is sweet and mildly warming, and it lacks a sharp alcohol taste.

*Making tinctures:* If you have gathered the herbs yourself, clean them by picking out damaged parts and brushing dirt off roots. Do not wash above-ground plant parts. Roots, stems, and bark need to be chopped. Place about 2 ounces of plant material in a pint jar. Fill the jar to the top with alcohol to lessen the possibility of spoilage. Cap the jar tightly and label it with the name of the herb, alcohol content, and the date. Store where it won't be exposed to direct sunlight, and give it a gentle shake every few days. If you see the liquid level going down, top off the jar with some more alcohol.

The moon exerts ongoing effects on the Earth, including the level of oceans and the growth of plants, as well as our own internal regulatory mechanisms and our hormones. It is also said to influence tincture making. It may therefore be beneficial to honor the effects of the moon by allowing our tinctures to work for at least one complete moon cycle, going from one new moon to the next, or preferably for a full six weeks, from one new moon to the full moon six weeks later.

After two to six weeks, strain the alcohol tincture from the plant material. This usually requires some vigorous wringing of the herbs in cheesecloth or cotton muslin to extract as much of the liquid as possible. Pour your tincture into well-labeled glass jars or tincture bottles (the jars need not be filled to the top) and store in a cool, dark place such as a pantry or the refrigerator.

Dosage of a tincture depends on the herbs used, the condition being treated, and the person's age and weight. Usually between 5 and 25 drops are taken four times a day. Store tinctures out of reach of children as an overdose might make them sick. Tinctures remain good for a minimum of two to three years.

*Making liniments:* These are tinctures prepared for external use in the treatment of muscle and ligament trauma. They tend to contain herbs that act as local stimulants (for example, angelica, cinnamon, wintergreen, cayenne, and calendula) in order to bring deep warmth to the affected area and disperse blood congestion to reduce bruising. The alcohol (use vodka or another 100-proof alcohol) makes them quick absorbing and penetrating. Prepare as for tinctures, or add essential oils to an alcohol base. Apply by rubbing enough into the skin to cover the sore or bruised area. Do not use on broken skin.

### OIL BASES

Herbal oils, salves, and ointments can be made at home. Essential oils are highly concentrated plant extracts that cannot easily be made at home and are rarely used internally because their strength can be fatal. I have occasionally suggested the use of essential oils in this book as external remedies, and caution you to store them out of the reach of children.

*Herbal oils* are vegetable oils in which herbs have been infused. They are different from essential oils, which are derived by extracting large volumes of concentrated, active chemical ingredients from plants. Herbal oils are used in the treatment of sore muscles, sprains, aches, infections, and irritated skin, as well as for massage. Many herbal oils mentioned in this book can be used on broken skin, although arnica oil cannot.

To make an herbal oil, fill a clean and totally dry jar with dry herbs. Now fill the jar to the brim with oil. Almond, olive, and sesame oils are the most commonly used, but any vegetable oil is acceptable. Store at room temperature in partial sunlight for one to four weeks. Some herbs, such as garlic and rosemary, will keep well in oil for the longer time span, while other herbs, particularly the more delicate plants and plant parts such as chickweed and rose petals, will begin to spoil after a week. Hot weather will cause the plants and oil to spoil more quickly, whereas plants extracted in a cool environment will keep longer before you decant them. Direct light and heat should be avoided. Infuse and store on a surface that will not be damaged by any oil seepage that may occur. At the end of the given time period, strain well and store in a cool, dark place or refrigerate. Oils will keep for up to a year or more, and are considered good as long as they have not turned rancid. A rancid oil has a peculiar smell that is distinctly different from either the smell of the fresh oil or the plant being steeped. If you suspect that your oil has turned, discard it and begin anew.

*Salves* are used for healing skin injuries: wounds, burns, stings, rashes, sores, and the like. Salve can be made a few different ways, all of which are effective. This first method is preferable because it requires less time than the others, thereby retaining more of the subtle properties of the herbs. Prepare an herbal oil from your desired ingredients, then pour it into a small pot. To this add grated beeswax, 1 tablespoon per ounce of oil. Heat over a low flame until the wax is melted. To test for readiness, put a small amount onto a teaspoon and place it in the refrigerator. After a minute, it will harden to its finished consistency. Salve should be firm and solid but not so hard that it won't melt into your skin. If the consistency is correct, pour your salve into small jars, cool to room temperature, cover, and store. If your salve is too soft, add more beeswax; if it is too hard, add more oil.

A second method is to place about an ounce of herbs and $1/3$ cup of oil in a small pot. Simmer for 2 hours on a very low flame with the pot covered. Add a bit of oil if necessary, and watch carefully to avoid scorching. After cooking, strain the herbs well through a cotton cloth or cheesecloth, squeezing as much of the oil as possible out of the plant material. You may need to let the oil cool before this can be done. Clean the pot and dry it (discarding the used plant material), then pour the oil back in, adding a couple tablespoons of grated beeswax. Melt this over a low flame, stirring constantly. Check for readiness as in the first method, then bottle and store.

Another method requires less watching. Mix 4 ounces of oil, 1 ounce of herb, and $1/2$ ounce of beeswax in an ovenproof pot. Cover the pot and bake the mixture for about three hours at 250°F. Strain through cheesecloth, bottle, and store.

Salves will keep for a couple of years if stored in the refrigerator, about a year if not. To extend the life of your salve to the full two years, add 1 teaspoon of vitamin E oil or 1 to 2 tablespoons of an herbal tincture per 4 ounces of salve (while still warm, before bottling). Any herbal tincture will work, as it is the alcohol that helps preserve it, but to increase the healing qualities of your salve, use a tincture with either skin-healing or antimicrobial properties. Echinacea and calendula tinctures make good choices for use in herbal salves.

**Ointments** are prepared exactly like salves, but less beeswax is used in order to obtain a softer product. Cutting the amount of beeswax by half should yield a desirable consistency.

When you experiment in your kitchen pharmacy, above all enjoy yourself. Of course it is best not to be wasteful, but don't worry if you make a mistake and have to discard something. Compost piles are very forgiving. Try to be patient and learn from your mistakes. Be persistent; the rewards are worth it!

# Common and Latin Names for Herbs in This Book

Many plants may have the same common name, and any given plant may have a number of common names. A plant's Latin name (also known as the "botanical" or "horticultural" name) is its internationally recognized name. When purchasing herbs, check their Latin names to ensure that you are using the correct plants in your herbal preparations.

Alfalfa: *Medicago sativa*
Anise: *Pimpinella anisum*
Astragalus: *Astragalus membranaceus*
Bayberry: *Myrica cerifera*
Beth root: *Trillium spp.*
Black cohosh: *Actaea racemusa, syn., Cimicifuga racemosa*
Black haw: *Viburnum prunifolium*
Black walnut: *Juglans nigra*
Blessed thistle: *Cnicus benedictus*

Blue cohosh: *Caulophyllum thalictroides*
Borage: *Borago officinalis*
Bupleurum: *Bupleurum falcatum*
Burdock: *Arctium lappa*
Calendula: *Calendula officinalis*
Catnip: *Nepeta cataria*
Chamomile: *Anthemis nobilis; Matricaria chamomilla*
Chasteberry: *Vitex agnus-castus*

Chickweed: *Stellaria media*
Cinnamon: *Cinnamomum zeylanicum*
Cleavers: *Galium aparine*
Comfrey: *Symphytum officinale*
Cramp bark: *Viburnum opulus*
Dandelion: *Taraxacum officinale*
Dong quai: *Angelica sinensis*
Echinacea: *Echinacea angustifolia*
Elder: *Sambucus nigra*
False unicorn: *Chamaelirium luteum*
Fennel: *Foeniculum vulgare*
Fenugreek: *Trigonella foenum-graecum*
Flax seed: *Linum usitatissimum*
Gentian: *Gentian officinalis*
Ginger: *Zingiber officinale*
Ginseng: *Panax quinquefolium*
Goldenseal: *Hydrastis canadensis*
Hawthorn: *Crataegus oxyacantha*
Hops: *Humulus lupulus*
Irish moss: *Chondrus crispus*
Kudzu: *Pueraria lobata et thunbergiana*
Lady's mantle: *Alchemilla vulgaris*
Lady's slipper: *Cypripedium pubescens*
Lavender: *Lavandula officinalis*
Lemon balm: *Melissa officinalis*
Lemon grass: *Cymbopogon citratus*
Licorice: *Glycyrrhiza glabra*
Liferoot: *Senecio aureus*
Lime (linden) blossom: *Tilia europea*
Lobelia: *Lobelia inflata*
Marshmallow: *Althaea officinalis*
Meadowsweet: *Filipendula ulmaria*
Motherwort: *Leonurus cardiaca*
Myrrh: *Comiphora molmol*
Nettle: *Urtica dioica*
Oatstraw: *Avena sativa*
Parsley: *Petroselinum crispum*

Partridge berry: *Mitchella repens*
Passionflower: *Passiflora incarnata*
Peony: *Paeonia* spp.
Peppermint: *Mentha piperita*
Plantain: *Plantago major*
Red clover: *Trifolium pratense*
Red raspberry: *Rubus idaeus*
Rehmannia: *Rehmannia glutinosa*
Rose: *Rosa canina*
Rosemary: *Rosmarinus officinalis*
Sage: *Salvia officinalis*
Sarsaparilla: *Smilax officinale*
Saw palmetto: *Serenoa serrulata*
Shepherd's purse: *Capsella
   bursa-pastoris*
Skullcap: *Scutellaria laterifolia*
Slippery elm: *Ulmus fulva*
Spearmint: *Mentha viridis*
Spikenard: *Aralia racemosa*
St. John's wort: *Hypericum perforatum*
Thyme: *Thymus vulgaris*
Usnea: *Usnea barbata*
Uva-ursi: *Arctostaphylos uva-ursi*
Valerian: *Valeriana officinalis*
Vervain: *Verbena officinalis*
White oak: *Quercus alba*
Wild yam: *Dioscorea villosa*
Witch hazel: *Hamamelis virginiana*
Wood betony: *Betonica officinalis*
Yarrow: *Achillea millefolium*
Yellow dock: *Rumex crispus*

# Resources ⚘

THE FOLLOWING ORGANIZATIONS AND COMPANIES provide high-quality services and are reputable resources in the midwifery and herbal communities. Inclusion here, however, does not necessarily imply endorsement all of the opinions, products, or services provided by these companies, and is not a direct referral to any individual practitioners.

## MIDWIFERY AND HERBAL ORGANIZATIONS

### American Botanical Council (ABC)

6200 Manor Rd.
Austin, TX 78723
(512) 926-4900
www.herbalgram.org

ABC is a nonprofit educational and research organization dedicated to providing reliable, scientifically sound information about medicinal herbs to health-care professionals and the public.

### American Herbalists Guild (AHG)

1931 Gaddis Rd.
Canton, GA 30115
(770) 751-6021
www.americanherbalist.com

The American Herbalists Guild was founded in 1989 as a nonprofit educational organization to represent the goals and voices of herbalists. It is the only peer-review organization in the United States for professional herbalists specializing in the medicinal use of plants. AHG membership consists of professionals, general members (including students), and benefactors.

### Association of Labor Assistants & Childbirth Educators (ALACE)

PO Box 390436
Cambridge, MA 02139
(617) 441-2500
www.alace.org

ALACE is a nonprofit educational organization and support group for doulas, labor assistants, and childbirth educators.

### Association for Pre- & Perinatal Psychology and Health (APPPAH)

340 Colony Rd.
Geyserville, CA 95441
(707) 857-4041
www.birthpsychology.com/apppah/
index.html

APPPAH was founded in 1983 by Toronto psychiatrist and psychologist Thomas R. Verny, M.D., D.Psych., F.R.C.P.C., as a forum for individuals from diverse backgrounds and disciplines interested in psychological dimensions of prenatal and perinatal experiences. Typically, this includes childbirth educators, birth assistants, doulas, midwives, obstetricians, nurses, social workers, perinatologists, pediatricians, psychologists, counselors, researchers, and teachers at all levels. One does not have to be a professional, however: all who share these interests are welcome to join.

### Birthing the Future

PO Box 1040
Bayfield, CO 81122
(970) 884-4090
www.birthingthefuture.com

This is the "baby" of Suzanne Arms, author of *Immaculate Deception*. Its purpose is to inspire, foster, and advocate vision and practical models for the healing and well-being of life on this planet, with an emphasis on birth and midwifery. Beautiful photographs and birth posters.

### Citizens for Midwifery

PO Box 82227
Athens, GA 30608-2227
(888) 236-4880
www.cfmidwifery.org

This organization serves as the national clearinghouse for consumer groups supporting midwifery and educates the public about the advantages of the midwife's model of care.

### Depression After Delivery (DAD)

4756 University Village Place NE #253
Seattle, WA 98105-5021
(888) 404-7763
www.behavenet.com/dadsgwa

DAD is a national support organization that provides self-help education, information, and referral for women and families coping with blues, anxiety, depression, and psychosis associated with the arrival of a baby.

### Doulas of North America (DONA)

PO Box 626
Jasper, IN 47547
(888) 788-DONA
www.dona.org

DONA is an international association of doulas who are trained to provide the highest quality emotional, physical, and educational support to women and their families during childbirth and postpartum. DONA is the premier doula organization founded by Marshall Klaus, M.D., Phyllis Klaus, John Kennell, M.D., Penny Simkin, and Annie Kennedy in 1992. Evidence-based certification programs are offered for both birth doulas and postpartum doulas. Membership in DONA includes nearly 4,500 birth and postpartum doulas.

### Foundations in Herbal Medicine

PO Box 4544
Albuquerque, NM 87196
(888) 857-1976
(505) 266-2160 fax
fihm1@aol.com
www.fihm.com

The Foundations in Herbal Medicine course, created by Tieraona Low Dog, M.D., also an herbalist, provides an integrated perspective on the use of herbal medicine that is based on sound scientific principles and longstanding herbal wisdom.

### International Cesarean Awareness Network (ICAN)

1304 Kingsdale Ave.
Redondo Beach, CA 90278
(310) 542-6400
(310) 542-5368 fax
www.ican-online.org/resources
/links.htm

The International Cesarean Awareness Network, Inc. (formerly Cesarean Prevention Movement) is an international, nonprofit organization that was founded by concerned parents and professionals in June 1982. The threefold purpose of this organization is to lower the rising cesarean rate through education, to provide a forum where women and men can express their thoughts and concerns about birth, and to provide a support network for women who are healing from past birth experiences and for those who are preparing for births.

### International Childbirth Education Association (ICEA)

PO Box 20048
Minneapolis, MN 55420
(612) 854-8660
www.icea.org

ICEA is an internationally recognized organization that provides excellent resources for childbirth educators. It offers a comprehensive catalog of books on pregnancy, birth, and related topics, and also serves as a resource center for this information.

### La Leche League International

1400 N. Meacham Rd.
Schaumburg, IL 60173-4808
(847) 519-7730
(800) LA-LECHE
www.lalecheleague.org/contact.html

La Leche League is an international, nonprofit, nonsectarian organization dedicated to providing education, information, support, and encourage-ment to women who want to breastfeed. All breastfeeding mothers, as well as future breastfeeding mothers, are welcome to come to meetings or call leaders for breastfeeding help. La Leche also provides health-care professionals with continuing education opportunities and the latest research on lactation management.

### Midwives Alliance of North America (MANA)

4805 Lawrenceville Hwy., Ste. 116-279
Lilburn, GA 30047
(888) 923-MANA
www.mana.org

This is a national midwifery organization dedicated to women's freedom and reproductive health. With members all over the globe, MANA is a good contact if you are trying to find or become a midwife.

### National Certification Commission for Acupuncture and Oriental Medicine (NCCAOM)

11 Canal Center Plaza, Ste. 300
Alexandria, VA 22314
(703) 548-9004
www.nccaom.org

NCCAOM is a nonprofit organization established in 1982. Its mission is to promote nationally recognized standards of competence and safety in acupuncture and Oriental medicine for the purpose of protecting the public.

### North American Registry of Midwives (NARM)

5257 Rosetone Drive
Lilburn, GA 30047
(888) 842-4784
www.narm.org

NARM is an international certification agency whose mission is to establish and administer certification for the credential "Certified Professional Midwife."

### United Plant Savers (UpS)

PO Box 420
East Barre, VT 05649
(802) 479-9825
www.unitedplantsavers.org

United Plant Savers is a grassroots membership organization and encourages those interested in native medicinal plants to join. Members receive a wide offering of benefits including a membership package of useful information, a semiannual newsletter, opportunities to receive free native plants and seeds, discounts to UpS-hosted conferences, and the ability to apply for a grant to sponsor a community planting project. Members are encouraged to participate in different ways to help "Plant the Future."

### Waterbirth International Global Maternal/Child Health Association, Inc.

PO Box 1400
Wilsonville, OR 97070
(503) 673-0026
www.waterbirth.org/index2.html

Waterbirth is a project of the nonprofit public benefit corporation Global Maternal/Child Health Association. It has been assisting women and their families discover the benefits of laboring and giving birth in water since 1989. It offers unique services to parents and practitioners alike. Look at the website to gain an understanding of the gentle birth choice of laboring and giving birth in water.

## MIDWIFERY, PARENTING, AND HERBAL PUBLICATIONS

### Compleat Mother

PO Box 209
Minot, ND 58702
(701) 852-2822

A magazine about pregnancy, birth, and breastfeeding. Very honest and uncompromising.

### Doula Magazine for Mothers

PO Box 71
Santa Cruz, CA 95063-0071
(831) 464-9488
www.santacruzguide.com/page.cgi/
    pages/970114/97011430.html

This magazine includes articles on pregnancy, birth, parenting, natural health care, toddlers, and more. Always a nurturing read.

### The Farm

42, The Farm
Summertown, TN 38438
(616) 964-3798

A wealth of excellent birth videos, a world-renowned birthing center, and publishers of *Spiritual Midwifery* by Ina May Gaskin.

### HerbalGram

American Botanical Council
6200 Manor Rd.
Austin, TX 78723
(512) 926-4900
www.herbalgram.org/herbalgram

An excellent and informative magazine that keeps abreast of scientific studies in herbal medicine.

### Herbs for Health Magazine

741 Corporate Circle, Ste. A
PO Box 4101
Golden, CO 80401
www.interweave.com

*Herbs for Health* is a popular herb magazine with articles written by serious herbal practitioners. Great for those who want to know more about herbs, but not at an academic level.

## Journal of the American Herbalists Guild

1931 Gaddis Rd.
Canton, GA 30115
(770) 751-6021
www.americanherbalist.com

This is an academic journal on clinical botanical medicine issues. The executive editor, Aviva Romm, is a practicing midwife and clinical herbalist.

## Midwifery Today

(800) 743-0974
www.midwiferytoday.com

*Midwifery Today* is a resource that offers a quarterly journal for midwives, nurses, doulas, childbirth educators, doctors, parents, parents-to-be, and anyone who wants to learn more about pregnancy, labor, and birth.

## Mothering Magazine

PO Box 1690
Santa Fe, NM 87504
(800) 984-8116

Perhaps the oldest of the alternative parenting magazines in the United States, *Mothering* seeks to honor and celebrate pregnancy, birth, parenthood, and children. *Mothering* celebrates the experience of parenthood as worthy of one's best efforts and fosters awareness of the immense importance and value of parenthood and family life in the development of the full human potential. As a readers' magazine, they recognize parents as the experts and provide truly helpful information upon which parents can base informed choices.

## BULK HERBS, HERBAL PRODUCTS, BOOKS, AND SUPPLIES

### Avena Botanicals

219 Mill St.
Rockland, ME 04841
(207) 594-0694
www.avenainstitute.org

Deb Soule grows and prepares her own medicinal preparations from herbs especially for women. The mail-order catalog offers more than 150 tinctures. The Institute also offers on-site education programs in herbal medicine.

### Bushy Mountain Bee Company

(800) BEESWAX

Not an herb supplier, but a great source of pure beeswax for making salves.

### Cascade Health Care Products

1826 NW 18th
Portland, OR 97209
(503) 595-1720
(800) 443-9942
(503) 595-1726 fax
www.1cascade.com

A complete line of health products for pregnant women and midwives as well as many for babies and kids; good source of moxibustion supplies. The *Birth and Life* catalog offers a comprehensive selection of books on prenatal health, pregnancy, midwifery, and herbs. Their *Moonflower* catalog offers herbs, nutritional supplements, and homeopathic remedies.

### Frontier Cooperative Herbs

PO Box 299
Norway, IA 52318
(800) 669-3275

Bulk herbs and health and beauty products at wholesale prices.

### Herb Pharm

PO Box 116
Williams, OR 97544
(800) 348-4372
www.herb-pharm.com

The highest quality tinctures available, from a company that takes extraordinary pride in its products and values its customers.

### Herbalist and Alchemist

51 S. Wandling Ave.
Washington, NJ 07882
(800) 611-8235
www.herbalist-alchemist.com

Herbalist David Winston has a twenty-year history of commitment to making and providing the highest quality herbal products: herbal extracts, glycerine extracts, Chinese herbs, medicinal herbs, ayurvedic, and Native American herbs. David also offers an on-site educational program in botanical medicine.

### Homeopathic Educational Services

2124 Kittredge St.
Berkeley, CA 94704
(800) 359-9051
www.homeopathic.com

Offers a comprehensive catalog for those interested in homeopathy.

### Maine Seaweed Company

PO Box 57
Steuben, ME 04680
(207) 546-2875

Excellent sea vegetables harvested with complete respect for the health of the ocean.

### Redwing/Meridian

44 Linden St.
Brookline, MA 02146
(800) 873-3946
(800) 356-6003

A great source of herbs as well as lay and technical books on traditional Chinese medicine.

### Sage Mountain Herb Products

PO Box 420
East Barre, VT 05649

Offers herb products formulated by Rosemary Gladstar, a highly experienced herbalist. All of Rosemary's products, as well as her book *Herbal Healing for Women,* are highly recommended.

## MIDWIFERY AND HERBAL DISTANCE LEARNING PROGRAMS

### Herbal Medicine for Women

Aviva Jill Romm
1931 Gaddis Rd.
Canton, GA 30115
(770) 751-7548
Avivajill@aol.com

**PROFESSIONAL LEVEL:** for practitioners and health professionals interested in introducing or expanding their use of herbs in clinical practice.

**FOUNDATION LEVEL:** for childbirth educators, doulas, and those who want a solid introduction to herbal medicine for women's health.

A comprehensive course on therapeutic herbal medicine for midwives, physicians, clinical herbalists, nurse-practitioners, nurses, and other health-care professionals interested in the safe and effective use of botanical medicines for women.

• A blend of critically reviewed, evidence-based data, modern clinical experience, and traditional herbal wisdom.

• Includes high-quality, professionally presented written materials, audio and video components, and required reading, including *Herbal Medicine for Women's Health,* a textbook by Aviva Romm (Churchill, 2003).

• Self-paced modules with assignments individually reviewed by experienced advisors.

• Lessons cover therapeutic applications of individual herbs, clinical conditions, and case reviews on topics extending from menstruation through childbearing to menopause.

### Ancient Art Midwifery Institute

PO Box 788
Claremore, OK 74018
(918) 342-2926
www.ancientartmidwifery.com

Ancient Art Midwifery Institute was established in 1981 as the Apprentice Academics Midwifery Home Study Course. Since then, it has enrolled more than 1750 students and revised the curriculum. The institute's three-year home-study course provides a well-respected academic foundation in the science of midwifery.

### Art and Science of Herbalism

PO Box 420-M
East Barre, VT 05649

Rosemary Gladstar, founder of the California School of Herbal Studies, is a pioneer woman herbalist and author of numerous booklets on herbs for women, men, and children. She offers a correspondence course in herbal studies.

### Hygieia College

40 North State St.
Joseph, UT 84739
www.freestone.org/hygieia

Jeannine Parvati Baker is the founder of the Hygieia College program, which is "a college in the original meaning, that is in a grove of trees, which is a state of mind." Lessons are in womancraft, herbalism, and the art of midwifery. Baker is the author of a number of books, including *Hygieia: A Woman's Herbal* and *Prenatal Yoga and Natural Birth,* and a coauthor of *Conscious Conception.*

### Utah School of Midwifery

282 North State St.
Orem, UT 84057
(888) 489-1238
(801) 764-9068
www.midwifery.edu/history.html

The Utah College of Midwifery (UCM), formerly the Utah School of Midwifery, was founded in 1980. The college incorporated as a nonprofit organization in December 1998. The administration and faculty of UCM keep abreast of current educational and occupational development by being members of national and state midwifery and midwifery education organizations and serving on national and state committees and boards.

### Wise Woman Center

Susun S. Weed
PO Box 64-M
Woodstock, NY 12498
(914) 246-8081
www.susunweed.com

Susun Weed, the author of *Healing Wise, Wise Woman Herbal for the Childbearing Year,* and *Menopausal Years,* offers workshops and apprenticeships at her home and travels internationally on speaking engagements.

# Bibliography ❦

Achterberg, Jeanne. *Woman as Healer*. Boston: Shambhala Publications, 1991.

Allaire, Alexander D. "Complementary and Alternative Medicine in the Labor and Delivery Suite." *Clinical Obstetrics and Gynecology* 44, no. 4 (Dec 2001): 681–91.

Allaire, Alexander D., Merry-K Moos, Steven R. Wells. "Complementary and Alternative Medicine in Pregnancy: A Survey of North Carolina Certified Nurse-Midwives." *Obstetrics & Gynecology* 95, no. 1 (Jan 2000): 19–23.

Arms, Suzanne. *Immaculate Deception*. New York: Bantam Books, 1975.

———. *Immaculate Deception II: A Fresh Look at Childbirth*. Berkeley, Calif.: Celestial Arts, 1994.

Backon, J. "Ginger in Preventing Nausea and Vomiting of Pregnancy: A Caveat Due to Its Thromboxane Synthetase Activity and Effect on Testosterone Binding." *European Journal of Obstetrics and Gynecology and Reproductive Biology* 42 (Nov 1991): 54, 163–64.

Baker, Jeannine P. *Deep Ecology of Birth*. Monroe, Ut.: Freestone Publishing, 1991.

———. *Prenatal Yoga and Natural Birth*. Berkeley, Calif.: North Atlantic, 1986.

———. *Hygieia: A Woman's Herbal*. Monroe, Ut.: Freestone Publishing, 1979.

Baker, Jeannine P., F. Baker, and T. Slayton. *Conscious Conception*. Sevier, Ut.: Freestone Publishing, 1986.

Balacs, Tony. "Safety in Pregnancy." *International Journal of Aromatherapy* 4, no. 1 (spring 1992): 12–15.

Baldwin, Rahima. *Special Delivery*. Berkeley, Calif.: Celestial Arts, 1986.

Baldwin, Rahima, and Terra Palmarini. *Pregnant Feelings*. Berkeley, Calif.: Celestial Arts, 1986.

Ballantine, Rudolph. *Diet and Nutrition.* Honesdale, Penn.: Himalaya International Institute, 1978.

Bates, Barbara. *A Guide to the Physical Examination.* 3d ed. Philadelphia: J. B. Lippincott Co., 1983.

Beinfield, Harriet, and E. Korngold. *Between Heaven and Earth: A Guide to Chinese Medicine.* New York: Ballantine Books, 1991.

Bennett, Jennifer. *Lilies of the Hearth.* Willowdale, Ontario, Canada: Camden House Publishing, 1991.

Bing, Elizabeth, and Libby Colman. *Making Love during Pregnancy.* New York: Bantam Books, 1977.

Boston Women's Health Book Collective. *Our Bodies, Ourselves for the New Century.* New York: Simon & Schuster, 1998.

Brewer, Gail S., and Tom Brewer. *What Every Pregnant Woman Should Know: The Truth about Diet and Drugs in Pregnancy.* New York: Penguin Books, 1977.

Brinker, Francis. *Herb Contraindications and Drug Interactions.* 2d ed. Sandy, Ore.: Eclectic Medical Publications, 1998.

Brooke, Elizabeth. *Herbal Therapy for Women.* London, England: Thorsons, 1992.

Buckley, Kathleen, and Nancy W. Kulb. *Handbook of Maternal Newborn Nursing.* New York: John Wiley and Sons, 1983.

Cardini, Francesco, and Huang Weixin. "Moxibustion for Correction of Breech Presentation: A Randomized Control Trial." *Journal of the American Medical Association* 280, no. 18 (11 Nov 1998): 1580–84.

Carlsson, Christopher P., et al. "Manual Acupuncture Reduces Hyperemesis Gravidarum: A Placebo-Controlled, Randomized, Single-Blind, Crossover Study." *Journal of Pain Symptom Management* 20, no. 4 (Oct 2000): 273–79.

Cavanagh, Dennis, Ralph Woods, Timothy O'Connor, and Robert Knuppel. *Obstetric Emergencies.* Philadelphia: Harper and Row, 1982.

Cohen, Nancy W. *Open Season.* New York: Greenwood, Bergin, and Garvey, 1991.

Cohen, Nancy W., and Lois Estner. *Silent Knife.* New York: Greenwood, Bergin, and Garvey, 1983.

Corda, Murshida. *Cradle of Heaven: Psychological and Spiritual Dimensions of Conception, Pregnancy, and Birth.* Lebanon Springs, N.Y.: Omega, 1987.

Dale, Alisa, and Sheila Cornwell. "The Role of Lavender Oil in Relieving Perineal Discomfort Following Childbirth: A Blind Randomized Clinical Trial." *Journal of Advanced Nursing* 19, no. 1 (Jan 1994): 89–96.

Davis, Elizabeth. *Women's Intuition.* Berkeley, Calif.: Celestial Arts, 1989.

———. *Heart and Hands: A Midwife's Guide to Pregnancy and Birth.* Berkeley, Calif.: Celestial Arts, 1987.

Davis-Floyd, Robbie. *Birth as an American Right of Passage.* Berkeley, Calif.: University of California Press, 1992.

Dharmananda, Subhuti. *Treatment of Infertility and Miscarriage with Chinese Herbs.* Portland, Ore.: Institute for Traditional Medicine and Preventive Health Care, 1989.

———. *Your Nature, Your Health: Chinese Herbs in Constitutional Therapy.* Portland, Ore.: Institute for Traditional Medicine and Preventive Health Care, 1986.

Dick-Read, Grantly. *Childbirth without Fear.* New York: Harper and Row, 1979.

Dunham, Carroll. *Mamatoto: A Celebration of Birth.* New York: Penguin USA, Viking, 1991.

Ehrenreich, Barbara, and Deidre English. *Witches, Midwives, and Nurses: A History of Women Healers.* New York: Feminist Press at the City University of New York, 1973.

Eisenberg, Arlene, H. E. Murkoff, and S. E. Hathaway. *What to Eat When You're Expecting.* New York: Workman Publishing, 1986.

Ellingwood, Finley. *American Materia Medica, Therapeutics and Pharmacognosy.* 11th ed. Reprint. Sandy, Ore.: Eclectic Medical Publications, 1998.

Federation of Feminist Women's Health Centers. *A New View of a Woman's Body.* New York: Touchstone, 1981.

Felter, H. *The Eclectic Materia Medica, Pharmacology and Therapeutics.* 1922. Reprint. Sandy, Ore.: Eclectic Medical Publications, 1994.

Field, Tiffany, et al. "Labor Pain Is Reduced by Massage Therapy." *Journal of Psychosomatic Obstetrics and Gynaecology* 18, no. 4 (Dec 1977): 286–91.

Field, Tiffany, et al. "Pregnant Women Benefit from Massage Therapy." *Journal of Psychosomatic Obstetrics and Gynaecology* 20, no. 1 (Mar 1999): 31–38.

Fischer-Rasmussen, W., S. K. Kjaer, C. Dahl, and U. Asping. "Ginger Treatment of Hyperemesis Gravidarum." *European Journal of Obstetrics, Gynecology, and Reproductive Biology* 38 (Jan 1991): 19–24.

Flaws, Bob. *Free and Easy: Traditional Chinese Gynecology for American Women.* Boulder, Colo.: Blue Poppy Enterprises Press, 1986.

———. *A Handbook of Traditional Chinese Gynecology.* Boulder, Colo.: Blue Poppy Enterprises Press, 1987.

———. *The Path of Pregnancy.* Boulder, Colo.: Blue Poppy Press, 1993.

Foster, Steven, and J. Duke. *Eastern/Central Medicinal Plants.* Boston: Houghton Mifflin Co., 1990.

Francia, Luisa. *Dragontime: Magic and Mystery of Menstruation.* Woodstock, N.Y.: Ash Tree Publishing, 1991.

Frawley, David, and V. Lad. *The Yoga of Herbs.* Santa Fe, N.M.: Lotus Light, Lotus Press, 1986.

Frye, Anne. *Care during Pregnancy,* vol. 1 of *Holistic Midwifery: A Comprehensive Textbook for Midwives in Homebirth Practice.* Portland, Ore.: Labrys Press, 1995.

———. *Understanding Lab Work in the Childbearing Year.* New Haven, Conn.: Labrys Press, 1990.

Fulder, Stephen, and Meir Tenne. "Ginger as an Antinausea Remedy in Pregnancy: The Issue of Safety." *HerbalGram* 38 (Fall 1996): 47–50.

Gallo, Michael, and Maumita Sarkar, et al. "Pregnancy Outcome Following Gestational Exposure to Echinacea." *Archives of Internal Medicine* 160, no. 20 (13 Nov 2000): 3141–43.

Gaskin, Ina May. *Spiritual Midwifery.* Summertown, Tenn.: Book Publishing Co., 1980.

Gelis, Jacques. *History of Childbirth: Fertility, Pregnancy, and Birth in Early Modern Europe.* Boston: Northeastern University Press, 1991.

Gladstar, Rosemary. *Herbal Healing for Women.* New York: Simon and Schuster, 1993.

Goer, Henci. *Obstetric Myths versus Research Realities: A Guide to the Medical Literature.* Westport, Conn.: Greenwood, Bergin, and Garvey, 1995.

Goldsmith, Judith. *Childbirth Wisdom from the World's Oldest Societies.* New York: Congdon and Weed, 1984.

Grossinger, Richard. *Embryogenesis.* Berkeley, Calif.: North Atlantic Books, 1986.

Harrison, Michelle. *A Woman in Residence.* New York: Penguin, 1982.

Hazell, Lester. *Commonsense Childbirth.* New York: Berkley Books, 1976.

Hedegaard M. "Life Style, Work and Stress, and Pregnancy Outcome." *Current Opinion in Gynecology* 11, no. 6 (Dec 1999): 553–56.

Ho, C.-M., S.-S. Hseu, S.-K. Tsai, T.-Y. Lee. "Effect of P-6 Acupressure on Prevention of Nausea and Vomiting after Epidural Morphine for Post–Cesarean Section Pain Relief." *Acta Anaesthesiologica Scandinavica* 40, no. 3 (Mar 1996): 372–75.

Hobbs, Valerie. *Complications of Labor and Delivery.* Ann Arbor, Mich.: Informed Homebirth and Parenting, 1982.

———. *Herbs for Women: A Guide for Lay Midwives.* Ann Arbor, Mich.: Informed Homebirth and Parenting, 1981.

Hochstrasser, B., and P. Mattman. "Mainstream Medicine versus Complementary Medicine (Homoeopathic) Intervention: A Critical Methodology Study of Pregnancy." *Forsch Komplementarmed* 6, no. 6, suppl 1 (Feb 1999): 20–22.

Hoffman, David. *The Holistic Herbal.* Moray, Scotland: Findhorn Press, 1983.

Huxley, Laura. *The Child of Your Dreams.* Rochester, Vt.: Inner Traditions, Destiny Books, 1992.

Jensen, Margaret D., Ralph Benson, and Irene Bobak. *Maternity Care: The Nurse and the Family.* St. Louis: Mosby, 1981.

Jewell, D., and G. Young. "Interventions for Nausea and Vomiting in Early Pregnancy." In Jim P. Neilson, Caroline Crowther, Ellen Hodnett, Justus Hofmeyr, and M. Keirse, eds. *Pregnancy and Childbirth Module of the Cochrane Database of Systematic Reviews, The Cochrane Collaboration,* issue 2. Oxford, England: Update Software, 1997.

Katz-Rothman, Barbara. *The Encyclopedia of Childbearing.* New York: Henry Holt, 1993.

Keating, Angela, and Ronald Chez. "Ginger Syrup as an Antiemetic in Early Pregnancy." *Alternative Therapies in Health and Medicine* 8, no. 5 (Sept–Oct 2002): 89–91.

Kirschmann, John, and L. Dunne. *Nutrition Almanac.* New York: McGraw-Hill, 1984.

Kitzinger, Sheila. *The Complete Book of Pregnancy and Childbirth.* New York: Alfred A. Knopf, 1983.

————. *Education and Counseling for Childbirth.* New York: Schocken Books, 1979.

————. *Birth at Home.* New York: Penguin, 1979.

Klaus, Marshall, and John Kennell. *Bonding.* New York: Penguin USA, Plume, 1983.

Koehler, Nan. *Artemis Speaks: VBAC Stories and Natural Childbirth Information.* Occidental, Calif.: Jerald R. Brown, 1985.

Kushi, Michio, and Aveline Kushi. *Macrobiotic Pregnancy and Care of the Newborn.* New York: Japan Publishing, 1983.

La Leche League. *The Womanly Art of Breastfeeding.* New York: Plume, 1981.

Leboyer, Frederick. *Inner Beauty, Inner Light: Yoga for Pregnant Women.* New York: Alfred A. Knopf, 1978.

Liedloff, Jean. *The Continuum Concept.* Reading, Mass.: Addison-Wesley Publishing Co., 1977.

Litoff, J. B. *The American Midwife Debate.* New York: Greenwood Press, 1986.

Louden, Jennifer. *The Woman's Comfort Book.* New York: HarperCollins, 1992.

————. *The Couple's Comfort Book.* San Francisco: HarperCollins, 1994.

Low Dog, Tieraona. *An Integrative Approach to Women's Health.* Albuquerque, N.M.: Integrative Medical Education Associates, 2001.

Madaras, Lynda, and Jane Patterson. *Womancare: A Gynecological Guide to Your Body.* New York: Avon Books, 1984.

Magee, Laura A., Paolo Mazzotta, and Gideon Koren. "Evidence-Based View of Safety and Effectiveness of Pharmacologic Therapy for Nausea and Vomiting of Pregnancy (NVP)." *American Journal of Obstetrics and Gynecology* 185, no. 5 supplement understanding (May 2002): S256–61.

Mariechild, Diane. *MotherWit.* Trumansburg, N.Y.: The Crossing Press, 1981.

McClure, Vimala Schneider. *Infant Massage.* New York: Bantam Books, 1989.

McGuffin, M., et al. *Botanical Safety Handbook.* New York: CRC Press, 1997.

McIntyre, Anne. *The Herbal for Mother and Child.* Rockport, Mass.: Element Books, 1992.

Meek, Leslie R., Kristi M. Burda, and Erin Paster. "Effects of Prenatal Stress on Development in Mice: Maturation and Learning." *Physiology & Behavior* 71, no. 5 (Dec 2000): 543–49.

Meltzer, Donna I. "Complementary Therapies for Nausea and Vomiting in Early Pregnancy." *Family Practice* 17, no. 6 (Dec 2000): 570–73.

Mendelsohn, Robert. *How to Raise a Healthy Child in Spite of Your Doctor.* New York: Ballantine Books, 1984.

————. *MalePractice: How Doctors Manipulate Women.* Chicago: Contemporary Books, 1982.

Merchant, Carolyn. *The Death of Nature: Women, Ecology, and the Scientific Revolution.* San Francisco: HarperSanFrancisco, 1980.

Miller, Jonathan, and D. Pelham. *The Facts of Life.* New York: Penguin USA, Viking, 1984.

Mills, S., and K. Bone. *Principles and Practice of Phytotherapy: Modern Herbal Medicine.* Edinburgh, Scotland: Churchill Livingstone, 2000.

Mitford, Jessica. *The American Way of Birth.* New York: Dutton/Signet, 1992.

Montagu, Ashley. *Growing Young.* New York: McGraw-Hill, 1981.

Moskowitz, Richard. *Homeopathic Medicines for Pregnancy and Childbirth.* Berkeley: North Atlantic Press, 1992.

Murphy, Patricia Aikens. "Alternative Therapies for Nausea and Vomiting of Pregnancy." *Obstetrics & Gynecology* 91, no. 1 (Jan 1998): 149–55.

Niebyl, Jennifer R., and T. Murphy Goodwin. "Overview of Nausea and Vomiting of Pregnancy with an Emphasis on Vitamins." *American Journal of Obstetrics and Gynecology* 186, no. 5 supplement understanding (May 2002): S253–55.

Nissim, Rina. *Natural Healing in Gynecology.* New York: Pandora Press, 1986.

Noble, Elizabeth. *Essential Exercises for the Childbearing Year.* Boston: Houghton Mifflin Co., 1982.

———. *Childbirth with Insight.* Boston: Houghton Mifflin Co., 1983.

Noble, Vicki. *Shakti Woman.* San Francisco: HarperSanFrancisco, 1991.

———. *Uncoiling the Snake.* San Francisco: HarperCollins, 1993.

Nofziger, Margaret. *A Cooperative Method of Natural Birth Control.* Summertown, Tenn.: Book Publishing Co., 1979.

———. *The Fertility Question.* Summertown, Tenn.: Book Publishing Co., 1982.

Norheim, Arne Johan, Erik Jesman Pedersen, Vinjar Fonnebo, and Lillian Berge. "Acupressure Treatment of Morning Sickness in Pregnancy: A Randomised, Double-Blind, Placebo-Controlled Study." *Scandinavian Journal of Primary Health Care* 19, no. 1 (Mar 2001): 43–47.

Northrup, Christiane. *Women's Bodies, Women's Wisdom.* New York: Bantom Doubleday Dell, 1998.

Olds, Sally, Marcia London, and Patricia Ladewig. *Maternal Newborn Nursing.* Menlo Park, Calif.: Addison-Wesley, 1984.

Packer-Tursman, Judy. "Alternative Therapy Struggles to Bridge East-West Divide." *Washington Post* 10 Nov 2002. www.washingtonpost.com/wp-dyn/articles/A36744-2002 Nov10.html.

Panuthos, Claudia. *Transformation through Birth.* South Hadley, Mass.: Greenwood, Bergin, and Garvey, 1984.

Peterson, Gayle. *Birthing Normally.* Berkeley, Calif.: Mindbody Press, 1984.

Peterson, Gayle, and Lewis Mehl. *Pregnancy as Healing.* 2 vols. Berkeley, Calif.: Mindbody Press, 1984.

Price, Shirley. "Using Essential Oils in Professional Practice." *Complementary Therapies in Nurse Midwifery* 4, no. 5 (Oct 1998): 144–47.

Pritchard, Jack, and Paul MacDonald. *William's Obstetrics.* New York: Appleton-Century Croft, 1976.

Reeder, Sharon, Luigi Mastroianni Jr., and Leonide Martin. *Maternity Nursing.* Philadelphia: J. B. Lippincott Co., 1983.

Regutti, Amy. "Pregnancy Support with Acupuncture and Traditional Chinese Medicine." *Infused: The Community Pharmacy Newsletter* 4, no. 3 (June 2002): 1–3.

Rich, Adrienne. *Of Woman Born: Motherhood as Experience and Institution.* New York: W. W. Norton & Co., 1986.

Romm, Aviva. "Healing a Uterine Prolapse." *The Birth Gazette* 10, no. 3 (Summer 1994): 19–21.

———. *Natural Health after Birth.* Rochester, Vt.: Healing Arts Press, 2002.

———. *A Pocket Guide to Midwifery Care.* Freedom, Calif.: The Crossing Press, 1998.

———. "Treatment of Incomplete Miscarriage with Botanical Therapies and Continuing Reproductive Care." *Journal of the American Herbalists Guild* 2, no. 2 (Fall/Winter 2001): 16–17.

———. *Naturally Healthy Babies and Children.* Berkeley, Calif.: Celestial Arts, 2003.

Romm, Aviva, and Jonathan Treasure. "American Herbalists Guild Professional Member Botanical Therapeutics Survey: Vitex Agnus Castus." *Journal of the American Herbalists Guild* 2, no. 2 (Fall/Winter 2001): 27–31.

Roscoe, Joseph A., and Sara E. Matteson. "Acupressure and Acustimulation Bands for Control of Nausea Review." *American Journal of Obstetrics and Gynecology* 185, no. 5 supplement understanding (May 2002): S244–47.

Schwartz, Leni. *Bonding before Birth.* Boston: Sigo Press, 1991.

Sears, William, and Martha Sears. *The Birth Book.* Boston: Little, Brown and Co., 1994.

Shuttle, Penelope, and P. Redgrove. *The Wise Wound.* New York: Grove Press, 1986.

Slotnick, R. Nathan. "Safe, Successful Nausea Suppression in Early Pregnancy with P-6 Acustimulation." *Journal of Reproductive Medicine* 46, no. 9 (Sep 2001): 811–14.

Smith, C. A. "Homoeopathy for Induction of Labour." *Cochrane Database Syst Rev* 4 (2001): CD00339.

Stern, Robert M., Michael D. Jokerst, Eric R. Muth, and Chris Hollis. "Acupressure Relieves the Symptoms of Motion Sickness and Abnormal Gastric Activity." *Alternative Therapies in Health and Medicine* 7, no. 4 (Jul–Aug 2001): 91–94.

Stillerman, Elaine. *Mother Massage.* New York: Dell Publishing, 1992.

Strong, Thomas H. "Alternative Therapies of Morning Sickness." *Clinical Obstetrics and Gynecology* 44, no. 4 (Dec 2001): 653–60.

Stukane, Eileen. *The Dream Worlds of Pregnancy.* New York: Quill, 1985.

Taber, Ben-Zion. *Manual of Gynecologic and Obstetric Emergencies.* Philadelphia: W. B. Saunders Co., 1984.

Taylor, Dena. *Red Flower: Rethinking Menstruation.* Freedom, Calif.: The Crossing Press, 1988.

Thevenin, Tine. *The Family Bed: An Age-Old Concept in Child Rearing.* Garden City, N.Y.: Avery, 1992.

Tierra, Lesley. *The Herbs of Life.* Freedom, Calif.: The Crossing Press, 1992.

Tierra, Michael. *Planetary Herbology.* Santa Fe, N.M.: Lotus Light Publications, Lotus Press, 1988.

————. *The Way of Herbs.* Santa Cruz, California: Orenda/Unity Press, 1980.

Tiran, D., and S. Mack. *Complementary Therapies for Pregnancy and Childbirth.* London, England: Bailliere Tindall, 1995.

Tortora, Gerard, and Nicholas Anagnostakos. *Principles of Anatomy and Physiology.* New York: Harper and Row, 1984.

Tyler, Varro. *Herbs of Choice: The Therapeutic Use of Phytomedicinals.* Binghamton, N.Y.: Haworth Press, 1999.

Upton, Roy. "Chaste Tree Fruit (Vitex agnus castus)." *American Herbal Pharmacopoeia and Therapeutic Compendium.* Santa Cruz, Calif.: American Herbal Pharmacopoeia, 2001.

————. "Cramp Bark (Viburnum prunifolium)." *American Herbal Pharmacopoeia and Therapeutic Compendium.* Santa Cruz, Calif.: American Herbal Pharmacopoeia, 2001.

————. "Cranberry Fruit (Vaccinium macrocarpon)." *American Herbal Pharmacopoeia and Therapeutic Compendium.* Santa Cruz, Calif.: American Herbal Pharmacopoeia, 2002.

Varney, Helen. *Nurse Midwifery.* Boston: Blackwell Scientific Publications, 1980.

Verny, Thomas, and John Kelly. *The Secret Life of the Unborn Child.* New York: Dell Publishing, 1981.

Vutyavanich, Teraporn, et al. "Ginger for Nausea and Vomiting in Pregnancy: Randomized, Double-Masked, Placebo-Controlled Trial." *Obstetrics & Gynecology* 97, no. 4 (April 2001): 577–82.

Wagner, Marsden. *Pursuing the Birth Machine.* Camperdown, Australia: ACE Graphics, 1994.

Weed, Susun. *Healing Wise.* Woodstock, N.Y.: Ash Tree Publishing, 1989.

————. *Wise Woman Herbal for the Childbearing Year.* Woodstock, N.Y.: Ash Tree Publishing, 1985.

Weiss, Rudolf. *Herbal Medicine.* Gothenburg, Sweden: AB Arcanum, 1988.

Werner, David. *Where There Is No Doctor: A Village Health-Care Handbook.* Palo Alto, Calif.: Hesperian Foundation, 1977.

Wilkinson, Jenny M. "What Do We Know about Herbal Morning Sickness Treatments? A Literature Survey." *Midwifery* 16 (Sep 2000): 224–28.

Wilkinson, Susan, et al. "An Evaluation of Aromatherapy Massage in Palliative Care." *Palliative Medicine* 13, no. 5 (Sep 1999): 409–17.

# Index 🌱